CREATIVE TEACHING IN CLINICAL NURSING

CREATIVE TEACHING IN CLINICAL NURSING

Jean E. Schweer, R.N., B.S., M.S.

Professor of Nursing, Indiana University School
of Nursing at Indiana University—Purdue University,
Indianapolis, Indiana

Kristine M. Gebbie, R.N., M.N.

Assistant Professor, St. Louis University,
School of Nursing and Allied Health,
St. Louis, Missouri

THIRD EDITION

The C. V. Mosby Company

Saint Louis   1976

Library of Congress Cataloging in Publication Data

Schweer, Jean E
    Creative teaching in clinical nursing.

    Bibliography: p.
    Includes index.
    1. Nursing—Study and teaching.   I.   Gebbie, Kristine
M., joint author.   II.   Title.   [DNLM: 1.   Education,
Nursing. WY18 S412c]
RT73.S35 1976   610.73′07′11   75-31627
ISBN 0-8016-4377-5

VH/M/M   9   8   7   6   5   4   3

Preface

Creativity is an elusive happening, a chance encounter, a second of excitement, an event to remember. The fact that one can write a book about creativity does not reduce the creative act to something that can be taught and learned the same way one teaches and learns the multiplication tables. Settings and styles conducive to creativity can be learned, and one can become open to the possibility; eventually one takes the risk of trying a new combination or a different approach, of asking a new question, of stating a new conceptualization.

This third edition of *Creative Teaching in Clinical Nursing* is the first with dual authorship. In providing additional material and thought for this revision, I have had a challenging role. The risk of changing focus, adding opinion, and reinforcing facts is tied to the hope that those who have found this text useful over the past years will continue to do so. The major thrust is the same as that of the first edition. This brief preface is followed by an extensive quotation from the preface to that edition in order to introduce the goals of both authors. If this book results in increased potential for creativity in students and teachers of nursing, it will have been worth the risk.

"If you don't expect the unexpected, you will never find it." *Jurgen Moltmann*

Kristine M. Gebbie

From the preface to the first edition

The primary aim of this book is to assist the nursing teacher in exploring the concept of creativity as it applies to the functions of clinical teaching.

The purposes of this book are as follows:

1. To promote the concept of creativity as an existing integral, dynamic force within the total teaching-learning environment, depending on every teacher's ability to risk the self in using the creative potential to maximal advantage.
2. To emphasize the need for school of nursing educators and, particularly, clinical nursing teachers, to accept the challenge of change in order to keep pace with the rapidly developing patterns of education.
3. To acquaint those concerned in general with nursing education and, especially, teachers of clinical nursing, with the wide range of teaching approaches, technological advances, and educational communication media that are readily available and adaptable for use in the teaching of clinical nursing.
4. To emphasize the need for teachers of clinical nursing to capitalize on their creative abilities by using available time and equipment to their greatest advantage in planning clini-

cal learning experiences that provide students with individualized opportunities to learn through their own involvement in the teaching-learning environment.

Changes in higher education are taking place with frightening speed. Often that which seems idealistic today is already or soon to be reality. The danger lies in placing responsibility for the creative utilization of teaching techniques and innovations in the hands of teachers who lack the courage to accept the challenge to change. This change is basic to creative action! There is real danger that some of the proposals of our own nurse educators and some proposals in this book may never materialize because teachers do not have the sustained support they need to accept the challenge of change so necessary to approach teaching with a creative open mind.

I do not believe that the concepts presented in this book call for anything utopian. Teachers of clinical nursing do have a commitment to examine past and present practices in the light of the future, which is upon us and which for many began yesterday. Each teacher of clinical nursing has a potential for some degree of creativity in providing meaningful learning experiences for students. The degree and kind are dependent largely upon the individual, but often all that is needed are a few plantings of hybrids to eliminate the seeds of doubt, leading to a whole new approach to teaching.

Jean E. Schweer

Contents

Unit I   Foundations of teaching in clinical nursing

Let the great world spin forever
down the ringing grooves of change.

ALFRED LORD TENNYSON

1 Relationships between past, present, and future teaching programs in clinical nursing

HISTORICAL DEVELOPMENT OF CLINICAL TEACHING PROGRAMS IN NURSING EDUCATION

Examination of the periods of growth in the history of nursing education allows one to reflect on those concepts that shaped clinical teaching programs through the years and to use them as models for prediction of the kinds of programs likely to be developed in the future. These concepts frequently occur in rhythm with the pendulum of time. A concept appearing at a given time in history gradually becomes altered and takes on new meanings. At some later period many of the original elements of the same basic concept reappear in still another form to meet the current needs. A brief review of the historical development of nursing education in the United States reveals that some concept of clinical teaching has always been present in schools of nursing. Over the years concepts of clinical teaching have changed in terms of the prevailing philosophy held by schools of nursing regarding clinical teaching, the administration of clinical teaching programs, the functions of the clinical teacher, the designation of personnel to perform the functions of clinical teaching, the quantity and quality of clinical teachers, and the impact of the multiple pressures of the surrounding social system.

Beginning patterns of clinical teaching

With the establishment of the first three schools of nursing in the United States according to the Nightingale plan, nursing education possessed rudimentary elements of clinical teaching. The clinical experience was primarily an apprenticeship system in which students learned at the bedside from a more experienced nurse. In the beginning much of the teaching was done by the superintendent of the nursing school. As students progressed in the programs, they became the next available source of teachers for new student nurses. When these one-year programs were lengthened to two years, the students were designated as head nurses during the second year and were given the responsibility of teaching the first-year students. The great difference between the American school system and the Nightingale school system was in the quality of teaching. In the Nightingale plan nurses completing a one-year course remained under the jurisdiction of the school for three years. Those chosen as head nurses (teachers) were carefully screened and selected. In the American plan head nurses were selected during the second year according to their demonstrated abilities; however, this system often broke down so that, in effect, any nurse in the second year became a head nurse (teacher).

Another form of clinical teaching was seen in the system employed by many of the hospital schools, whereby students were sent into the homes to give bedside nursing care in exchange for a fee that reverted to the hospital. This practice was justified on the basis that it provided valuable educational experience in preparing students for private duty nursing. However, this system

3

was labeled undesirable when it was revealed that students were sent into the homes unsupervised, and experiences were often prolonged to allow protracted collection of the fees for the hospital!

It is difficult to determine exactly the extent to which clinical teaching and clinical teachers were present during this early period. Roberts cites records stating that Jane Delano held the position of instructor and assistant superintendent in 1890 at the University of Pennsylvania Hospital, and Isabel McIsaac, principal of the Illinois Training School for Nurses, is believed to have been the first to institute clinical demonstrations of nursing procedures in 1895.[1]

The success of these early schools was in reality the result of their affiliation with established hospitals offering a sufficient number of patients and varieties of conditions to provide adequate experiences for students. This vital factor was often overlooked by hospitals that were organizing schools of nursing for the primary purpose of providing improved nursing service to patients, giving little regard to the primary purpose—a well-prepared graduate nurse. As these hospital schools of nursing began mushrooming, it became apparent that the apprenticeship method of teaching was leading to undesirable practices. These were the result of such problems as insufficient time for skill development, insufficient opportunities for gaining the theoretical background information needed to apply theory to practice, and learning of skills that was limited to what could be perpetuated from one nurse to another.

Clinical teaching at the turn of the century

Shortly after the turn of the century a few outstanding nurse educators led the movement to remove nursing education from its apprenticeship status. The Johns Hopkins School of Nursing moved the instruction to the classroom and employed two full-time nursing arts instructors to teach procedure-centered demonstrations and practice. Other leading schools of nursing followed this pattern of appointing nursing arts instructors. One might wonder how these teachers became qualified to hold these positions. It was a general practice to appoint nursing arts instructors on the basis of their past performance skills and professional achievements without special preparation requirements. Since these women were appointed by virtue of their outstanding performance and vision regarding nursing and nursing education, it would be reasonable to assume that many of them had received additional preparation, whether by accident or design. This pattern of teaching did not become universal at this time, but schools of nursing using the apprenticeship concept of education continued to flourish. Too many schools operating on unsound financial and educational policies were unwilling or unable to appoint nurses "just to teach."

By 1915 most of the instruction had been removed to the classroom, thus allowing students freedom to practice procedures without harm to the patient. This approach created a new set of problems: the student's interest in learning waned as the personalized approach to patients in the hospital setting was lost; students lost the opportunity to observe symptoms of patients as described in the theory courses; the classroom procedures and equipment represented the "ideal" rather than the "real"; ineffective lines of communication between the classroom teacher and the head nurse who supervised the students on the wards caused the head nurse to lose interest in teaching; and the head nurse was often unaware of what was being taught in the classroom, causing a discrepancy between how the procedures were taught in the classroom and how they were performed in the hospital.

Widespread concern for these problems was recognized by nurse educators, as evidenced by several papers presented at the Twenty-Fifth Annual Convention of the National League of Nursing Education in 1919. The report of these proceedings contained three significant articles relating to clinical teaching. The article by Helen M. Wood, "The Value of the Clinical Method of Teaching in Nursing Schools and How it Can be Organized," expressed some of the concepts of clinical teaching during this era. Miss Wood's overall concept of clinical teaching was that of providing physician-conducted bedside clinics for teaching small groups of students to recognize symptoms through careful observation and to make comparisons with previously learned theoretical information.[2] A second article, by Parmelia Merman Doty, was "The Need of Cooperation Between the Head Nurse and Instructor." The author expressed concern for the development of the dichotomy of teaching functions between the head nurse and the instructor and described the need for closer cooperation between them in standardizing the teaching of nursing procedures.[3] In a third article, "How can We Make the Student's Practical Work Experience More Profitable from an Educational Standpoint?" Elizabeth Burgess expressed the need for making the student's clinical experiences educationally sound and offered some suggestions for providing conditions conducive to learning. A glimpse of the past as a reflection upon our present-day thinking can be better appreciated by the following quotations from the article:

The value of the practical experience should be emphasized in every possible way. It should be presented as of foremost value in her course. Instruction in the sciences should be presented as fundamental and contribtuory to the final accomplishment of better care of the patient rather than made an end in itself. The test of greatest importance should be that in the major subject of Nursing. Students should be stimulated by their daily experience not dulled by its routine, nor should they be regarded or allowed to think of themselves as a part of the machinery of the hospital.[*]

Miss Burgess might have been speaking to a modern audience when she stated:

The nurse instructor needs all of the knowledge she can obtain of the sciences, of psychology and pedagogy if she undertakes the teaching of the major subject in the curriculum.

A physician can give valuable instruction in anatomy and physiology; a bacteriologist, in bacteriology; the chemist and physician, in chemistry and materia medica; the dietitian, dietetics; all of which contribute to the necessary preparation of the student. The nurse instructor uses this instruction as the background for her teaching. Many lecturers on medical and surgical disease ignore the fact that emphasis should be placed on the nursing.

Nursing technique too is as frequently taught solely as a technical procedure without its reference to disease. We also find two errors frequently, that of teaching by demonstration, laying all the emphasis on skill in the accomplishment, and on the other hand little attention being given to the practice, the student studying the principles, the practice being left to a haphazard learning. The instructor should constantly aid the students to make the connection between class instruction and practical service.[*]

Time has not been sufficient to solve the problems she noted.

In reference to the sequence of arrangement of subject matter Miss Burgess stated the following:

The arrangement for class instruction in special subjects, and service in the departments, ought to be given in conjunction. . . . When this does happen the practical experience is teeming with educational value, especially if it is directed by the nurse instructor. Her work in the classroom is then so closely related to the ward that the students invariably make the connections. They are stimulated, interested and alive to the possibilities which the different services hold for them and intensely interested in the results of their efforts.[†]

During the 1919 meeting of nursing educators, round-table discussions were held. Reports of the group discussions further reflected the great concern of nursing educators for the provision of better teaching in terms of selection and development of

---

[*]Burgess, Elizabeth: How can we make the student's practical work experience more profitable from an educational standpoint? Twenty-Fifth Annual Report of the National League of Nursing Education, Baltimore, 1919, The Williams & Wilkins Co., p. 286.

---

[*]*Ibid.*, p. 287.
[†]*Ibid.*, p. 288.

teachers, improvement of teaching methods, and definition of teaching responsibilities. By 1922 the prevailing pattern of assigning the classroom instruction to full-time teachers and the clinical experience to the head nurse had regained its popularity. Echoes of a need for changing this basic pattern of teaching responsibility were heard when a number of speakers at the Twenty-Eighth Annual Convention of the National League of Nursing Education in 1922 raised issues and offered suggestions for improving clinical teaching programs. In her speech, "Clinical Teaching in Schools of Nursing," Beulah Crawford cited the suggestion originally made by members of the Nursing and Health section of the alumni of Teachers' College, whereby a clinical teacher would be developed who would work full time with students on the wards and report to the classroom instructors regarding the types of available experiences in order to correlate theory and practice more closely. It is interesting to note that while Miss Crawford praised this concept of the clinical teacher, she believed it to be a Utopian dream toward which all schools should aim. She proposed that, in the interim, clinical instruction could be accomplished through cooperative action of the classroom teacher and the head nurse by using the morning report each day to correlate clinical and theoretical information, by student participation in physicians' rounds and clinics, and by the case method of patient care followed by a written case study.[4] Advocating essentially the same methods, Mary S. Power discussed the importance of providing selected clinical experiences for students in "The Importance of Clinical Instruction for Nurses."[5] Perhaps the outstanding example of the kind of concern nurse educators were experiencing was expressed by S. Lillian Clayton in her speech, "The Place of the Teaching Supervisor in our Educational Program." She approached the subject by describing the teaching supervisor's qualifications, role, functions, and relationships with other administrative personnel. The

descriptions were based upon reports from various schools that had begun to utilize a teaching supervisor in the clinical teaching program.[6]

Although a number of schools were considering the use of a teaching supervisor, Bellevue Hospital School of Nursing is believed to have been the first to establish such a position, in 1922. It was started in the area of pediatrics, where the teaching supervisor organized equipment and made arrangements for classes and demonstrations using patients on the wards. With the help of a few others this program began to grow, so that by 1927 each clinical service was analyzed and a clinical teaching program was built around the clinical material available on the wards. This project is described in *Clinical Education in Nursing*, by Blanche Pfefferkorn and Marion Rottman.[7] In 1926 Bellevue Hospital School of Nursing created another position designated as a ward instructor. This position was created to relieve the head nurse of teaching responsibilities as the administration of ward activities continued to expand. The ward instructor was responsible for the students' orientation, instruction, and supervision on a full-time basis.

The establishment of the Yale University School of Nursing in 1922 was vital in changing some of the fundamental concepts about the practice of nursing as differentiated from the practice of medicine. The Yale University School of Nursing took the lead in altering the teaching pattern to include both the physical and psychological needs of patients. Of even greater significance was the transformation of the concept of the case-study approach from its prototype of the physician's case study to a patient-centered nursing care study. Although some other schools of nursing followed this pattern, these concepts were only another Utopia for most schools at this time. Schools and hospitals were not well enough staffed with head nurses, supervisors, or teachers to carry out additional teaching functions at the same time that they were responsible for an ever-increasing load of technical routines.

The effect of the Goldmark report of 1923 was not seen directly in clinical teaching. Its primary impact was to close those schools that lacked a sufficiently large and varied patient population, prepared faculty, and administrative strength to provide adequate education.

Period of adjustment

By the early 1930s there was a growing recognition that a new kind of person was needed to meet the demands of nursing service and to provide adequate clinical teaching programs for students; the common pattern of clinical teaching seemed to be that of the supervisor-teacher. Between 1933 and 1953 many of the changes relating to clinical teaching came about gradually. A cross-sectional view of this 20-year span of time reveals a wide variation in the quality and type of clinical teaching programs in schools of nursing. There were those schools that had no designated clinical teaching program, those that still relied heavily on the head nurse to perform the teaching functions for the clinical teaching program, and those that had graduated to the use of the supervisor-teacher. There were also a number of schools responsible for changing the clinical teaching pattern to that of placing the entire responsibility of the students with the ward teachers without additional administrative responsibilities. Ward teaching activities were defined by the 1937 curriculum guide as those organized clinics and conferences that are planned in connection with the clinical experience, a care study, and perhaps some formal classes.[8]

A common pattern of activities of the ward teacher went something like this: The ward teacher was assigned a group of students, often located in more than one unit; the ward teacher made herself available for assisting students in making nursing care safe according to whatever experiences were available at the time. When students on other wards needed assistance with situations they felt unprepared to handle, they called the ward teacher to the unit. In addition there were usually such daily activities as the following: ward rounds by physicians, a ten- to fifteen-minute ward class or morning circle after the morning report, and individual conferences to assist students in planning nursing care and in writing nursing care studies. Formal teaching usually consisted of supplementing the physician's lecture and clarifying issues as necessary.

By 1945 nurses were beginning to recognize that patients needed as much or more help in their social and emotional adjustment to their illness as they did in their physical care. The ward teachers, who were faced with these problems while supervising students, assumed the responsibility of planning for the integration of social and health aspects within the clinical teaching program. This brought about a change of approach in developing the nursing care plan to include a written plan for assisting the patient and his family to adjust to the restrictions of his illness and to understand his home care and the directions for prescribed home treatments. Along with this change came a shift in emphasis regarding patient-centered ward teaching: the establishment of group conferences in which the written plan of care of an individual patient was discussed in terms of the patient's needs, while group members contributed their knowledge in an effort to provide nursing measures to relieve the situation. The gradual restructuring of nursing practice to include such conferences occurred over the same period. In some teaching centers this kind of conference included contributions from the related disciplines in planning a more unified approach to patient care.

By midcentury a general framework for the development of a clinical teaching program in a school of nursing had been well established and had begun to be considered a necessary part of the total curriculum pattern. A major change regarding curriculum development in schools of nursing was heralded in 1950. The National League of Nursing Education renounced its responsibility for developing further revisions of the *Curriculum Guide for Schools of Nursing* and launched an all-out program to place the responsibility for curriculum development with the faculty members of individual schools of nursing. This change might well be labeled the "dawn of creativity" in curriculum building, since faculty members were encouraged to experiment with new ideas. Individuals vitally concerned with the development of sound clinical teaching programs, caught by the sparks of creative thinking, were challenged to experiment with the development of various clinical teaching programs to fit their individual school needs, yet worthy of scrutiny by the profession. It remains difficult for schools to take the accreditation guidelines as merely that and to prepare curricula creatively. All too often they behave as if a magic guide that assures success will be found.

Focus on the future

History reminds us that it is through the development, identification, and resolution of problems that progress is made. Our own nursing journals echo our ability to take issue with ideas that threaten our current educational practices. As a profession we seem to be at last moving forward to a point at which we take issue with current educational practices. This is the kind of initiative we need in assuming the responsibility of stimulating those creative elements from which the ideas of the future will come. Nursing journals are offering, as never before, a wealth of information regarding the kinds of clinical teaching programs representative of many types of curricula that have been tried by schools of nursing. As each approach is offered for perusal we grow a bit in terms of our willingness to share our work with others, our willingness to view the work of others with an open mind, our willingness to try our own experiments, and our willingness to

assume the initiative or sustain our efforts in moving forward with new ideas that will help shape our future. However, evidence exists that we do not put the knowledge gained by our colleagues into practice and that individual nurses insist on relearning by trial and error the same lessons mastered by others. Perhaps the key to redirecting the energy lost in this process is the guidance and example of the clinical nursing teacher.

EFFECTS OF THE CHANGING SOCIAL ORDER ON PATTERNS OF CLINICAL TEACHING

In part the direction of change in curriculum and clinical teaching patterns in schools of nursing is prescribed by the changing social order. The rapidity and occasional uncertainty with which these changes occur have been described repeatedly in current literature. Curricula in most settings, not only nursing, give, at best, token attention to such changes as population expansion, communications and transportation systems. scientific and technological advances, accumulation of knowledge, economic condition of society, contemporary youth culture, and social barriers.

Keene suggests:

College students, as never before, must be trained to think, to be afforded a means of establishing a sense of values, to become accustomed to living with suspended judgments, to be given an understanding that final and definitive answers were probably never man's lot and surely are not today. College students need to sense the evolutionary nature and significance of man's pursuit of truth, of the multi-causal factors which condition everything from the functioning of man's body to local, county, state, national, and international events. With such an educational approach, there is a strong possibility that they as individuals can become sufficiently flexible to investigate properly and assess the complex events with which our society is and will continue to be constantly bombarded.*

---

*Keene, C. Mansel: Such keen and delicate instruments, Teachers College Record **65:**255, Dec., 1963.

Continual investigation and evaluation of social change properly becomes the responsibility of society's educational systems and the individuals who make up that society. Nurse educators and clinical teachers must provide a learning environment that helps students to develop intellectual power embodied with flexibility and adaptability in facing new situations and solving new problems. The following cursory discussion concerns those social changes appearing to have a sizeable impact upon the directions clinical teaching programs may take.

Population expansion

As Reva Rubin has suggested,[9] one judges the greatness of a society in terms of the performance and achievement of its members rather than in terms of its numbers. Population changes are related to many social changes, such as war and peace, depression and prosperity, ignorance and knowledge, medical advances and stagnation, and national disasters and condition of economic and social welfare. The overall trend in population size has been upward, however.

Although census figures for the United States have shown a gradual but continuing decline in the annual population growth rate since 1957, the projected increased population rate for the 20 to 29 year age group, in which childbearing is most heavily concentrated, indicates a continued population expansion during these years.[10] Some other countries have yet to achieve even the slowing of growth. Closely related to this uncontrolled population growth is the problem of hunger, since food supplies have not increased at the same rate as the population. Health professionals have rarely considered the resolution of these intermingled problems as a clinical teaching responsibility. Pressure from society at large may lead to an increase in classroom education and caregiving experiences pertinent to the problems.

As a result of the increased birth rate between 1944 and 1957 and the increased life-span, all educators are faced with the immediate and future problems of providing more and better educational facilities for a young population that is rapidly approaching double proportions and has been predicted to triple by 1980. Futurists have begun to consider the eventual social impact of this "baby boom" as it becomes an "aged boom" and draws increasingly on social resources.

The combination of large numbers of persons representing a wide range of age groupings attempting to establish interpersonal relationships that hopefully will provide them with a satisfying way of life yields both positive and negative results. As the individual seeks to solve his problems in a complex social structure, he may need new approaches. The concept of group activities such as discussion groups, workshops, seminars, group projects, and group therapy has served a useful purpose in helping individuals to contribute effectively on a cooperative basis in a democratic society. Nursing schools have been no exception in accepting and using these approaches. However, as college enrolments become increasingly larger and student-faculty ratios expand, other approaches are needed if clinical teachers expect to stimulate creative thinking and direct it into channels of productivity that will enable students to make their unique contributions to clinical nursing.

Communications and transportation systems

Early American community life was strongly oriented toward deeply rooted interpersonal relationships established according to the customs, traditions, mores, and demands of the local inhabitants. As new industries and businesses grew and complex modern cities arose, so began the mobility of the population. Those who once experienced life as "big fish in a little pond" found themselves experiencing life as "little fish in a big pond." Thus began the trend toward exchanging one's social role from the distinctive patterns of closely knit community relationships for a depersonalized mode of life in an urban-suburban community.

Modern systems of communications and transportation share equally in the role of bringing individuals and nations together. Through such technological advances as communications satellites, national and international television and radio, wire news services, and other less dramatic but effective systems, information is being shared among the nations of the world. The ability to see and hear about the experiences of men everywhere through the medium of television is one of the most outstanding differences between present and previous generations. Television has become the main transmitter of information, as evidenced by the fact that a total of 81 million sets were in use before 1970.

Educationally we are beginning to utilize the potentials of some improved communications devices for gathering and disseminating scientific information. We now readily receive live telecasts of current events around the world through the use of communications satellites. There has been a rapid evolution in transmission techniques relative to global and interplanetary television communications. Many of these techniques are destined to become part of a system for receiving and disseminating live educational programs to and from all parts of the world. Progress is being made toward establishing nationwide and worldwide communications links so that diagnostic data gathered in one locale may be transmitted in a matter of minutes to computers for analysis and immediate return of results.

A simplified version of this system now exists whereby specialized telephone systems transmit communications between a particular physician and an expert in the field anywhere in the nation or world. Such systems can be linked to classrooms and laboratories for simultaneous teaching and discussion of the clinical process. In the vast field of medicine alone scientists are developing a variety of systems for storing, retrieving, and disseminating information. We have barely begun to appreciate not only the scientific advances made possible by such instrumentation but also the potential for harm which such advances carry. The latter includes the application of healing techniques without regard for personal choice of the patient or patient's family and the violation of privacy in the storage and retrieval of data. Nurses have yet to become aggressive in identifying or resolving such issues.

Our transportation systems have also provided a vast network of rapid, economical means of travel. Every year 35 million people in the United States move from one section to another, from one state to another. The continued improvement of modes of travel makes it inevitable that the future social structure of our nation will continue to change.

The constant movement of people creates other problems such as pressures exerted by family and friends who question the advisability of the move; pressures involved in the act of moving; anxieties regarding disruption of contact with friends, along with the need to seek new friends; loss of family unity; disruption of formal educational opportunities; language barriers; constant readjustment to the physical and environmental conditions; epidemiological problems; and lack of continuity in health care. We have not been able to assure, however, that there is a coordinated system of care for the mobile population or care that is easily accessible for those without the luxury of a private automobile.

The patterns of international understanding set by our statesmen are rapidly becoming a part of the total life of the citizens of the nation. World travel for the purpose of human understanding and world peace is becoming an important and integral part of life. Travel for its own sake will gradually lose its appeal to those young people who stand ready to shape the future of our nation. Judging from such patterns of international travel, it is entirely possible that the majority of students entering schools of nursing within the next two decades will have either traveled or lived in one or more other countries. Concomitantly the leaders in government, industry, business, and education will have experienced the opportunity to participate in the life activities of many nations. This kind of orientation to international understanding should have a profound influence upon the kind of leadership exercised in administering the affairs of our nation. Appreciation of the truly global nature of many health problems remains limited, particularly since many of the more virulent contagious diseases have been at least partially controlled.

The clinical teacher must possess a personal philosophy that recognizes a responsibility for contributing to the well-being of the world population. Understanding the meaning of different values and customs of people everywhere makes the clinical teacher responsible to apply this knowledge in two dimensions: (1) understanding the student as an individual affected by this new and changing social order and (2) assisting students in understanding patient behavior as a function of this same system, varied according to their individual values, customs, and anxieties.

The utilization of the latest communication and transportation systems also has a profound effect on the methods used to teach students more efficiently and effectively, as described in Chapter 8.

Scientific and technological advances

Technological advances based on new scientific knowledge have occurred in greater numbers in the past 20 years than in all other years of mankind's existence. It is estimated that the facts learned by today's youth will have become obsolete by the time they are 30 years old. The continuing trend toward mechanization has revolutionized the labor force and the work procedures of those professionals who provide improved services for a growing population. Many routine, repetitive tasks can be accomplished by the use of electronic devices, freeing professional personnel to function at a much higher level of competency. Nurses, on the whole, seem to have either attempted to ignore the new technology by resisting the introduction of new systems and equipment or have overresponded by "nursing the machines" rather than the people they (and those machines) serve. In the implementation of a machine-based system (for patient care or education), critical questions are whether or not the need for the technology is real, and whether or not the energy investment in technology will result in recognizable improvement in reaching desired goals in patient care.

The Hospital Information System used by Children's Hospital, Akron, Ohio, serves as an example of the direction automation is taking to minimize the clerical tasks of the nurse and other health workers. The system utilizes an automatic data processing computer to handle a large volume and wide variety of information for storage and retrieval as needed. Manual entry units and printers are available in each nurses's station, radiology department, dietary department, laboratory, central supply room, operating rooms, recovery rooms, pharmacy, and the outpatient department. When the machines are programmed for *maximal use*, one set of orders *properly* recorded will be activated by each department involved in supplying the necessary equipment and information for completing the orders. Drugs, meals, laboratory procedures, diagnostic tests, roentgen rays, surgery, formula feedings, therapy schedules, and charge slips are handled in this manner. Other uses of the data processing equipment include securing admission data, preparation of condition and census reports, and daily physicians' summary sheet providing up-to-date information for each patient's chart. Thus, one simple operation of the manual entry unit eliminates the need for the Kardex, medicine cards, various requisitions, hand-written reports and charge slips, and myriads of other details now attended to by nursing personnel. The properly skeptical reader will realize, however, that the preceding is true only when the italicized conditions are met. As many know, there is no mix-up quite like a computer mix-up!

Regardless of oft-voiced opinions, automatic devices can never replace the human relationship between patient and nurse. Whenever repetitive and manual skills can be handled automatically, humans are free to act as decision makers in close relationships with patients. Freeing nurses from desk tasks to patient-centered tasks is not merely a means to an end, that end being "care." It is an end in itself—the caring relationship that is the essence of nursing. The fulfillment and satisfaction gained from such a nurse-patient transaction can be only as great as the ability demonstrated by the nurse. This means that while the clinical teacher teaches students what they need to know about the intricacies of operating the equipment and interpreting observed results, the student must also learn how to interweave the features that are necessary to a supportive relationship. The professional manages the delicate balance of scientific and technological necessities, the individual patient's unique needs, and the constraints of the system.

Accumulation of knowledge

Changes in educational standards, a rapidly increasing number of people creating new knowledge, and the quest for vast amounts of technical knowledge have resulted in a continued growth of a great storehouse of knowledge. Technological devices have provided exhaustive information-retrieval systems; valuable information can be stored on tape and microfilm; government agencies, armed forces, and private companies have prepared exhaustive files on research reports and made them available for reference; and there are at least 100,000 national and international technical and scientific journals in circulation.

As one means of coping with the explosion of knowledge and its impact on human behavior, educators as well as others have turned to specialization. Specialization began with the concept of the division of labor. Managers in business and industry discovered that isolating specific areas for intensive study for purposes of accelerating technological advances and making task assignments according to a specific job increased the daily refinement of the job and the total output of work. Aspects of the specialization process have filtered into the professional fields, as witnessed by the wide range of specialized dentists, lawyers, engineers, social workers, physicians, nurses, and educators. Nurses need little to remind them of the infinitesimal division of labor within the hospital setting. Although there are some areas in the hospital that rightfully call for the services of the true specialist in a given profession, the division of labor has the impact of treating patient care as an assembly line, with the goal being to provide so many baths per hour or beds made per day. The end result is apparently to serve more patients quickly but with little thought given to the degree of expertness with which each person should be functioning.

In clinical teaching we have borrowed the specialization approach from industry and higher education. Industry taught us that skills could be perfected more rapidly and more patients could be served if students were given repetitive assignments until a task was learned, with each new assignment becoming increasingly more difficult. As enrollments increased along with the knowledge explosion, clinical teachers borrowed specialization concepts from higher education. The clinical teacher, often a "self-taught expert" in the field, spoke and acted with authority regarding a particular specialized clinical field, relying on other authorities in other fields when additional information was needed. Current practice emphasizes soundly based expertise in some subfield of nursing as a proper prerequisite for faculty members.

The prevailing pattern of clinical teaching in schools of nursing has been one of specialization according to the traditional medical content areas. There is a growing trend for schools of nursing to reevaluate the kinds of programs they have developed in terms of the type of professional person needed by today's society.

Many schools are beginning to restructure their entire curricular patterns in ways that offer a challenge to every clinical teacher who is vitally concerned about the nursing profession. Those leaders who have revamped clinical programs in nursing did so as the result of two major discoveries regarding the tradition-bound, stereotyped, quasi-specialized approach to clinical teaching. These discoveries were as follows:

1. Except in rare instances the clinical teacher designated as the expert in a specific clinical area did not have a sufficient educational background to operate as a specialist in the respective field. On the other hand those clinical teachers who possessed highly specialized educational backgrounds too frequently failed because they lacked the general education knowledge needed to communicate with students in terms of a wholistic approach to patients.

2. Much of the learning about patient care crossed boundaries from one clinical area to another. Thus, clinical teachers often failed to teach students to develop a concept of the patient as an individual with many-faceted problems relating to a variety of clinical areas. There is a growing realization that one can teach the basic concepts of health and illness applying to all patients. Such an approach requires an expert clinical teacher to assist students in applying previously learned general concepts to the nursing care of patients regardless of the medical diagnosis.

The truly expert clinician in a specialized field of nursing usually functions quite differently from the clinical teacher but should be considered a valuable asset to any clinical teaching program. By reciprocal agreement the clinical nursing specialist and the clinical teacher can complement each other's work in the enrichment of the kind of learning experiences made available to the students. Now is the time for nursing educators to determine who are the true specialists of nursing and how they can best serve to enrich the clinical teaching programs.

Affluence and finance

The relative affluence of many nursing students and years of seeming prosperity have made it difficult for many students to understand and appreciate the impact of economics on health and health care. Rising salary scales for nurses, coupled with the seemingly remote connections between a patient's bill and a nurse's paycheck, have masked the fact that, even in affluence, many people are too poor to be healthy. With the end of prosperity in recession or depression, the optimistic picture of American health may be an easy bubble to burst. As special recruitment programs have gained momentum, health professions have aquired members who know from experience that health care is not a cheap, accessible commodity.

Affluent as our social system may have appeared, there has been a great reluctance to publicly fund health care for all citizens. Many of the barriers are political, related to altering a well-entrenched power structure centered around the entrepreneurial sale of health care by physicians. Aside from the balance of power, however, good health care for all is costly, although we have not accumulated all the data necessary to compute costs. Each program enacted to serve a special group (such as Medicare for the elderly) has cost far beyond original estimates. Although this excess is partly caused by abuses, it is also because the ostensible affluence has been used to mask the needs of many.

The slow process of social change is illustrated in the following predictions made in the 1960s regarding what would be accomplished by 1975:

1. By 1975 the country will reach a new peak of affluence with the production of goods and services passing the $1,000 billion mark.
2. Expansion of private enterprise will also continue to grow, probably in a movement to counterbalance government welfare programs.
3. In less than 20 years a minimum income may be assured for all.
4. The ultimate success of government welfare programs is dependent upon action taken by individual large cities to relieve such things as poverty, substandard housing, urban blight, racial discrimination, industrial waste, air pollution, general decay of sectors of the city, and unequal opportunities for education and health programs.
5. Cultural deprivation will be overcome as every family member is given an opportunity to attend formal and informal educational programs and is given access to good books, music, and art.
6. School segregation will no longer be a problem; every child will be guaranteed fifteen years of free public education from kindergarten through two years of college. There also will be available four-year college scholarships for qualified applicants.
7. By 1975 insurance covering most major medical costs will be available to most Americans.
8. By 1980 the life expectancy will rise to 73 years, but older persons will have more enjoyment from life by being allowed to taper off working time rather than retiring at a given age limit.
9. Many communicable diseases will be eliminated.
10. The use of complicated devices such as the artificial heart, kidney dialysis, and other similar experimental devices will be made available to all as public and private programs pool their resources to these ends.[11]

Few today would be so bold as to predict the achievement of all these goals.

Social barriers

The affluence of our society has brought about a highly competitive mobility for the achievement of social status as measured by the degree and kind of attainment of material goods such as clothing, housing, food, club membership, vacations, world travel, sporting activities, and the like. The confusing experiences of adjusting to a whole new set of social class values are just beginning as we continue to strive to live up to our declared commitment to individual freedom and development.

Of particular significance to nursing education is the manner in which women and men are compared according to leadership abilities in today's society. The so-called masculine or feminine traits usually ascribed to the male and female roles have been the results of social conditioning. As a result, internal conflicts arise as both the male and female seek to fulfil their personal goals of entering a truly challenging world but are forced into conformity by entering a field that historically has been considered the prerogative of the male or the female and has been cast as a predominantly masculine or feminine role.

In the United States, as in the rest of the world, two factors seem to be responsible for maintaining the nursing profession as a predominantly female occupation: (1) the feminine role as defined by society has been equated with the tasks related to nursing, and (2) pay scales for nurses generally have been set according to the lesser pay standards accorded women.

Society's persistence in equating nursing with women has created such problems as the following:

1. The female is often beset by conflicting ideas regarding her role as a woman in the profession and in her

relationships with others. Women are described as tending to rate other women as overdemanding, manipulative, competitive, and hypercritical. These impressions may generate feelings of insecurity so that the one in command tends to exercise authority in going by the rules and expects others first to be loyal to her, then to the job to be done.

2. The traditional concept of masculinity still persists, making it difficult to interpret the role of the male in a field so predominantly composed of females. Thus, the conflicting concept of roles limits the number of men who would like to pursue their new-found-but-not-yet-accepted role in the profession of nursing.

3. The existence of negative attitudes of men concerning the job capability of women is evidenced in many realms and contributes to our failure to recruit more men into the field of nursing. It may also account for the prevalence of problems that relate to nurse-doctor and nurse-administrator relationships.

4. The broadened career opportunities for both men and women make recruitment competition stiffer. The stability of a health career in the unstable job market has worked to the profit of all health careers, however.

5. A large percentage of nurses are women experiencing the socially difficult and challenging combination of traditional family responsibilities and a professional career. There is pressure on both educators and employers to recognize these changes and to accommodate them.

Nurse educators must begin to think in terms of providing professional leadership that strengthens the image of the nurse, recognizing the reality of the situation and the nurse's ability to identify the self needed to function effectively.

Another social concern in nursing today is the inclusion of nontraditional members. Al-though federal funds are available for providing economic assistance for the education of nurses, the nursing profession is just beginning to seek out the disadvantaged as a group and to help them enter professional nursing education programs. A report in 1969 by Osgood[12] and another in 1970 by Yates[13] give evidence that it is both desirable and possible to provide professional education opportunities for the disadvantaged without jeopardizing the admission and graduation standards or the quality of instruction for a given institution. Through federally funded projects nurse educators have provided equal opportunity for the disadvantaged by: (1) providing financial aid to the individual; (2) assisting secondary schools to provide academic programs for those potentially interested in nursing; (3) assisting interested students in seeking post–high school study to better prepare them for entrance to schools of nursing; (4) providing tutorial assistance prior to entrance to a nursing program and throughout the program as necessary, and (5) providing a flexible nursing curriculum, allowing the disadvantaged to proceed at a rate designed to meet their levels of ability. To reach the special kinds of needs of the disadvantaged with a relevancy that links nursing to their own realm of understanding requires creative nursing educators who are committed to social action.

General educators have recognized the need for planning curriculum patterns that provide opportunities for individuals to think effectively in situations highly charged with personal involvement. If indeed nursing represents the large degree of personal involvement to which it lays claim, it is difficult to avoid recognizing a degree of involvement in problems of the social system at large. From that it follows that nursing education should provide students with the opportunity to examine various facets of social issues in order to deal realistically with the current basic social problems. Clinical teachers must be aware of their own biases in planning learning experiences, and they must continue to develop an awareness and understanding of the prevailing socioeconomic problems and their inevitable effects upon the learning abilities of students.

Clinical teachers will need to learn how to use every ounce of creative talent in planning appropriate learning experiences to help students with wide variations in backgrounds discover and develop themselves to their fullest potential. Such an approach may loom as a virtual impossibility to some; for others it holds the promise of creating a whole new way of providing an educational program for those who come from deficient backgrounds.

Clinical teaching programs will need to give prime consideration to the planning of learning experiences that promote opportunities for students to develop skills in establishing effective and satisfying interpersonal relationships through the process of self-awareness, self-understanding, and self-acceptance. They also must reflect a philosophy of individual freedom that avoids constraints based on masculine or feminine roles, systems of class or racial hierarchy, or biases about age. Clinical learning experiences should be kept flexible enough to allow students to discover and learn how to cope with the value system of patients representative of both sexes and a wide range of ages, social classes, races, and religions. Such a clinical teaching program calls for an approach that offers opportunities for students to examine many facets of each issue and express their negative and positive feelings before making value judgments relative to the current social problems as they affect the health and welfare of our society.

Total curriculum planning

In curriculum planning, clinical teachers should reexamine these facets of the changing social order relative to their ultimate effects on the kind of students entering the school of nursing. We must build curricula that will utilize the greatest talents of the teachers and release the creativity of the

students by allowing them the opportunity to add to their current knowledge without limiting the possibility of their discovering new concepts of professional competence and personal fulfilment. We dare not waste valuable time by perpetuating the practice of teaching those concepts already known to most students or by attempting to teach "everything" without regard for the changing world in which we live. Another important aspect of curriculum planning relates to the types of facilities that will be utilized to handle the new kinds of health care problems for increasing numbers of patients. The eradication of many communicable diseases, the increased longevity at both ends of the age spectrum, the increased availability of medical care insurance plans, the availability of facilities for long-term care, the centralized regional health centers or clinics, the home-care programs, the intensive care units for complicated illnesses, and the widespread use of the heart pump, kidney dialysis, and other such devices, along with the possibility of a dozen new approaches by next year, call for adjustments in the curricula to provide nurses with the experiences necessary to meet these changing needs. Once the objectives are established, the learning experiences to accomplish the goals can be provided within any of a number of the available facilities such as the intensive care unit, the various wards of the hospital, the outpatient clinics, the home-care program, the chronic disease hospital, the nursing home, the regional community health center, or any number of community agencies and services.

Planning teaching programs in clinical nursing

The clinical teaching program of any school should be planned as a direct outgrowth of that faculty's understanding of the scope of nursing today *and* of the major predictable changes within that scope. The "and" is often a problem: all too frequently it is the scope of nursing yesterday and the major innovations of today that are considered in the planning process. Recent incorporations into clinical experiences have included care of groups of patients, care for those on monitoring and life supporting mechanical devices, care for those with chronic illnesses, especially older persons, and care for the healthy to keep them well. Few programs have determined how to adequately provide clinical or classroom teaching that observes the changing system in which care is given, or observes the newly validated professional stance of the nurse.

The problem-centered approach to the nursing care of patients continues to be used with abandon, often leading to a stereotyped kind of learning situation for students. As a result, the search is on for finding better ways of helping students make meaningful applications of background knowledge to the solving of patient-centered problems. A dynamic approach to problem-centered nursing care requires a nurse who has, in addition to a sound basic knowledge of health and illness from multiple angles, a working knowledge of the prevailing socioeconomic situation including the average range of income representative of occupations and professions; the existing degree of affluence; the progress made by city, county, and federal government agencies to relieve poverty, substandard housing, urban blight, racial discrimination, cultural deprivation, inequality of educational opportunities, and air pollution; the availability of community health centers and kinds of services provided; the kinds of health programs provided by official and nonofficial agencies; and the availability of provisions for covering the cost of medical care and eligibility requirements. As the patients' problems are identified, the nurse can draw on this information in many distinct ways, including: (1) identifying those socioeconomic and health and welfare resources that the patients possess and (2) using the knowledge about existing health and welfare facilities and services to help patients identify and utilize the kinds of available resources that would be most effective in supplementing their resources during the process of rehabilitation.

Nursing and nurse educators must waste no talent, skills, or creative ability in the development of students' potentials. A quest for quality and equality necessitates respect for the individual regardless of age, sex, social, cultural, or economical status.

EMERGING PATTERNS OF CLINICAL TEACHING PROGRAMS IN NURSING

One of the problems facing nurse educators is that of providing clinical teaching experiences geared to the different purposes inherent in each of the three types of basic professional nursing education programs. Educators must be willing to take a new look at these different programs, depart from the use of the same well-known approaches, and determine ways and means of planning clinical teaching experiences that are in agreement with the objectives of a given type of program and within the realm of possibility in terms of specified time limits and maximum utilization of human and material resources.

It seems reasonable to assume that there are at least as many patterns of clinical teaching programs as there are schools of nursing. Each type of educational program includes general kinds of learning experiences needed to fulfill its purposes; the rights and responsibilities for planning a complete curriculum of which the clinical teaching program is an integral part lie with the individual school. In subsequent chapters there will be discussions about planning, selection, and organization of clinical learning experiences; planning and supervision of patient care experiences involving various skills; planning clinical experiences to meet varying levels of student achievement; adaptation of teaching tools and methods for use in clinical teaching; and evaluation of progress in the clinical learning experience. But the *ways* in which these elements are manipulated to fashion a clinical teaching program in accord with the objectives of the total curriculum of a given school determine its success or failure.

The following descriptions of emerging patterns of teaching in clinical nursing are intended as representative examples of voluminous amounts and kinds of innovations with which schools are experimenting. Because of the rapidity with which programs grow and the fluidity with which they change, it is necessary to use a generalized presentation without identifying a particular pattern with any specific school of nursing.

Clinical teaching programs in diploma schools of nursing

The diploma program aims to prepare graduates to use basic scientific principles in giving nursing care and in planning for the care of patients; many schools also prepare students to direct other members of the nursing team. The graduate receives a diploma in nursing without a college degree and is eligible for licensure as a registered professional nurse. Diploma programs are usually established by hospitals and provide theory and clinical experiences related to nursing care of patients in general hospitals.[14]

Continuing pressure, most recently in the report of the Lysaught Commission on Nursing,[15] has been used to urge diploma schools toward associate or baccalaureate degree programs. Many of these schools have altered their curricula in these directions without making the necessary formal educational and institutional changes. Diploma schools of nursing receive much support because they continue to coincide with the image of nursing held by a preponderance of society. Although diploma schools of nursing have survived and flourished through nearly a century of professional growth and progress and continue to supply a large percentage of the graduate nurses to the profession, there is a growing recognition of the need to redirect their efforts to develop innovative, educationally sound programs that meet the changing health needs of society.

Diploma schools of nursing have progressed from a philosophy of hospital-physician controlled nursing service apprenticeship to a philosophy more congruent with student-centered educational principles. Total curriculum reorganization has brought about changes in the patterns of clinical teaching programs such as the following: (1) time spent in the clinical experience is controlled and planned to meet students' learning needs; (2) there is a reduction in the repetitive practice of nursing techniques; (3) theory and its application in the comparable clinical experiences are taught concurrently; (4) clinical teachers assume the responsibility for the students' learning experiences—making student assignments, supervising students in patient care, and assisting them to develop nursing care plans to meet the total needs of patients; (5) more emphasis is given to the development of skills in understanding human behavior and interpersonal relationships; (6) clinical experiences are planned to allow sufficient time for students to analyze patient behavior; and (7) clinical teachers and students work in close relationships with one another in assessing patient needs and planning appropriate nursing action. Although there are recognizable differences in the purposes between the diploma school of nursing and the baccalaureate degree school of nursing, the processes of clinical teaching in the majority of diploma schools of nursing parallel those of the collegiate schools of nursing. For those "quality" diploma schools of nursing one is hard-pressed to describe patterns of clinical teaching that differ greatly from collegiate schools. Alternate suggestions are that the *patterns* of clinical teaching described for the collegiate schools of nursing be studied and appropriately adapted to the philosophy and goals of the clinical teaching programs of the diploma schools of nursing, or that diploma schools whose educational structure is indistinguishable from that of college programs move to become accredited within colleges.

The future direction of curriculum and clinical teaching patterns in these schools will be determined by the schools themselves. They need to make no apologies for their programs; what *is* needed is an "operation bootstrap," in which each diploma school of nursing *honestly* evaluates its total resources to determine the nature, breadth, and level of nursing education it *can* provide. The diploma school that is so armed can move toward an orderly implementation of the kind of program it *can honestly* provide—be it collegiate, associate degree, or other—with pride and dignity. Such a program will reap the rewards of making a truly valuable, educationally sound contribution to nursing education, nursing, and society.

Clinical teaching programs in associate degree schools of nursing

The associate degree program aims to prepare graduates who can function under supervision as beginning staff nurses to give direct nursing care to patients and to collaborate with other nursing and health team members in providing individualized nursing care. The graduate receives an associate degree and is eligible for licensure as a registered professional nurse. These programs are usually established in junior or community colleges. The two-year curriculum pattern provides a continuum of concurrent courses in liberal arts, general education, and nursing courses that are broad in scope and usually include clinical experiences in medicine, surgery, obstetrics, pediatrics, and psychiatry.

The basic philosophy of the junior or community college, the nature of the objectives of the nursing program, and the student population it tends to attract give rise to the need for clinical teachers with vision to devise ways and means of providing stimulating, appropriate, and economical clinical experiences for students.

A problem-solving approach to the teaching of nursing knowledge is organized according to two basic concepts: (1) identification of broad basic nursing problems shared by all patients and (2) identification of the basic nursing functions needed to cope with these problems in providing nursing care for patients. This broad-fields approach cuts across all clinical categories of patients and incorporates aspects of pharmacology and diet therapy relating to the particular nursing problems being pursued. The focus of learning is on knowledgeable and skillful application of scientific principles to the performance of prescribed nursing techniques: identifying simple nursing problems and providing nursing measures to relieve the problems. Repetitive performance of procedures is kept to a minimum on the premise that students who understand the scientific principles underlying patient problem areas readily learn to perform specific procedures in a given hospital on becoming graduate nurses.

The student population tends toward heterogeneity; it is composed of men and women representing a wide range of ages, some who have already raised a family and some who are widowed, some who have had protracted practical life experiences in caring for the ill, and some who are seeking to fulfill their lifetime dream of "always wanting to be a nurse." The choice of an associate degree program may often be based on time or money needs rather than career goals or the content offered. In the majority of programs these students pursue their education while remaining in their own home environment; many continue to carry on their husband-wife or mother-father roles. As a result, the clinical teacher has the responsibility for providing a wide variation in the progression of learning experiences commensurate with the individual student's background knowledge.

Time limits imposed by these schools necessitate planning for the maximal use of those clinical facilities available for providing the best clinical learning experiences. The selection of these facilities is based on the concept of the laboratory experience as a means of meeting specific objectives such as to gain new knowledge and understanding through the performance of a particular experiment. A variety of facilities such as hospitals, clinics, physicians' offices, nursing homes, public health agencies, or other comparable agencies serve as the laboratory for the clinical experiences. The clinical teachers accompany the students to these selected laboratory facilities and guide them in the necessary clinical learning experiences until they achieve the desired educational objectives. Technological advances and constant discovery of new knolwedge make it imperative that clinical teachers assume sustained responsibility for monitoring the health care fields to assure that the technical skills taught are relevant to current nursing and medical practice. The limited time spent by students in each specific experience makes it necessary for each teacher to have a broad clinical educational base. In the course of one academic year, a teacher may function in two, three, or more settings, often quite different from one another.

Although some schools tend to follow a traditional pattern of designating specified days and time periods to be spent in the hospital or community agencies each week, many schools are devising more flexible ways and means of gearing the availability of clinical experiences more closely to the needs of the students. Since the general pattern of clinical teaching usually involves a closely knit nursing faculty working together to supervise the clinical experiences, the use of flexible scheduling patterns is accomplished by developing clinical programs around the regularly scheduled general education courses. Demonstrations of basic skills can be taught to large numbers of students by using closed circuit television systems followed by independent study and practice sessions. The use of tape recordings and programmed instruction devices offers students opportunities to master some basic content as out-of-class study assignments and releases valuable time for

the practice of more complicated clinical learning activities.

Some schools have discovered that the group approach to the simultaneous learning of a number of related skills can be successful. This group approach makes better use of available experiences for a number of students while permitting them to progress at their own rate of learning by moving them from one group activity to another according to individual needs. Several students may pursue a particular skill or problem with a patient while another group concentrates on still another problem area for the same patient. During this approach some students can use their time to observe their peers or others in the practice of basic technical skills and in nurse-patient relationships and attempt to analyze the results.

There are those who decry the use of this group method of assignment by claiming that it fragments the patient and does not allow the student to view the patient as a whole. But the secret of success for this approach, and others as well, lies solely in the ability of the clinical teacher. Not only is it necessary to plan ways of assisting students to develop a wholistic concept of human beings as individuals in a state of health or illness, but it is the responsibility of the instructor to work with the patients to ensure that the learning process of the student does not have a detrimental effect on the patients. Such planning involves the use of a variety of informal group conferences with the students. The preconference before each laboratory period provides opportunity for establishing the objectives for the total nursing care needed by the patients and for defining specific objectives of the individual student. During the clinical experience individual or group discussions or both are held as the need arises in order to help students in the interpretation of significant patient data and analysis of patient care. After the laboratory period the postconference discussion is concerned with evaluation of the patient's problems and the application of principles related to the problems and the corresponding nursing care. Involvement in the discussions also leads to increased ability of the student to relate more effectively to others in the groups and to evaluate the effectiveness of the contribution each student made to the whole in providing total nursing care for the patient.

To realize the maximum from such a demanding and challenging program the clinical teacher must have clearly defined objectives for clinical experiences and be capable of providing for individualized, carefully selected learning experiences. Like any teacher, the clinical faculty member in such a program must also possess an expert level of skill in providing professional nursing so that students have a role model as well as guidance and information. Students must be active participants in all clinical learning experiences, seek opportunities to further their own knowledge, and engage continuously in reflective thinking to apply learned basic principles to patient care problems related to technical nursing measures.

Clinical teaching programs in baccalaureate degree schools of nursing

The baccalaureate degree program aims to prepare graduates to plan, direct, provide, and evaluate nursing care to patients in a variety of settings; to demonstrate and interpret nursing care to others; to function as public health nurses; to fill leadership positions; and to enter graduate study in nursing. The graduate receives a baccalaureate degree in nursing and is eligible for licensure as a registered professional nurse. These programs are established by colleges and universities. The curriculum includes courses in liberal arts, biological and physical sciences, social sciences, and an upper division major in nursing. Theory and clinical experiences are offered in all clinical areas including public health nursing. Students entering this program represent two distinct backgrounds: (1) basic

nursing students having no previous background in the nursing major and (2) registered nurse students representing a wide range of background experiences in the nursing major.

The baccalaureate program lends itself to curriculum experimentation because of many factors such as the following: widespread development of new schools of nursing puts them in positions to innovate; administrative control is vested in an educational institution; liberal education courses are readily accessible; a wide range of physical facilities, resources, and services is available from the university; opportunities are available for securing the services of highly qualified university faculty members; and the length of the program allows for more opportunities for experimentation and for flexibility in scheduling.

While the traditional pattern of organizing clinical teaching programs according to distinct clinical services appears to meet the needs of some collegiate schools of nursing, other schools are beginning to experiment with different approaches. In some cases the faculty identify a number of core concepts drawn from the physical, biological, and social sciences in accord with the philosophy and objectives of the school. Then the clinical teaching program is organized to provide a longitudinal approach in the application of those broad concepts to increasingly complex, progressive experiences in the various clinical areas. A variation of this pattern utilizes a well-defined set of basic concepts regarding health and illness and their effects on patients congruent with earlier philosophical statements on nursing. The emphasis of the clinical teaching remains on the relationship between the concepts learned and the actual problems presented by the patient, regardless of the medical diagnosis. Although students are usually assigned to various clinical services on a rotation basis, the learning focus is on the basic application of concepts and principles of pathophysiology, psychology, sociology, and nutrition and the use of problem-solving techniques in assisting patients in terms of nursing. No deliberate attempt is made to teach the concepts in terms of medicine, surgery, pediatrics, obstetrics, or psychiatry.

However, it is difficult to lessen the use of the well-entrenched medical services approach. The tradition of a theoretical framework and our socialized deference to the physician's viewpoint often mean that the "new" approach is merely the same content poorly disguised by a few different words (for example, teaching traditional orthopedics as "mobility impairment" rather than covering a complete range of physical, social, and psychological immobility). This kind of situation calls for a clinical teacher who can adapt to a dual role and a multiplicity of clinical nursing situations.

Clinical supervision in the newer approach is usually confined to a group of students assigned to a particular clinical area; the clinical conferences consist of a group of students representing a variety of clinical areas and serve to coordinate the concepts in their application to the problems of patients representing a wide range of health and disease states.

The use of these patterns of variations often calls for a team teaching approach, which can be accomplished in a number of different ways:

1. All clinical teachers can work together as a team in supervising the students. During individual and group discussions the clinical teachers having the best background can be used effectively in helping students with problem-solving situations arising from a particular area at a given point in time.

2. Certain portions of the program can be taught by a master clinical teacher, with other clinical teachers supervising groups of students. All of the clinical teachers work as a unit in planning the total program and in auditing or contributing to the teaching sessions of the master teacher.

3. Specialists in other fields such as mental health consultants, nutritionists, social service workers, chaplains, and public health workers can contribute to the total clinical teaching team in a variety of ways. With the development of clinical nursing specialists at the master's and postmaster's level, the specialist in a clinical field such as heart disease is in a strategic position to function as a consultant to students and clinical teachers by assisting them with complicated nursing care measures and clarifying applications of scientific principles related to providing expert nursing care. Increasingly, members of clinical faculty are engaged in practice at the master clinician level, and thus are able to fill this role themselves.

The impact on nursing exerted by various social legislation programs has prompted many schools to plan clinical experiences on a broader base in order to accomplish the goals of the clinical teaching program. Clinical settings are being expanded to include hospitals, regional community clinics, nursing homes, chronic disease hospitals, well-child clinics, nursery schools, special education programs, physicians' offices, and a variety of other such agencies or institutions. For programs in which not all students receive clinical experience in each of these agencies (and there is a tendency for this to become the pattern), follow-up conferences with mixed groups of students representing each kind of setting can serve as the locus for all students to learn how to adapt nursing care to meet the needs of patients in these various settings.

Early experiences in direct patient care tend to promote student thinking in terms of task-centered nursing care rather than the desired patient-centered nursing care, because the patient's expectations of the nurse are not commensurate with the nurse's ability and because the student's primary concern is to live up to the patient's expectations. This resulting anxiety-laden performance by students and the ultimate effects upon the patients have led some schools to reexamine criteria used to determine selection of beginning assignments for students. Such an approach requires clinical teachers to evaluate the degree of care needed by patients in terms of ensuring patient safety, and then to determine the amount of knowledge and degree of skill needed by the student in order to overcome the fear of failure in safely meeting the patient's needs.

Another highly charged initial experience is that involving student-patient relationships. Having had only limited experience in the practice of nurse patient relationships, the student concentrates on the successful accomplishment of the task and tends to disregard the patient's behavioral response. To overcome this problem, some schools have provided observation laboratories whereby the student observes nurse-patient interaction and may enter into relationships with patients without being identified as a nurse. This arrangement offers numerous possibilities in helping the student communicate effectively with patients without being required to assume the nurse role before being equipped with enough self-understanding to assess psychological needs of patients and begin to understand their resultant behavior, or before becoming comfortable with the necessary psychomotor skills.

The problem of length of time needed to master designated skills in the clinical situation is being given careful scrutiny by many schools of nursing. There is a growing trend toward determining how programs can be planned to allow students to progress at their own rate rather than within a circumscribed time period. Such an approach is first dependent on the ability of the faculty to define those specific behaviors to be accomplished in order to meet the goals of a given course. When these behaviors have been established, the first important step has been taken. The clinical teacher can then determine whether the individual student is ready to move on to other tasks or whether additional help is needed in the accomplishment of the desired behaviors.

One means of planning the length of learning experiences in accord with the individual student's abilities is the use of independent study devices in schools of nursing. These are showing promising results; however, more time is needed to allow for validation studies to determine the long-term effectiveness of this approach. For those who cannot provide complete independent study units, clinical teachers can devise their own programmed instruction units for certain task learning along with methods of scheduling students to use the existing laboratories at varying times. Such an arrangement allows the student to engage in independent practice until ready to apply the knowledge or skill in the actual clinical situation.

Further elimination of repetitive clinical experiences can be accomplished by allowing for flexibility in scheduling students from one clinical unit to another as often as necessary during the daily experiences in order to provide the student with the most valuable and needed learning experiences. Serious consideration should be given, however, to the impact on the continuity of the relationship a patient experiences if students rotate daily or weekly.

Providing patient-centered clinical conferences is another aspect of flexible scheduling that has been found to provide more meaningful learning experiences for students. Historically these conferences have been scheduled and "taught" according to the pattern set for the week or even the month. Now the clinical conference is scheduled and planned according to the kinds of nursing care problems that arise from the student's daily clinical experiences. The conference discussions are kept dynamic by the clinical teacher, who must be alert to the kinds of problems that arise as students work with patients. The timing for the conferences must be *as the need exists;* when the need no longer exists, it no longer requires discussion. The students experiencing the problem must become involved in the discussion in terms of how they recognized and handled the problem. The clinical teacher's role becomes that of the devil's advocate; that is, the clinical teacher assumes a challenging, questioning role and manipulates the discussion so that the student can utilize knowledge, adapting it to explain new and different situations and to solve new and different problems. Such an approach also implies that the clinical teacher is secure enough to encourage independent action by the student and allow flexibility in the pursuit and application of knowledge by the student.

OUT OF THE PAST—INTO THE FUTURE

A myriad of sociological and technological changes have shaped the development of nursing education and passed into history. In over a century of American nursing (1873 to 1973) we have experienced and anticipated some of the most advanced and far-reaching technological and social changes ever envisioned. How, then, do these past and present patterns of clinical teaching affect future clinical teaching programs? As the light reflects the shadows, so the past reflects the shape of things to come, if not the details. To be prepared to meet the inevitable changing patterns of clinical teaching, we must discipline ourselves to become flexible enough to welcome and accept change. We must be willing to examine and analyze new situations in light of what we have known in the past, until they take on new and significant meanings in solving problems as they arise.

Out of the past. Repeatedly we have raised the question, "Who is the clinical teacher?" The head nurse, nursing arts instructor, ward supervisor, ward teacher, and finally the clinical instructor have performed a variety of functions in assuming the role of the clinical teacher in schools of nursing. There has been a continual shifting from one level of person to another in an effort to find the one who was in the best position to know and who also had the time to devote to the proper education of the students. *Into the future.* Current and predicted future educational patterns demand that the first criterion of who shall be the clinical teacher should be determined by who is the best qualified. As the whole educational system becomes elevated, we must look for the best qualified person to offer expert teaching. The clinical specialist may assume this responsibility either as a collaborative function or as a sole function; the head nurse or supervisor may also be a clinical specialist and may assume the clinical teaching functions; or the common pattern known today may remain except that the clinical teacher will be an expert in a clinical specialty in addition to functioning creatively as a clinical teacher.

Out of the past. Through the years there have been many variations in the patterns of designating responsibility of teaching the theoretical information in the classroom and the supervision of the "practice" portions of the program in the hospital setting. The present system of clinical teaching tends to remove more and more theory from the formal classroom setting and to place it in the live clinical situation. *Into the future.* As class enrollments grow, this same pattern will be refined and become relied upon more heavily; it is the method of implementing the pattern that will change. For example, the concept of team teaching uses this same basic method, but the creative clinical teachers will work together to produce many variations that should be highly successful. The multimedia approach and the use of electronic teaching aids will facilitate teaching basic theoretical information to large groups of students and team teachers working with small groups in the clinical situations to provide the necessary clinical nursing experiences.

Out of the past. The recognition by some of the earliest schools of nursing that student experiences in nursing practice could be extended into the home care of patients failed to survive as a standard practice because the goals were in terms of hospital needs rather than student needs. But the basic concept was revived as schools of nursing developed curricula that included supervised experiences in public health nursing. *Into the future*. The inevitable growth of health and social welfare programs, along with the change in kinds of health problems, offers opportunities for providing clinical experiences in a broader variety of settings such as centralized regional health centers, home-care programs, nursing homes, chronic disease hospitals, and research centers. Broadening the scope of resources to provide clinical experiences needed to meet the objectives of the program offers a wide range of background knowledge that may well be needed by tomorrow's nurse. Such an approach also gives rise to the need for clinical teachers having these kinds of specialized knowledges and skills to work cooperatively with teachers who may be well prepared in a given clinical speciality but ill equipped in system, theory and role behaviors to function effectively in these emerging kinds of health centers.

Out of the past. Since the beginning of the earliest schools of nursing, conflicts between nursing education and nursing service often centered upon the disparity between the teaching of nursing care in the classroom and the kind of nursing care actually being practiced in the hospital setting. This problem has continued to exist in varying degrees and in one form or another in almost every school of nursing in the United States. *Into the future*. Creation of integrated nursing service—educational organizations, through increased use of dual appointments, provides an avenue for elimination of the "we" versus "they" syndrome that so frequently affects communications between schools of nursing and places where nurses are employed. The obvious gaps between the two and their effects on student learning make it imperative that this problem be solved as soon as possible.

Out of the past. The basic concept of bedside clinics or ward rounds conducted

by physicians as a means of clinical teaching has continued to survive in one form or another. *Into the future*. This basic concept will take on a new dimension as physicians, nurses, social workers, and other health team members strive toward a working relationship built upon teamwork that respects the role played by each individual in contributing to the total needs of patients. As a result, the interdisciplinary conference will serve its function of improvement of patient care while taking on new significance as a teaching tool for nurses and other members of the health team.

Out of the past. The case method of assignment, the nursing care plan promoting individualized patient care, and the nursing care study transformed clinical learning experiences from procedure-centered learning tasks to patient-centered nursing care. *Into the future*. By the time automation has its greatest impact on hospital nursing services, students and graduate nurses alike will have more time to devote to the bedside management of patient-centered nursing care. There should be a continuation of a patient-centered approach to nursing care, but the methods for providing such care may be varied. For example, the increased numbers of patients seeking health care may well change the current method of student-patient assignment. Greater emphasis will be on learning how to manage a group of patients in terms of helping them reach a state of self-actualization. This concept could emerge from the very kind of learning the students experience if in their clinical experiences they have more freedom for their own self-actualization. Such an approach calls for flexibility in allowing students to select a basic problem related to the clinical theory and to select their own group of patients for study, consulting with the clinical teacher as necessary to work out a plan of care that is within the framework of the total program yet allows for the students' self-actualization.

Out of the past. The basic preparation of professional nurses has continued to be on one level—staff level positions in nursing—for so many decades that it is difficult to determine just how and when the various levels of nursing practice came into existence. Even more difficult to ascertain has been the development of curricula designed to educate nursing personnel to meet specific levels of performance in the practice of nursing. While we have attempted to develop curricula for diploma schools of nursing, associate degree schools of nursing, and baccalaureate degree schools of nursing, no clear line distinguishes one level of education from another. Nursing history reminds us that successive attempts have been made by far-sighted leaders in our profession, but no significant steps were taken to change the basic patterns of our educational programs. *Into the future.* We have at our disposal at least two recent landmark documents along with a number of new approaches to nursing education being advocated by those who have a commitment to the future direction of nursing and the concomitant direction nursing education must take to provide the high quality patient care needed and demanded by our nation. The first landmark was the adoption of the first Position Paper on the Educational Preparation for Nurse Practitioners and Assistants to Nurses, by the ANA Board of Directors in 1965, providing organized nursing with a set of values and beliefs regarding nursing and its implications for nursing and nursing education.

The second landmark document emerged from The National Commission for the Study of Nursing and Nursing Education, established in 1969 by the ANA and the NLN. The Commission was charged with the responsibility for conducting a national survey of changing practices and educational patterns and the projection of future probable requirements in professional nursing needed to provide high quality patient care. The preliminary report and recommendations set forth by the renowned Lysaught report early in 1970 have given rise to a renewed effort to find satisfying and enduring solutions to the multitude of problems related to supply and demand for nurses, nursing roles and functions, and nursing education and nursing careers.[15] Unlike the previous studies of this nature, the Commission is undertaking the task of putting its recommendations into practice. This means that nurses, individually and collectively, are assuming responsibilities at national, state, and local levels in an attempt to bring about changes in nursing education and in patterns of nursing practice, and to enlarge the base of financial support for nursing education and for recruitment of personnel needed to provide high quality nursing care. The rate of change has been slow, however, and many practicing nurses seem unaware of the potential for overall improvement in nursing education and practice.

Nurse educators also continue to pursue new directions for nursing education such as: rationale for the theoretical base of nursing practice; the career ladder concept; the open curriculum; the expanded roles of the nurse; the implications of physicians' assistants for nursing and nursing education; and the nurse as a specialist or a generalist at the graduate level.

New concepts and values such as these are often in conflict with those well-established attitudes, roles, and concepts inherited from generations living in a vastly different world. A long, hard look at the kinds of changes taking place, combined with an imaginative and knowledgeable approach to meet the current situation, is necessary if individuals are to fulfill themselves both personally and professionally, ultimately contributing to the growth of the nation and a better world.

REFERENCES

1. Roberts, Mary M.: American nursing history and interpretations, New York, 1954, Macmillan, Inc.
2. Wood, Helen M.: The value of the clinical method of teaching in nursing schools and how it can be organized, Twenty-Fifth Annual Report of the National League of Nursing

Education, Baltimore, 1919, The Williams & Wilkins Co.

3. Doty, Parmelia M.: The need of cooperation between the head nurse and instructor, Twenty-Fifth Annual Report of the National League of Nursing Education, Baltimore, 1919, The Williams & Wilkins Co.
4. Crawford, Beulah: Clinical teaching in schools of nursing, Twenty-Eighth Annual Report of the National League of Nursing Education, Baltimore, 1922, The Williams & Wilkins Co.
5. Power, Mary S.: The importance of clinical instruction for nurses, Twenty-Eighth Annual Report of the National League of Nursing Education, Baltimore, 1922, The Williams & Wilkins Co.
6. Clayton, S. Lillian: The place of the teaching supervisor in our educational program, Twenty-Eighth Annual Report of the National League of Nursing Education, Baltimore, 1922, The Williams & Wilkins Co.
7. Pfefferkorn, Blanche, and Rottman, Marion: Clinical education in nursing, New York, 1932, Macmillan, Inc.
8. Committee on Curriculum of the National League of Nursing Education: a curriculum guide for schools of nursing, New York, 1937, National League of Nursing Education.
9. Rubin, Reva: This I believe, Nursing Outlook **14:**55, July, 1966.
10. Long, Luman H., editor: The world almanac, New York, 1970, Newspaper Enterprise Associates, Inc.
11. Cohen, Wilbur J.: Social policy for the 1970's, indicators, Washington, D. C., 1966, Department of Health, Education and Welfare.
12. Osgood, Gretchen: Dimensions of involvement, Nursing Outlook **17:**53-55, Sept., 1969.
13. Yates, Judith: Breakthrough in Minnesota, American Journal of Nursing **70:**563-565, March, 1970.
14. National Commission for the Study of Nursing and Nursing Education: Summary report and recommendations, Am. J. Nurs. **70:**279-294, Feb., 1970.
15. Lysaught, J. P.: An abstract for action, New York, 1970, McGraw-Hill Book Co.

SUGGESTED READINGS

Abdellah, F. G., and others: New directions in patient-centered nursing, New York, 1973, Macmillan, Inc.

Alfano, Genrose, and others: Nursing in the decade ahead, American Journal of Nursing **70:**2116-2125, Oct., 1970.

Bennis, Warren G.: The temporary society, Journal of Creative Behavior **3:**233-242, Fall, 1969.

Brodt, Dagmar: Excellence or obsolescence, Nursing Forum **9**(1):19-26, 1970.

Brown, Amy F.: Curriculum development, Philadelphia, 1960, W. B. Saunders Co.

Bullough, V., and Bullough, B.: The emergence of modern nursing, ed. 2, New York, 1969, Macmillan, Inc.

Christman, Luther: What the future holds for nursing, Nursing Forum **9**(1):12-18, 1970.

Conant, Lucy: Closing the practice-theory gap, Nursing Outlook **15:**37-39, Nov., 1967.

Dickey, F. G.: Accreditation and social change, NLN Publication no. 15-1475, Department of Baccalaureate and Higher Degree Nursing, pp. 1-10, 1973.

Dineen, Mary: Current trends in collegiate nursing education, Nursing Outlook **17:**22-26, Aug., 1969.

Friedan, Betty: The feminine mystique, New York, 1963, W. W. Norton & Co., Inc.

Galbraith, John K.: The affluent society, New York, 1958, The New American Library, Inc.

Galeener, Janet: Providing more meaningful clinical experiences through group or multiple student assignment, Journal of Nursing Education **5:**29-31, April, 1966.

Gerzon, Mark: The whole world is watching, New York, 1969, The Viking Press, Inc.

Goldmark, Josephine: Committee for the study of nursing education, New York, 1923, Macmillan, Inc.

Hangartner, Carl: The responsibilities of universities and colleges for the educational preparation of professional nurses, Journal of Nursing Education **4:**19-27, Jan., 1965.

Harty, Margaret: Trends in nursing education, American Journal of Nursing **68:**767-772, April, 1968.

Heidgerken, Loretta E.: Teaching and learning in schools of nursing, Philadelphia, 1965, J. B. Lippincott Co.

Henderson, Virginia: Excellence in nursing, American Journal of Nursing **69:**2133-2137, Oct., 1969.

Kelly, Nancy: The student voice in curriculum planning—threat or promise, Nursing Outlook **17:**59-61, April, 1969.

Kramer, Marlene: The new graduate speaks again, American Journal of Nursing **69:**1903-1907, Sept., 1969.

Lewis, Edith: The associate degree program, American Journal of Nursing **64:**78-81, May, 1964.

Lysaught, Jerome P.: From abstract to action, New York, 1973, McGraw-Hill Book Co.

Miles, Matthew: Education in the '70s; some predictions, Teachers' College Record **65:**441-454, 1964.

Montag, Mildred L.: Utilization of graduates of associate degree nursing programs, Journal of Nursing Education **5:**5-9, April, 1966.

Moore, Marjorie: The professional practice of nursing, Nursing Forum 8(4):361-373, 1969.

Noy, Pinchas: The "youth protest" and the "age of creativity," Journal of Creative Behavior 4: 223-233, Fall, 1970.

Nursing students in campus protest, Nursing Forum 8(2): 117-142, 1969.

Ozimek, Dorothy: The preparation of a generalist, Nursing Outlook 16:28-29, Dec., 1968.

Pellegrino, Edmund: Rationale for nursing education in the university, American Journal of Nursing 68:1006-1009, May, 1968.

Powell, John Walker: Communication, technology and education, Adult Leadership 17:302-304, Jan., 1969.

Ramphal, Marjorie: Needed: a career ladder, American Journal of Nursing 68:1234-1237, June, 1968.

Reinkemeyer, Sister Agnes: New approaches to professional preparation, Nursing Forum 9(1): 27-40, 1970.

Richards, Jean F.: Integrating a clinical specialist into a hospital nursing service, Nursing Outlook 17:23-25, March, 1969.

Shetland, Margaret: Teaching and learning in nursing, American Journal of Nursing 65:112-116, Sept., 1965.

Stein, Rita F.: Perspectives and patternments in contemporary nursing knowledge, Education Horizons 57:61-68, Winter, 1968-1969.

Stevens, B. J.: Adapting nursing education to today's student population, Journal of Nursing Education 10:15, April, 1971.

Tyler, Ralph: Curriculum—challenge for experimentation, Nursing education—creative, continuing, experimental, New York, 1966, National League for Nursing, pp. 3-10.

Vaillot, Sister Madeine Clemence: Nursing theory, levels of nursing, and curriculum deveolpment, Nursing Forum 9(3):234-249, 1970.

Wood, L.: Proposal: a career plan for nursing, American Journal of Nursing, 73:832-835, May, 1973.

2 Establishing the frame of reference

CLARIFICATION OF TERMS

To identify the frame of reference used throughout this book, it is necessary to clarify the relationships between teaching and creativity and the ultimate relationships between creative teaching and creative teaching in clinical nursing. The words *creative clinical teaching,* laden with value judgments, make it virtually impossible to illustrate or "label" all aspects of creativity inherent in the teaching of clinical nursing. The nature of this book charges the writer with the responsibility for allowing the readers to use their own "creative thinking" talents in analyzing the discussion of creativity concepts relative to the clinical teaching process, and for guiding their thinking in terms of a wholistic approach in the application of creativity to teaching in clinical nursing.

What is teaching?

The functions of teaching in general education and in specialized fields such as nursing education have often been analyzed and stated by various professional groups and individual faculty members, but there appears to be no one universally agreed upon definition of teaching. Although there is a tendency toward relying on connotations of that which is "good" teaching, a simple definition of teaching should be concerned with the *acts* of teaching regardless of their quality. In establishing a frame of reference on which to build concepts of creative teaching in clinical nursing, we have not included in the stated definition of teaching decision-making functions relative to curriculum development; the definition is concerned with the *acts of teaching.*

Teaching is the facilitating or arranging of experiences within the learner's world in a way that helps him find meaning and purpose. *Teaching is* the act of communicating in a variety of ways with the individual or group or both at the actual point of the learner's experiences so that he can reach his unique potential. *Teaching is* the act of setting the stage and shifting the scenery so that the learner makes differentiations and organizes parts and wholes into new and meaningful patterns. *Teaching is* the greatest of all human tasks after learning.

What is creativity?

Creativity in and of itself is not new; it is the placement of concepts of creativity in a particular context that is new. In the Judeo-Christian tradition only God was creative, any notion that man could be creative was considered blasphemous. Not until about three centuries ago did there emerge the concept of human beings as creative in thought and action. The recognition of this concept brought about the gradual realization of the tremendous unsuspected potentialities of human beings, the nature of human resources, and the meaning of respect for the individual. There followed a long period of time in which the word *creative* was equated with the description of those acts within the realm of artistic talents; little regard was given to any deeper significance of the term in relation to teaching.

The year 1950 seemed to mark the beginning of a movement to gain deeper understandings of the creative process as it applied to human activities in certain areas of science, industry, business, psychology, and psychiatry. As the value of practical applications of these understandings was reported educators began to meet together to examine the substance of the creative process and its practical application to the realm of teaching. As a result, the elements of creativity have been described with diversity by a number of authorities from various fields. However, one must remember that the effectiveness of helping students reach their creative potential hinges largely upon the teacher's attitudes toward creativity. Close examination of some of the definitions reveals certain qualifying factors that tend to limit the application of the term *creativity;* others have taken a more liberal point of view. This latter viewpoint offers a more flexible base of operation for providing creative teaching programs in clinical nursing. Thus the selection of the definition of creativity to serve as the frame of reference for this book was adapted from that offered by Alice Miel.*

Creativity is a quality inherent within every individual. *Creativity is* exhibited by the individual in amount and kind according to the principles of individual differences. *Creativity is* a deliberate act of an individual to relate previously unrelated experiences in a manner that produces something *new to him,* is satisfying to the self, and is useful to him in a constructive manner.

What is creative teaching?

The teacher must maintain environment conducive to creative thinking. Every learning situation provides the teacher with this opportunity to use a creative approach in dealing with changing conditions. The relative degree of creativity produced by a wholistic approach is difficult to assess, but the effects are subtle and of lasting value because the teacher understands and utilizes the characteristics, attitudes, and

habits inherent in the act of creative teaching.

Creative teaching is approaching each teaching experience as a new and unique assignment, which demands understanding and concern for the individual students and the utmost knowledge and skill in working with the subject matter. *Creative teaching is* recognizing failure in one course of action as cause for immediacy in devising other means of transmitting the knowledge, skill, or attitude to be learned or appreciated. *Creative teaching is* knowing when to use previously established but effective routine approaches to problems and when to reject habitual responses as patterns of teaching for more constructive approaches. *Creative teaching is* fostering self-respect and self-discovery in the learner. *Creative teaching is* providing unlimited opportunities for individuals and groups to assume responsibility for furthering their own learning experiences.

What is teaching in clinical nursing?

Nursing education has the advantage of having readily available sources of actual life situations for providing students with rich clinical learning experiences in which to practice patient-centered nursing care. Today as never before there are unlimited opportunities for learning offered by various clinical services, outpatient clinical services, and specialized services in general and specialized hospitals; community nursing service agencies; neighborhood health centers; extended care facilities; nursery schools; physicians' offices; and occupational health programs in industry. Any respectable definition of teaching in clinical nursing must of necessity include the same basic elements that have been so aptly described by eminent nurse educators concerned with clinical teaching. Such basic elements include the following: clinical teaching constitutes the heart of the nursing curriculum; clinical teaching involves planning, organizing, teaching, supervising, and evaluating students' direct experiences in patient care; clinical teach-

---

*Miel, Alice, editor: Creativity in teaching, Belmont, Calif., 1961, Wadsworth Publishing Co., Inc.

ing provides students with an opportunity to make application of theoretical knowledge to provide improved, patient-centered nursing care. These concepts serve as the basis for the following definition, which is used as the structural frame of reference throughout the book.

Teaching in clinical nursing is the vehicle that provides students with the opportunity to translate basic theoretical knowledge into the learning of a variety of intellectual and psychomotor skills needed to provide patient-centered quality nursing care.

What is creative teaching in clinical nursing?

In accepting the previously stated definition of creative teaching, it is clear that the task of the clinical teacher is to apply those concepts of *creative teaching* to the particular tasks of *teaching in clinical nursing.* The clinical teacher who assumes the responsibility for teaching a given number of students in the clinical situation is in a vulnerable position to practice varying degrees of creative teaching every day. Assuming that such teaching is based on theoretical background and on available clinical resources, the very environmental conditions for providing clinical experiences change from patient to patient, from day to day, and even from one time of day to another. Concomitantly no student responds to the learning situation exactly the same as any other student by virtue of different backgrounds of knowledge, experiences, and other learning variables. Other extraneous factors operating at a given point in time also affect the teacher's choice of response in handling the learning situation. The creative teacher in clinical nursing is concerned with the individual patient and the individual student, uses the scientific knowledge of medicine and human behavior available to examine the previous and existing factors present in the learning situation, and responds to the occasion through the use of constructive action that allows students to assume

responsibility for their learning in accord with their capabilities. Thus, the definition of creative teaching in clinical nursing is drawn from the application of the acts of teaching, creative teaching, and teaching in clinical nursing.

Creative teaching in clinical nursing is the art of applying the components of creative teaching to every act involved in the teaching of clinical nursing. *Creative teaching in clinical nursing is* accomplished by the teacher who uses the concepts of creativity as resources for greater thought and new avenues of approach to the problems of daily clinical learning.

Who is the creative teacher in clinical nursing?

To describe the creative teacher in clinical nursing would be at once repetitious and premature, since it would involve a summary of the preceding definitions translated into specific descriptive qualifications that will be discussed more fully in a later chapter. Rather, the following poem is offered to invite your further thoughtful consideration of the question: *Who is the creative teacher in clinical nursing?*

He was my teacher*

Ralph W. Seager

He harrowed minds with curving question
   marks,
Teaching as much outside the book as in;
He'd listen out the window for spring larks,
Postponing Euclid's chalky discipline.

He kept the bur of "Why?" beneath the tail
Of every sluggard slouched down in his seat,
Our spines came straight—we did not dare to
   fail,
And we survived by thinking on our feet.

He was my teacher—wise—yet hard as knots,
I tried to pick him loose and so undo him.
But he was miles ahead of all my plots:
I've found instead that he has tied me to him.

---

*Seager, Ralph W.: Cup, flagon and fountain, © 1965 by the author, published Wake-Brook House, Coral Gables, Fla., p. 65. Used by permission.

NEED FOR UTILIZATION OF CREATIVE TEACHING APPROACHES
In emerging patterns of professional nursing education

While schools of nursing have been busy experimenting with electronic and technological advances affecting methods of teaching, nursing service agencies have become equally involved in the transformation of procedural aspects of patient care. The nurse has been freed of some of the traditional responsibilities as the result of such innovations as electronic diagnostic devices; electronic monitoring devices; automation of preparation, handling, and disposing of equipment and supplies; and computerized record systems. As this shift in responsibilities occurs, there develops an imperative need for learning new technical skills along with a need for even greater depth of understanding of human behavior in order to continue to provide quality nursing care to patients, albeit with the help of machines.

In nursing education there is a continuous flow of reports of curriculum experimentation. The following two distinct patterns seem to emerge: (1) revising curriculum patterns to include learning experiences needed to assist the nurse in developing those dimensions of skills and intellectual thought needed to keep pace with the rapidly growing field of automated medical science and its effects on society and (2) planning and implementing teaching innovations that could considerably enhance the potential for fostering student-centered learning. As schools of nursing plan for the utilization of television instruction, programmed learning devices, multimedia approaches, independent study plans, computer laboratories, flexible scheduling and grouping, and team teaching, it is imperative that those involved in the teaching be more than "transmitters of knowledge." The task of the teacher no longer centers on telling or showing students what they should know or how they should do a task; rather it becomes one of guiding the students through problem-solving types of materials that have been prepared by experts. As a particular subject is studied, it is presented to students in terms of central problems to be explored by them. Students are expected to work through the problems as they see them according to the evidence supplied through the educational materials and to develop and test their own hypotheses. Herein lies the test of creative ability of the teacher! The creative teacher's purpose is to *guide* the students *through* the problem, assisting them to build and test their own hypotheses without fear of being judged either right or wrong by the teacher. The creative teacher must recognize that each student may use a different analytical approach to solving the problem and that some will not know how to go about it without considerable assistance. Students soon learn that they do not seek direct answers regarding content from the teacher. For the teacher to substitute a reply that has learning value in assisting the students to find their own answers while maintaining their self-respect requires more creativity than to supply the answer the students seek.

The clinical teacher must also know about or have an exceedingly fine background regarding the prepared educational materials; many teachers will find themselves involved in the preparation of such materials. Effective use of these devices and approaches will allow more time for the teacher, but the time should be spent in planning learning experiences that will more clearly meet the students' individual needs. The use of an approach to learning heavily reliant on mechanization calls for the planning of frequent small group sessions with students so that they can maintain their contact with and benefit from the master teacher as well as from each other. Teachers' creative talents will be reflected in the way they handle discussion groups so that they supplement and enrich that information gained by other means.

This problem-solving approach is not

new to nursing, nursing education, or nurse educators, but it is the *way* in which it is used that is so vital to the self-actualization of the learner. Its purpose is to encourage the analytical and imaginative powers of students as they engage in the task. There is no seeking "the right" answer (that which the students have learned is expected by the teacher). Instead the creative teacher must provide an atmosphere that promotes learning while simultaneously assisting the students individually and in groups to evaluate their proposed solution to the problems and preserving the dignity of the individual.

In emerging patterns of teaching in clinical nursing

With the emphasis on new curriculum patterns and multimedia teaching approaches, what happens to those direct learning experiences alluded to in the clinical teaching programs? How does the creative teacher fit into clinical teaching programs using a skill-oriented approach to a patient-centered setting?

That which has been said regarding the need for creative teaching in the field of nursing education aptly applies to the more specialized teaching functions in the clinical nursing setting. Perhaps of greatest importance is the consistency with which clinical and other teachers utilize their creative talents so that students, whether in a formal classroom setting or in a clinical setting, know that their actions and ways of thinking, methods used to solve problems, and proposed hypotheses will be reviewed, corrected, and expanded without being arbitrarily judged right or wrong by the teacher. The creative clinical teacher, who has shown consistency in being receptive to ideas of the students and has offered ideas only as alternatives to be pursued along with many others, has created an atmosphere of freedom nurturing the professional and personal growth of students. Within the clinical nursing situation, students who have had the opportunity to learn in this kind of environment interpret the meaning of freedom in terms of the following:

1. Meeting the patient's interactive and support needs more as a fellow human being than as an automaton—students are comfortable, relaxed, and interested in others within the situation; they enter into an expressive relationship with the patient rather than simply ministering to the physical needs of the patient in order to "get the job done."
2. Making a nursing assessment in terms of feeling free to express their ideas or "hunches" regarding the needs of patients, and free to modify existing restrictions, policies, and rules (within the realm of safety to the patient and others) to best meet the patients' needs.
3. Using imagination in trying new approaches to patient care.
4. Recognizing the need to change their course of action and taking the necessary steps to make the needed change.

As students see that their own ideas are accepted and treated with the same objectivity as those of others, including the clinical teacher, they begin to see the complementary relationships between their own ideas and those of others. The creative clinical teacher must determine ways and means of guiding the progressive development of skills in critical thinking needed by students in learning to make valid judgments about the ideas they have expressed. As a result, the students recognize those concepts as resources to be used to further enrich their own understandings and to help others in the clinical situation.

Perhaps one of the greatest tasks with which the creative teacher in clinical nursing is faced is that of dealing constructively with differences of performance abilities of students. To date those methods that have most often been tried have created as many new problems as they have purported to solve. Thus, there remains an important challenge to the creative clinical teacher— how can one deal constructively with differences of ability without classifying students into rigid categories of inferiority and superiority? The following are closely related subproblems also offering a challenge to the clinical teacher: How can one deal with the wide range of individual differences in performance abilities without creating feelings of defeat by the less able and feelings of superiority by the competent? What standards of performance ability can be used to determine the mastery of skills? How much is enough experience for each individual? How is evaluation of performance accomplished when students proceed to learn at their own rate?

We do know that greater creative behavior in individuals can be stimulated by helping them to release whatever creative potential they possess. Frequently such ability has been repressed by educators to the point that the individual could not recognize his full potential, let alone realize it. Once this barrier is removed, the learner can be helped to the level of self-actualization and resultant creative action. Nowhere in nursing is there so much fertile field for growth and development of creativity than in the area of clinical nursing. If, indeed, we believe in the concept that persons possess seeds of creativity, we must provide the environment that will nourish and permit the growth of those seeds to maturity. *It would seem, then, that from the clinical teacher's viewpoint, creativity begets creativity!*

SUGGESTED READINGS

Alamshah, William: The conditions for creativity, Journal of Creative Behavior 1:305-313, July, 1967.

Brown, Amy F.: Clinical instruction, Philadelphia, 1949, W. B. Saunders Co.

Brown, Amy F.: Curriculum development, Philadelphia, 1960, W. B. Saunders Co.

Bruner, Jerome S.: On knowing, New York, 1965, Atheneum Publishers.

Creativity and learning, Daedalus 3:527-763, Summer, 1965.

Deroche, Edward: Creativity in the classroom, Journal of Creative Behavior 2:239-241, Fall, 1968.

Doppelt, Jerome E.: Definitions of creativity, Transactions of the New York Academy of Sciences 26:788-793, May, 1964.

Foster, Florence P.: The human relationships of creative individuals, Journal of Creative Behavior 2:111-118, Spring, 1968.

Gabig, Mary G., and Lanigan, Barbara: Dynamics of clinical instruction in nursing education, Washington, D. C., 1956, The Catholic University of America Press.

Gardner, John W.: Self-renewal, New York, 1965, Harper & Row Publishers.

Guilford, J. P.: Creativity: yesterday, today, and tomorrow, Journal of Creative Behavior 1:13-21, Spring, 1966.

Heidgerken, Loretta E.: Teaching and learning in schools of nursing, Philadelphia, 1965, J. B. Lippincott Co.

Hinton, Bernard L.: A model for the study of creative problem solving, Journal of Creative Behavior 2:133-142, Spring, 1958.

Maslow, Abraham H.: Toward a psychology of being, New York, 1962, D. Van Nostrand Co.

Michael, William, editor: Teaching for creative behavior, Bloomington, Ind., 1968, Indiana University Press.

Moustakas, Clark: Creativity and conformity, New York, 1967, Van Nostrand Reinhold Co.

Muse, Maude B.: Guiding learning experiences, New York, 1950, Macmillan, Inc.

Power, E. J., and others: Being a creative faculty member is more than . . . teaching, NLN 1972 Workshop, NLN Publication no. 16-1417, Council of Diploma Programs, pp. 1-74, 1973.

Renz, Paul, and Christoplos, Florence: Toward an operational definition of giftedness, Journal of Creative Behavior 2:91-96, Spring, 1968.

Taylor, Calvin W., editor: Widening horizons in creativity, New York, 1964, John Wiley & Sons, Inc.

Taylor, Calvin W., and Barron, Frank, editors: Scientific creativity: its recognition and development, New York, 1963, John Wiley & Sons, Inc.

Toffler, Alvin: Future shock, New York, 1970, Random House, Inc.

Torrance, E. Paul: A new movement in education: creative development, Lexington, Mass., 1965, Ginn and Co.

3 Interpretation of the creative process

If we truly seek to keep creativity alive, we must continue to nourish the conditions in which creativity flourishes. An understanding of the basic elements of the creative process helps us to recognize creative behavior as it occurs, to examine our own approaches and responses to the learning situation, and to provide a learning environment that includes those ingredients that nourish creativity and starve conformity.

The creative process as described here has its origin within the self. The end product of the creative act, whether an idea, object, invention, court of action, or performance, is dependent on the self and the degree to which one activates his capacities to form new relationships with the environment. There is no definite *degree* of creativity except in the eyes of the creator. In some views there is no good or bad creativity; those qualities are assigned to the product according to the way in which it is used. For example, the discovery of atomic fission can be seen as a neutral act of creativity. Its alternate applications in atomic weapons or in the cure of disease may be valued as bad or good depending on one's value system and perspective.

Many ways and means of describing the creative process have been devised, revealing many similarities and some differences according to the particular philosophical orientation. The publication edited by Alice Miel[1] has been used to serve as the frame of reference for describing the creative process and its implications for creative teaching in clinical nursing.

ASPECTS OF THE CREATIVE PROCESS

The four major aspects of the creative process are (1) openness, (2) focus, (3) discipline, and (4) closure.[2]

Openness

The term *openness* refers to the deliberate act of allowing one's self to entertain new, unstructured thoughts about a current issue or problem. It is the letting down of the barriers of prejudice and rigidity to allow freedom of thought. The open person engages in a process of continually seeking information from all sources. To enter into this first step of creativity is perhaps the most crucial of all; it means one must reduce the socially supportive and protective defenses and allow the *complete* self to be open to experience in a less structured way before formulating any theories to interpret the ideas.

When openness exists, there is a break in the stimulus-response pattern, which allows freedom for detailed perception of the stimulus without rapid response based on rigidity and predetermined beliefs. At this stage one remains open to ambiguous ideas and continues to collect and examine diversified information without passing judgment on it. Historical and biographical data about a number of artists and scientists considered creative reveal that it is possible to be open receptively to a singular phase of experience that ultimately produces a creative piece of work along singular lines. However, an openness involving awareness of that which exists at the moment within the context of one's total experience leads to a more socially and personally constructive form of creativity.

The teacher who is secure enough to risk the self by serving as a model in the practice of openness fosters a learning environment conducive to creative thinking. The teacher *invites* students to raise isues having wide range implications for discussion. The teacher *allows* students to present various questions for study. The teacher is *supportive* and *nonjudgmental* in the approach to the discussion of the questions raised. The teacher allows enough time for a generous sampling of *contributions to be made from the group.* The teacher *expects* to exchange ideas or experiences as a result of creative interaction with students. In short the creative teacher provides a supportive, nonjudgmental, unhurried environment in which students are allowed to explore a number of avenues of inquiry about a particular problem in order to learn how to develop an open mind and consider a number of possibilities before pursuing a course of action. The creative teacher is aware that learning is continuous and that students are often excellent teachers themselves. The creative teacher avoids the all-too-frequent message: "Discuss all you want but finish where you began." This freedom to explore within one's limits and abilities charges the learner with responsibility for self-growth in seeking experiences leading to creative responses.

Focus

Openness makes data available; focus begins the process of translating significant pieces of data into meaningful patterns. The end product is the result of the individual's interaction with the environment. The ability to continue to focus on data in creative ways is dependent on past experience, present situation, and perceived future potential. A person may use openness and focusing alternately before reaching a new combination or idea that can be shared or used.

The concept of freedom that implies that for every right accorded the individual there is an equal responsibility can be used as a common ground of understanding to foster the development of this process of creativity in the learning situation. Freedom of expression can be nurtured in a manner that allows the learners to develop their own focus and to define the direction in which their ideas are leading them. For example, the teacher should allow students to report their experiences as *they* experienced them rather than supply them with preplanned ideas. Here again the teacher plays a vital role in providing a supportive environment that allows students to take intellectual risks, make speculations based on inconclusive information, and probe deeper into the problem through a continuous evaluation process until they focus their findings in terms of their relevancy to the total learning situation. Many teachers who can accept the risk-taking nature of creative learning in the classroom have difficulty accepting it in the clinical practice setting. The line between patient safety and essential student freedom is a fine one.

Discipline

Once openness and focus have been achieved, disciplined production begins. Creative individuals produce in a self-disciplined manner; having set a focus as the standard for identifying the means of reaching their ultimate goals, their action is disciplined to accomplish that focus. Creative individuals are first answerable to themselves; therefore, they set their own unique patterns of self-discipline in order to complete a creative idea or product that can be judged according to its original focus. Creative teachers, however, are answerable to their students; teachers of a clinical discipline are further accountable to their own patients and to their students' patients.

Ideally, at this stage of the creative process the teacher should provide the facilities, equipment, and uninterrupted time needed to allow the students to use a self-disciplined approach to creative action; unfortunately this concept of fostering creative ability in students is often viewed as being unrealistic. But the teacher who is truly concerned about finding a practical way of providing the necessary ingredients for creative thinking does not need to wait for these "ideal" conditions. The teacher who knows the students, recognizes their individual differences, and accepts each according to individual merits can offer them encouragement on an individual basis and can provide flexibility in the daily time scheduling of educational experiences. The teacher should also recognize that students soon learn to make their own adjustments to self-discipline. A pattern of work established by a given student should be considered adequate for that student if it brings results; a different pattern may be more effective for another student. Often students need only the teacher's encouragement and confirmation of their ideas for working out their own plans of action for the task they have set themselves. The truly creative teacher's task lies in consistently fostering and interpreting to others the concept of self-discipline and its relationship to assisting students to fulfill their commitment to their focus and ultimately meeting their own self-actualization goals. The interpretation may not only apply to students; the teacher may also be called on to justify individual learning plans to senior faculty and administrators.

Closure

The final stage of the creative process that brings the project or idea to completion is represented by that point at which the creator has met *his* criteria for the project, thus completing the task. The closure act may reveal the creator's tremendous achievement of self-discovery; it may reveal limitations suggesting that either the project be abandoned or the course of action be directed toward a more fruitful and satisfying adventure. A creative act is considered complete when the creative person "feels" that *his* product is finished, regardless of the reason; this decision must be made by the creator or else the product is not truly *his* creative work.

Creativity is at once a demanding, frustrating, satisfying experience. The teacher who understands the motivational and behavioral patterns of individual students can be instrumental in guiding them through this creative process, which leads them into making their own judgments regarding the completion of the product or activity. Where the creative process occurs within the context of a human laboratory such as a health care setting, the closure may be limited by the constraints of others involved in the system.

Creativity or problem-solving

In retrospect these processes of creativity may well cause one to ask, "How does this process of creativity differ from that of problem-solving as used in nursing?" The underlying steps of creativity and problem-solving do parallel each other; the difference lies in the process of self-actualization that *must* be present for the final product to be creative. The problem-solving process may result in a creative product, but it will definitely result in a solution. The creative process, however, is not always linked to an identifiable problem to be solved. The degree to which the processes of problem-solving are in truth processes of creativity is dependent not only on the kind of learning environment and example provided by the teacher but also on the student's own ability.

APPLICATION OF ASPECTS OF THE CREATIVE PROCESS TO CLINICAL TEACHING

How do these four components of the creative process relate to creative teaching in clinical nursing? Specific application of the process of creativity to teaching in clinical nursing situations is best illustrated by using an example structured on the following assumptions:

1. That the problem to be studied is *the provision of nursing care to patients having problems of pain.*

2. That the clinical teacher is responsible for a small group of students in the given nursing setting and that it is a setting in which the teacher is accepted as a competent, creative practitioner of nursing.

3. That the clinical teacher is responsible for supervising the students' clinical experiences, including making the application of theoretical materials to the clinical situation.

4. That the teacher understands and utilizes the process of creative thinking in functioning as a teacher in the clinical nursing setting.

5. That the students have had ample opportunity to pursue such theoretical aspects of the pain phenomena as mechanisms of biological responses to painful stimuli; physiological concepts of pain; psychological concepts of pain; pain perception and resultant reactions based on one's previous experience with pain, cultural attitudes about pain, pain threshold, and preexisting physiological conditions; medical management of pain; assessment of patients in pain; and planning and providing nursing care to manage pain and pain perception based on a nursing diagnosis.

With these assumptions in mind the following examples illustrate how the four aspects of the creative process can be applied to teaching in the clinical nursing setting, giving the student the opportunity to grow through self-actualization in the process of translating the basic theoretical knowledge of the pain phenomena into the learning of a variety of intellectual and psychomotor skills related to providing patient-centered, quality nursing care.

Openness

Openness—the process of deliberately allowing students to entertain new, unstructured thoughts about a current issue or problem. The clinical teacher invites the students to raise questions that they believe need to be studied on the subject of pain. The students might raise such questions as the following: What are the characteristics of pain as experienced by patients? Why do different patients react to to pain as they do? What kind of pain is most often associated with specific diseases? How do patients describe pain? Does pain occur more frequently at certain hours of the day or night? How do age, sex, race, and religion affect the individual patient's reaction to pain and how do they differ in the ways in which they communicate these reactions to pain? What medications seem to be most effective in relieving pain? Are certain medications more effective for certain kinds of pain? How can we accurately describe and report pain? What nursing measures seem to have the greatest effect on relieving pain? How do individual patients vary in response to nursing measures used to relieve pain? When students raise questions already answered in available nursing or basic science research, the data should be made available so that they can pursue knowledge that has not been more than adequately explored already.

The creative teacher in clinical nursing sets goals to be met in the study of the pain phenomena and its implications for the planning of nursing care measures to meet the needs of patients but recognizes that students who are provided with the opportunity to explore a variety of inquiries about pain and consider a number of possibilities for clinical experiences not only may meet these same goals but may identify and reach additional ones. Thus, planning for clinical experiences regarding pain begins with a student-centered discussion in which the clinical teacher provides supportive, intellectually critical assistance while allowing a number of possibilities to be considered before selecting and pursuing a course of action.

Focus

Focus—the process of making a deliberate attempt to refine the data into a structural pattern that will represent the individual's interaction with the environment.

The role of the clinical teacher now becomes that of assisting each student to define the direction to be pursued in light of the original questions raised. For example, two students may seek to identify the common characteristics of pain and the nursing action most successful in relieving the identified characteristics. One student may wish to select clinical experiences involving a group of patients with common medical diagnoses; another may wish to select patients at random. As students identify the kinds of clinical experiences needed, the clinical teacher provides an environment suited for obtaining these experiences. The clinical teacher assists students in reporting their findings as *they perceive them*. In helping students work through the problems, the teacher raises questions based on the students' original plan and focus of operation, expressing and evaluating their findings in terms of the implications of their ideas to the goals of the learning situation. The creative teacher in clinical nursing allows the students to recognize and accept their own failures but is available to focus the process in another direction. Acceptance of failure is particularly difficult for the beginner. The creative teacher can help by sharing personal experiences and subsequent actions with students, as a means of opening students to a realistic understanding of the complex nature of a profession such as nursing.

Discipline

Discipline—the process of accomplishing one's committed focus through self-disciplined actions. Having provided the students with opportunities to determine what they need to know and how selected learning experiences will help them to focus their ideas into constructive outcomes, the creative clinical teacher must continually provide a learning environment that fosters self-discipline. While the clinical teacher cannot allow students to pursue their problems without regard for meeting the educational outcomes of the course, much individualized instruction is needed to produce self-disciplined learning. If the clinical teacher has allowed the student to select the problem of identifying the common characteristics of pain and the nursing action most successful in relieving them and to suggest that a random sampling of patients be used for the clinical experience, it follows that the clinical teacher must offer guidance in assisting the student to pursue this task through the self-actualization process.

The scheduling of class and clinical hours, the length of each clinical experience, the number of patients cared for each day, the frequency of conferences or demonstrations, must to some extent be individualized for each student. Self-discipline regarding ideas to be pursued or rejected and concepts to be considered or adopted is difficult to achieve in a setting where all external discipline is provided by a rigid educational system.

The clinical teacher's task in fostering self-disciplined action is two-dimensional: (1) to assist students to fulfill their commitment to their own focus and (2) to promote and interpret the concept of self-discipline to others so that students may function in an environment that fosters self-actualization.

Closure

Closure—the point at which the creative process is terminated in accord with the criteria set by the student. If closure is to come from the students, the clinical teacher must help them reflect on their progress from time to time. For the student who chose to study the identification of common characteristics of pain and the nursing action most successful in relieving them using a random sampling of patients, the clinical teacher raises questions designed as a self-help device in determining the student's progress. The creative clinical teacher raises questions such as the following: How much information do you have that suggests some answers to the original question that you raised? How much additional information or time do you think you need to answer your problem? What changes should you make in the scope of selection of patients in order to answer the question satisfactorily? How completely can you answer the question in relation to the time you have to work with this problem? What new avenues of thought have been revealed by your findings? How does your current knowledge relate to some previously learned concepts and also apply to the present problem? How do your findings relate to future nursing problems? Questions of this type asked periodically by the clinical teacher help the students determine their ultimate goals and clarify their thinking as they attempt to work through their own problems. Even though in the eyes of the teacher the question does not appear to be answered adequately, the important factor in the completion of the creative act is that it represents the best that the individual believes can be done at the time and provides direction for future acts.

Not every attempt at creativity will result in an identifiable "creation," something that can be touched or shared or appreciated by others. In some cases creativity results in failure—the total absence of findings or a discovery—which is opposed to the goal that the attempt was intended to meet. At other times creativity results in a person reconfirming, in his own way, an accepted method or idea. The teacher who demands a new discovery from every student may be as detrimental to the student's professional growth as one who punishes any deviation from tradition.

Providing a teaching environment that fosters creativity

Creativity is determined by the act of the whole individual. Each teacher will identify creative approaches to the teaching of clinical nursing; however, the following suggestions may prove helpful in attempting to provide an environment that fosters creativity.

The creative teacher in clinical nursing supports self-respect and self-confidence, which provide the self with the capacity to respect, trust, and love others.

The creative teacher in clinical nursing plans daily toward long-term goals but deliberately leaves many avenues open to allow freedom of expression by the students. The planning of learning experiences includes arranging for the kinds of facilities and equipment required to meet the expressed needs of the students. There is a give-and-take relationship between students and teachers; some suggestions come from individual students; some come as a result of one student making suggestions to another student; and some come from the teacher. If the teacher lacks a specific skill necessary to a student and can identify another who can better serve as a role model, arrangements for individual preceptorship or observation can be made.

The creative teacher in clinical nursing provides an atmosphere of freedom of expression in individual and group relationships with students. The teacher expects the unexpected and is able to "stretch" the mind in seeking ways and means of helping students to do likewise in finding suitable answers to problems arising out of the daily clinical experiences.

The creative teacher in clinical nursing has the deepest respect for the inherent rights and responsibilities of individual students. The teacher puts forth effort to become personally acquainted with individual students in order to be sensitized to the kinds of behavior that trigger positively and negatively charged actions and reactions. The clinical teacher who knows the students can direct group discussions so that the dignity and worth of the individual are preserved and can provide for freedom of expression of "new" ideas. At the same time the clinical teacher must take into account such things as the ability of other students to assimilate the "new" idea—its possibilities for further considerations and its worth in terms of what it really represents; the curiosity shown by some; the flat rejection given by those who say it will not work; and the ability of some to visualize the effectiveness of the idea and manipulate it to fit their own ideas. Allowing these communications to flow freely yet constructively may be the beginning of a whole new line of creative activity by any one member of the group.

The creative teacher in clinical nursing is rewarded as each student generates an idea, is allowed to keep it alive, and works it through to a self-satisfying conclusion. For those creative ideas appearing to be ill timed, the clinical teacher gives support while explaining why it is impossible to pursue them at that point. By that very act the clinical teacher may later experience the satisfaction of seeing a student's dream become a reality.

The process of becoming a thinking, practicing nurse evolves as the creative teacher uses every opportunity to stretch boundaries of conformity into freedom. The student who is free opens the mind to let in new ideas upon which to focus thought and action. Freedom of thought with acceptance by the teacher gives rise to freedom of expression and action by the student. As the risk of giving more of self in terms of ideas, solutions to problems, or new products becomes less and less of a threat, the student becomes more and more concerned and involved with people, objects, and situations. With each new involvement the personal commitment becomes intensified, and the emergence of one's full potential is reflected by successive creative acts.

Whether it be from the perspective of the teacher or the learner, the common denominator of the creative process is *freedom.*

REFERENCES

1. Miel, Alice, editor: Creativity in teaching, Belmont, Calif., 1961, Wadsworth Publishing Co., Inc.
2. Foshay, Arthur W.: The creative process described. In Miel, Alice, editor: Creativity in teaching, Belmont, Calif., 1961, Wadsworth Publishing Co., Inc.

SUGGESTED READINGS

Aichlmayr, Rita: Creative nursing, Journal of Nursing Education 9:19-27, Nov., 1969.

Alamshah, William H.: The conditions for creativity, Journal of Creative Behavior 1:305-313, Summer, 1967.

Alamshah, William H.: Creative living, Journal of Creative Behavior 4:123-130, Spring, 1970.

Bowers, B. H.: Promoting creativity in nursing education, Hospital Progress 52:64-65, Feb., 1971.

Davis, Gary: Training creativity in adolescence: a discussion of strategy, Journal of Creative Behavior 3:95-104, Spring, 1969.

Goldberg, Minerva J.: Films on creativity do they exist? Journal of Creative Behavior 4:190-209, Summer, 1970.

Guilford, J. P.: Creativity: retrospect and prospect, Journal of Creative Behavior 4:149-168, Summer, 1970.

Hughes, Harold K.: The enhancement of creativity, Journal of Creative Behavior 3:73-83, Spring, 1969.

Lipson, L. F.: Creating a learning environment, Journal of Nursing Education 11:4-9, Aug., 1972.

Michael, William B., editor: Teaching for creative endeavor, Bloomington, Ind., 1968, Indiana University Press.

Torrance, E. Paul: Education and the creative potential, Minneapolis, 1963, University of Minnesota Press.

Unit II   Climate for creative teaching in clinical nursing

This above all: to thine own self be true,
And it must follow, as the night the day,
Thou canst not then be false to any man.

SHAKESPEARE

4 Administrative framework for creative teaching in clinical nursing

By implication one might assume from the recurrent theme of this book that the teaching of clinical nursing is an entity unto itself. However, the teaching of clinical nursing, like any other phase of teaching, is an integral part of the total educational program offered by a given school of nursing. To examine it in its proper perspective, discussion is focused on the teaching of clinical nursing as it relates to the total creative teaching-learning process.

It is an established administrative principle that any school has the responsibility of providing its teachers with enough information to help them identify their responsibilities, to consider ways and means of contributing to the total purposes of the school, and to identify channels of communications to follow in carrying out their functions within their particular teaching area. As Gibson points out, a truly educational institution possessing a self-governing, scholarly faculty should not be hampered by being expected to adhere to strict line responsibilities and relationships shown by organizational charts. Competent personnel recognize the need to work with those individuals who can best bring intelligence and experience to bear on the solution of a problem that produces the desired results, rather than resorting to a set plan of organization neatly drawn up for instant referral. This is not to say that organizational charts are unnecessary. They do provide a point of reference for maintaining proper relationships between administrative officers, department heads, faculty, and staff officers.[1] Because administrative organizational patterns are highly individualized to meet the particular purposes of the institution and the students it serves, no attempt is made to describe or recommend administrative organizational patterns, or to classify functions of teaching personnel by virtue of their source of appointment. Rather, the discussion is focused on the fundamental belief that the development of a favorable climate for learning is dependent on: (1) administrative responsibilities for providing a climate conducive to creative teaching in clinical nursing and (2) the establishment of working relationships between the teacher of clinical nursing and others concerned with the education of nurses.

ADMINISTRATIVE CLIMATE CONDUCIVE TO CREATIVE TEACHING IN CLINICAL NURSING

It is acknowledged that a school exists for the purpose of education and welfare of the students it serves though there may be other purposes. These may include the advancement of scientific or professional knowledge, the provision of services to certain populations, or the supply of additional manpower for local, regional, or national needs. School of nursing administrators recognize their primary responsibility as that of education of students although they are often explicit about additional health goals along the lines mentioned. The administrator is placed in a position of being many things to many persons. Proper facilities and a sound curriculum are necessary, but they cannot guarantee an effective educational program for the students. The degree to which teachers in a given school of nursing have opportunities to release their creative potentials in teaching, practice, and research has a direct effect on the quality of the educational program.

This philosophy is further substantiated by a joint statement on government of colleges and universities formulated by the American Association of University Professors, American Council on Education, and Association of Governing Boards of Universities and Colleges in 1966. It describes more fully the kinds of shared responsibility and cooperative action among university board members, administration, faculty members, and students deemed necessary for the preservation of the integrity of institutions of higher education.[2] The administrator who seeks to serve the students well must assume responsibility for the "care and nurture" of the faculty in order to release their creative potential. Administrators cannot "make" creative teachers by the mere act of telling them they are free to be creative. The administrative responsibility is to *create conditions that nourish and reward creative teaching*. There must be enough freedom to challenge individual creative potential and enough order to supply the support needed for the self-actualizing process leading to the creative act. The democratic climate supports this view, leading to the suggestion that administrative practices based on the democratic concept should release creative potentials of the faculty.

The use of democratic principles as guides to administrative organization imposes rights and responsibilities on the total faculty organization; neither the administrator nor the faculty can be classified as slaves, that is, those whose actions are determined by goals established by another. It does mean that faculty members should be involved in determining philosophy, purposes, and programs, but that executive decisions should be centered in a few administrative persons. When faculty members either are expected to or voluntarily assume a myriad of detailed administrative functions, they are robbed of the time needed to release their creative talents in strengthening the total

educational program. If, however, a faculty attempts only to teach and tries to avoid all administrative work, it may discover constraints being placed on the teachers because decisions have been made in which the faculty had no voice.

School of nursing administrators seeking to provide a climate for creative teaching must exercise a control function and a releasing function in the "care and nurture" of the faculty. The control is to assure their sharing in the work load appropriately, including the decision-making; the release is from administrative and organizational tasks that distract from teaching. Only when individual faculty members learn to accept both the rights and responsibilities of implementing an educational program in terms of the creative potential abilities of the *total faculty* will the faculty be operating to its maximum potential for creative education. Therefore the following description of conditions to be provided by the administrator in fostering creative teaching applies equally to the classroom teacher, the clinical nursing teacher, and others contributing to the total teaching program.

1. *Teachers need an organizational structure that provides them with reasonable privileges and limitations.* Teachers are motivated to express their creative talents when they know that there is an existing chain of command for channeling their suggestions or requests, when they know that limits will be enforced but with consideration for individual differences, and when they know that the administrative officers are in touch with what is going on and will act as spokesmen for them in implementing their ideas.

2. *Teachers need to feel accepted and recognized.* Respect *by* administrative officers breeds respect *for* them. Teachers need to know that, regardless of their position within the organizational framework, they can express their ideas as individuals and will find someone who will listen to them, respect their ideas as representative of their own worth, and reward them with praise or recognition. Acceptance, recogni-

tion, and reward serve as the lubricants of self-expression.

3. *Teachers need to maintain their expertise.* A person is employed on a faculty because of recognized expertise, but continuous practice is needed to maintain that level. For the clinical faculty of a nursing school, the expertise is in providing nursing care to specific groups of patients. The organizational structure of the school must not allow and encourage nursing practice that separates the nurse from this intended function. Practice may be related to research studies or to testing new approaches but should clearly be apart from that practice done while supervising students.

4. *Teachers need to have access to resources contributing to new ideas about teaching.* Creative ideas often are germinated through the use of educational communication media, observation of "new" approaches to teaching, conferences, speakers, demonstrations, or study groups. A single observation of one of these means often initiates new ideas to be pursued in implementing an improved means of teaching a particular aspect of nursing or triggers an idea leading to an extensive research project, vastly changing the approach to the teaching of a total area of clinical nursing. By the same token, when teachers have ready access to these resources, they are motivated to experiment with ideas utilizing these or other similar resources.

5. *Teachers need to be encouraged to discover alternative ways of teaching.* An institution that operates on the basic conviction that change is inevitable and that encourages change, not for the sake of change but for the improvement of the teaching programs, is richly rewarded by those having the vision to look ahead and the courage to experiment with new approaches. Teachers functioning within this kind of environment move from the realm of "working around" problems to that of "working through" problems and dissatisfactions, opening up new vistas in learning experiences that foster student creativity. Administrators must be able to provide expert advice and support in pursuing such action.

6. *Teachers need the freedom of selecting, planning, and implementing their own ideas.* Even though there is a curriculum pattern to follow in terms of meeting the desired objectives, teachers need the freedom to vary their methods and approach from day to day or term to term in meeting the desired outcomes within the given time period. An environment of freedom to select, plan, implement, and evaluate ideas in justifiable terms fosters creativity as a natural course of action in the daily teaching experience.

7. *Teachers need to know that resource persons are available for help when needed.* When teachers know that they are free to seek expert help when needed to experiment with an idea, they are more willing to proceed because they have someone to support them. The administrator, however, must take the necessary precautions to avoid forcing ideas or help on teachers for the sake of producing something new in lieu of allowing the teacher to seek self fulfilment. Some administrators are so eager for progress that they themselves propose ideas more rapidly than they can be assimilated and with little regard for the teacher's willingness or ability to pursue them.

8. *Teachers need to be kept informed regarding activities of others in the total effort to improve the teaching program.* Teachers need to be kept informed of every stage of change so that they are ready to contribute positively to it when the need arises. Knowing what others are doing also stimulates the individual teacher's desire to devise new ways and means of changing his teaching program.

ORGANIZATIONAL RELATIONSHIPS BETWEEN CLINICAL NURSING PROGRAM AND TOTAL SCHOOL OF NURSING

As stated previously, a democratic administrative structure may be one that most readily supports the appropriate mix of freedom and control in an academic setting. In considering the structure of a school of nursing, the administrative framework for clinical nursing programs can be viewed in terms of their relationships to organization of the total curriculum and the working relationships between the clinical nursing teachers and the total faculty.

Teachers holding the responsibility for planning and implementing clinical nursing programs in each given area of the curriculum also share responsibility for total curriculum building in a two-dimensional relationship. The curriculum plan for a given clinical nursing area must show a horizontal and vertical relationship to (1) those nursing theory courses that are its counterpart and other supportive courses and (2) each of the clinical nursing courses comprising the total curriculum. It is obvious that the establishment of these relationships demands that teachers work as a team to establish the goals for providing a total learning situation for the student. Clinical nursing teachers need the freedom to communicate with one another in a pattern that will avoid fragmentation, repetition, or omission and will integrate learning experiences from one clinical area to another. The *pattern* of communication is not nearly as important as the *act* of communicating. The goal is to provide a curriculum that motivates students to creative learning behavior.

Inherent in each clinical area are some common understandings and skills to be learned or applied in new relationships from one clinical area to another. The multiplicity of ways and means of planning and teaching these clinical nursing experiences* supports the emerging concept of cooperative planning to meet the demands placed on the faculty by expanding enrollments, knowledge explosion, and educational technological innovations. Clearly clinical teachers cannot conduct clinical teaching programs independently of one another. They need opportunities to use their creative abilities in planning and implementing clinical nursing programs to meet the specific desired behavioral

---

*A full description of these methods appears in Chapter 8.

outcomes in an environment that fosters interdepartmental communications leading to cooperative, coordinated, creative teaching in clinical nursing.

ORGANIZATIONAL RELATIONSHIPS BETWEEN CLINICAL NURSING PROGRAM AND NURSING SERVICE AGENCIES

There was a time when full control over educational programs was exercised by caregiving institutions. Awareness of the limitations this placed on learning led to many instances in which there was no direct connection between the school and the service setting. In these cases the educators had no control over patient care provided, and those engaged in providing service prescribed none of the content of the educational setting. Since the 1960s, facilities such as medical centers encompassing both a school of nursing and a large hospital have explored integration of service and education through creation of dual appointments. The director of nursing in such a setting has line authority over both education and care. On a smaller scale many schools and service facilities share one or more master clinicians who function as both faculty members and care-givers. No matter what the organizational structure, it has become abundantly clear that cooperation and collaboration between those providing care and those preparing people to be care-givers are essential to maintain a high level of professional nursing for the public.

Commonly, there is a separation of school and care-giving agency. The school of nursing exists for the primary purpose of the education of students; the nursing service agency exists for the primary purpose of providing patient care. The clinical nursing teacher would do well to apply the words of Carl Sandburg, "Everybody is smarter than anybody," in establishing a pattern of relationships with others that will release the creative potential so vital to the development of a dynamic clinical nursing program. The potential for learning in a given clinical situation is directly proportional to the quality of the faculty present, the level of understanding that the faculty has of the goals and skills of the practitioners in the agency, the degree to which personnel in the situation accept students, the degree to which the personnel understand the total educational program, and the quality of nursing care that is practiced in the situation. The clinical nursing teacher must assume responsibility for working cooperatively with all levels of personnel involved with patient care. The pattern of following free-flowing, two-way organizational line communications regarding the clinical nursing program is sound procedure. At the level of operation involving direct student experiences in nursing care activities, the clinical nursing teacher should be allowed the freedom and accept the responsibility for communicating directly with all levels of nursing personnel, all members of the health team, community health, education, and welfare personnel, administrative personnel, and personnel in the supporting services in bringing about cooperative, intelligent action to solve problems affecting student learning experiences and patient care. In most clinical nursing situations these coordinated activities center around the head nurse or the equivalent position. The teacher will seize every opportunity to solicit this person's cooperation in the selection of clinical experiences and in the supervision and evaluation of students. Accountability for planning clinical experiences and supervision and evaluation of students are vested in the clinical teacher, but the coordinated action of the clinical teacher and others within the clinical setting are of inestimable value in establishing an environment for creative learning. For example, the clinical nursing teacher should consistently seek feedback from medical and nursing service agencies, providing specific data based on concrete evidence and suggested improvements regarding existing gaps between the quality of · patient care desired and that being provided. Reciprocal communications regarding the faculty members' observations of agency personnel and practices are equally appropriate. The gaps between nursing education and

patient services become considerably narrowed, and the ultimate results benefit both students and patients.

To foster creative teaching in clinical nursing, the administrative organization pattern must provide for free flow of communications up and down the hierarchical scale as a means of gaining access to necessary persons when support and resources are needed to carry forth the creative ideas. But, in addition, the basic philosophy of the school of nursing and nursing service agencies must embrace the concept of respect for the individual as a contributing, responsible member of the organization, allowing for flexibility in the establishment of spontaneous, cooperative working relationships as well as accountability for results.

Implementation of the clinical nursing program depends on: (1) the ability of administrative officers to develop collaborative relationships with those persons whose interests are directed toward providing creative, innovative approaches to the teaching of nursing and (2) the patterns of relationships between the nursing program and the organization of nursing service agencies providing facilities for clinical experiences.

To maintain an environment that fosters teacher creativity, the school of nursing administrator must exercise creativity in helping teachers to find themselves, to discover ways of making their own teaching become alive, to provide the guidance needed in making the decisions that remove the barriers to creativity, and to provide the controls and support needed to help them. Creativity in education is a perpetual challenge that follows a chain of events emanating from creative administration to creative teaching, leading to learning that prepares students for creative living.

REFERENCES

1. Gibson, Raymond C.: The challenge of leadership in higher education, Dubuque, Iowa, 1964, William C. Brown Co., Publishers.
2. American Association of University Professors, American Council on Education, and Association of Governing Boards of Universities and Colleges: Statement on government of colleges

and universities, American Association of University Professors Bulletin **52**:375-379, Winter, 1966.

SUGGESTED READINGS

Arrangements between institutions of higher education and agencies which provide learning laboratories for nursing education, N.L.N. Publication no. 15-776, Council on Baccalaureate and Higher Degree Programs, pp. 1-8, 1973.

Bensman, P.: An example of community planning for nursing education, Journal of Nursing Education **11**:23-28, Jan., 1972.

Bevis, E. O.: Curriculum building in nursing: a process, St. Louis, 1973, The C. V. Mosby Co.

Brown, Ray E.: Judgment in administration, New York, 1966, Blakiston Division, McGraw-Hill Book Co.

Corona, D. F.: College education tailor-made for registered nurses, Arizona State University, American Journal of Nursing **73**:294-297, Feb., 1973.

Eberle, Robert: Personnel management for change and innovation in education, Journal of Creative Behavior **3**:277-283, Fall, 1969.

Gordon, M., and others: A systematic approach to curriculum revision, Nursing Outlook **22**:306-316, May, 1974.

Gregory, Carl: The management of creative personnel, Journal of Creative Behavior **3**:271-276, Fall, 1969.

Gregory, Carl: The management of intelligence: scientific problem solving and creativity, New York, 1967, McGraw-Hill Book Co.

Hargreaves, A. G., and others: Maintaining academic freedom, American Journal of Nursing **71**:1590-1592, Aug., 1971.

Mercadante, Lucille: Education for service—the challenge, Nursing Forum **8**(2):151-159, 1969.

Merton, Robert: The social nature of leadership, American Journal of Nursing **69**:2614-2618, Dec., 1969.

Pierik, M. M.: Joint appointments: collaboration for better patient care, Nursing Outlook **21**:576-579, Sept., 1973.

Shanks, Mary D., and Kennedy, Dorothy A.: Administration in nursing, New York, 1970, Blakiston Division, McGraw-Hill Book Co.

5 The teacher of clinical nursing as a creative individual

Discussion of the desired characteristics of behaviors of the creative teacher in clinical nursing must be considered in terms of relevance to two important variables: (1) the existence of creative potential in every human being in terms of kind and degree and (2) the existence of a diversity of contradictory or inconsistent traits inherent in individuals exhibiting varying degrees of creativity.

The potential for creativity exists on a continuum as a relative characteristic of each individual, negating the notion that a person is either creative or noncreative. Numerous studies regarding the characteristics of creative individuals reveal no single, consistent pattern that can be used as a prototype of the creative person. On the contrary, research findings disclosing contradictory and inconsistent behavioral patterns indicate that there is need to consider the inconsistent and contradictory behavioral patterns exhibited by individuals in accord with their degree of creative potential.

THE CREATIVE TEACHER OF CLINICAL NURSING
The creative teacher of clinical nursing as a person

Students evaluate what the teacher says by comparing it with what the teacher does and is. The role model provided by the teacher's personal characteristics, attitudes, ideals, and clinical competencies is frequently emulated by the students. The prevailing atmosphere in the clinical setting, together with the role models of the clinical teachers and other nursing personnel, is a vital force in setting the learning pace in the clinical nursing environment.

As a person, the creative clinical nursing teacher is one who does the following:

1. Possesses a conceptual model to guide his own thinking and actions. Such a model is derived from many sources developed gradually from early childhood and continuing throughout life. Inherent in such a model is the ability of the teacher to place high priorities on freedom to act, respect and tolerance for individual differences, compassion for others, and support of those less mature.

2. Utilizes his full potential through a positive, realistic understanding and acceptance of self. The creative teacher who has learned to handle self-feelings constructively is better equipped to help others in the clinical setting and to help students work through their feelings as they become productive, creative learners.

3. Possesses a sensitivity and responsiveness to people, ideas, and events. Development of this talent involves a multisensory approach to the analysis of actions, ideas, and events. Creativity grows out of being able to recognize, understand, and approach day-to-day experiences by listing and observing verbal and nonverbal actions and interactions involving people, ideas, and events. As a result, the creative clinical teacher perceives a wide range of possibilities for responding with open-mindedness to the ideas and behaviors of others.

4. Exhibits an inner security in dealing with those high-risk situations evolving from the inevitable daily changes and

adjustments inherent in the teaching-learning process. The same feelings of security and self-confidence necessary for functioning as a productive member of society are requisites for functioning comfortably, productively, and creatively in the unpredictable, changeable clinical learning situation.

5. Recognizes the need for continued learning as a necessary ingredient for developing and perfecting his own creative approaches to teaching when challenges arise and new frontiers of learning appear. The creative teacher recognizes and accepts the idea that he can, and indeed does, learn with and from his colleagues and students as well as from testing and implementing his own ideas. The very act of recognizing and accepting one's own potential for creative teaching implies a commitment to continuous learning. The creative clinical teacher as a person responds positively to the exploration of new ideas, integrating previous knowledge with new discoveries to add enjoyment and vitality to everyday adventures in life and learning.

Professional qualifications and preparation of the creative teacher in clinical nursing

The purpose of this book is not to prescribe but to describe a frame of reference from which to make inferences regarding desirable professional qualifications for creative teachers of clinical nursing. Currently there are two distinct schools of thought regarding the professional education of teachers in nursing (with the first predominating): (1) that the clinical nursing teacher needs a clinically oriented background of preparation and (2) that the clinical nursing teacher needs a functionally oriented background of preparation. The basic beliefs regarding these two approaches are reflected by the varying degrees of preparation and experiences in specialized areas required by individual educational institutions; the ultimate establishment of such criteria remains the prerogative of each educational institution. The following general requirements are usually considered essential in determining qualifications of faculty members seeking positions as teachers in clinical nursing.

Professional degree requirements. The teacher in nursing should have completed a program of study in nursing beyond that which the students will attain upon graduation. To meet the minimal requirement of a master's degree in nursing, previous educational background should consist of a baccalaureate degree in nursing that included a broad base of physical, biological, and psychosocial sciences; theory and experience in the assessment of preventive and therapeutic health care needs leading to provision of nursing care for patients in all age categories, in a variety of health care settings and with a variety of health problems; and sufficient leadership skills to work with other health team members in implementing plans of care for patients and their families. The master's degree in nursing should offer concentrated advanced theory and experience in an area of clinical specialization that includes a variety of courses and experiences in related fields providing scope to the total specialized area. Advanced courses in the physical and biological sciences are essential to the practice of nursing in the specialized clinical areas, as are the social sciences in providing further insights into understanding human behavioral aspects of clinical nursing. If the teacher is expected to contribute creatively to the teaching of clinical nursing, there should also be some provision made for the study of such fundamental courses as philosophy of education, psychology of learning, statistics, principles of teaching, fundamentals of research, and evaluation techniques.

Current facts and figures regarding the number of nurses holding doctoral degrees compared with the number needed to fill teaching positions in nursing programs indicate that the demand far exceeds the supply. However, there is a growing trend toward making the minimal education requirement for nursing teachers that of postmaster's study leading to doctoral preparation, especially for those teaching at the master's level or beyond.

Professional competence. The teacher of clinical nursing not only must be knowledgeable regarding the given area of clinical specialization but must also know how to use it, demonstrating excellent technical skill based on content knowledge. The teacher in clinical nursing serves as a model for the students in every act involving patient care. Only the expert nurse who enjoys relating to patients and providing high-quality nursing care through the application of scientific principles can qualify as the model needed for students to follow in meaningfully applying theoretical information to direct patient care.

Professional experience. It is frequently held that the teacher who has had some previous experience in a practice setting is better equipped to teach clinical nursing. On the other hand the teacher in clinical nursing who has the desired academic preparation and the personal characteristics to meet the challenges of the situation should not be penalized by lack of previous experience. Opportunities can be provided for the inexperienced to continue to develop as practitioners while beginning to instruct others. It must be remembered that inexperienced teachers have one advantage over the experienced—they do not have to unlearn ways of teaching that are no longer appropriate. They often bring a fresh, new approach to the learning field resulting from their own recent student experiences. The truly creative, experienced clinical teacher will welcome the opportunity to work with a beginning teacher because of the mutual benefits to be gained.

Professional responsibility for continuing learning. Creative teachers of clinical nursing remain so only when they continue to update their knowledge and experience with the rapidly changing medical, nursing, and educational practices. Additional knowledge and experience are pursued by various means of continuing education from the beginning of life and are nurtured by each level of education until it becomes a built-in automatic response of the educated nurse seeking to function creatively as a teacher in the clinical nursing setting.

Creativity in teaching clinical nursing is directly related to the teacher's ability to blend professional and personal qualifications into a capacity to care—about the self, the students, the patients, and clinical nursing.

TEACHING EFFECTIVENESS REFLECTING CREATIVITY

It would be presumptuous to assume that the teacher of clinical nursing is creative by virtue of possessing the desirable characteristics and professional qualifications. Rather, it is the *way* in which the individual teacher *uses* these characteristics and qualifications that determines the degree of creativity responsible for effective teaching. The degree and kind of creative teaching in clinical nursing are directly proportional to the teacher's degree of self-concept, knowledge of content, clinical competence, and ability to establish satisfying working relationships with students, peers, nursing service personnel, medical and paramedical personnel, and other community agency personnel.

The self-concept

The previous chapter advanced the concept of providing a challenging environment as a necessary requirement for creative teaching. Once this is provided, it becomes the teacher's role, if willing, to risk the self in pursuing new or untried approaches to teaching or nursing. While it seems redundant to belabor the currently popular theme that self-understanding is the key to understanding of others, it would be equally remiss to ignore it in relationship to the teacher. The way in which a teacher approaches the multitude of problems inherent in the teaching of students depends on the *person as a teacher.* The teacher who seeks to understand the impact of what is happening in his inner life can develop awareness that helps expand and change his self-concept. Self-acceptance can provide the teacher with a realistic understanding of the self as a professional person who can be shared; the teacher is responsive to what is happening to others and recognizes the need for flexibility in the ever-changing relationships between the self and others. Jersild reminds us that this ability to accept others by virtue of accepting and drawing upon one's own emotions as resources represents compassion in its highest form and is an absolute condition of self-acceptance.[1] Most psychologists agree that the concept of self is the product of gradual development from early childhood through years of experiences in an adult world. Although it must be remembered that the self-concept can be negative, this discussion is limited to the development of a positive self-concept that is compatible with the concept of dynamic, creative teaching. The individual teacher who can share experiences or draw on them in the understanding of students can provide an excellent role model for the developing professional "self" of students. The use of the person as therapeutic agent is important in all nursing situations, and teaching this effectively is a principal challenge to the creative clinical teacher.

As the teacher in clinical nursing develops a sense of self-awareness and peer-awareness leading to compassion, a pattern of professional behavior evolves. Maslow describes creativity resulting from this self-actualization process as being radioactive—emitted to all of life regardless of problems or persons involved, making some things grow while being wasted on others.[2] The creative teacher possessing this kind of self-concept reflects an image of one who (1) teaches with confidence; (2) views the self and others as continually being in the process of growing professionally and personally; (3) enjoys teaching in clinical nursing and is proud to be counted in the profession; (4) maintains a satisfying peer relationship while holding to ideals and practices; (5) focuses full attention on the goals to be accomplished while performing the teaching functions, giving little thought to personal goals related to material gains or ego-centered rewards; (6) uses unique teaching approaches or techniques rather than copying others or apologizing for inadequacies; and (7) enters into each teaching experience with the enthusiasm of the big-game hunter and the caution and cunning of the hunted.

The self-concept is unique to each individual. The development of a self that reaches out toward others with respect and compassion for the self and others is dependent on each teacher's ability to face and to find the self while growing as a mature, compassionate individual.

Knowledge of content

An integral part of developing the self-concept is linked to one's knowledge of content, coupled with one's knowledge about community and world affairs. It is not enough just to know that which is required to be taught. For clinical teaching to survive with any degree of creativity, the teacher must have sufficient mastery of content to (1) understand basic science principles and relate them to clinical nursing problems, (2) understand nursing science theories and practices relevant to the specific clinical area, (3) apply knowledge to practice situations easily and productively, (4) know how historical patterns of scientific achievements have shaped and continued to shape our present medical and nursing practices, and (5) continue to broaden the basis for action by regular study and review of professional and related literature.

The relationship between the teacher's background of knowledge and ability to function creatively can be likened to the computer system; that is, the final outcome and desired results are directly proportional to the amount and kind of information input. The more breadth and depth of knowledge a teacher possesses, the more opportunities there are to establish new associations among known items of information leading to new responses, ideas, or performances. It also removes many barriers, allowing freedom for imaginative thinking, expression of ideas, and opportunities to test ideas, to evaluate their effectiveness, and to determine how they can apply to other situations. The teacher who possesses and uses information about the total world of daily living adds greater dimensions to the development of the student as a total person in a professional milieu. The rapidity of growth in technological advances affecting the health professions necessitates a student-teacher partnership in learning together as these theoretical discoveries become realities in the clinical nursing situation. The freedom to explore these innovations and share them with one another can make the discovery of new knowledge a joy and a source of fulfillment to both student and teacher.

Clinical competence

It has long been known that the student constructs a set of ideals relative to the role of the professional nurse, the role and responsibilities of the nurse in the community, and the professional responsibilities and privileges of the nurse that parallel the example set by teachers and graduate nurses with whom the student has contact. Every teacher-student contact produces some kind of learning as a result of the student's constant evaluation of the teacher by comparing *what the teacher does and is with what the teacher says.* Thus, it can be seen that the teacher of clinical nursing must be a role model of expert professional nursing care. While this is by no means a new concept in *principle,* it is relatively new in *practice.* Nursing literature, themes of nursing meetings, graduate education, and postgraduate programs reflect the existing struggle for developing ways of ensuring clinical competence for teachers in schools of nursing. This competence is not only to be evaluated at the beginning of an academic career; continuous practice and review must also be fit into the career pattern.

As Quint has so aptly stated, the profession of nursing is a high-risk occupation.[3] The creative teacher in clinical nursing must be willing to risk the self in providing an environment that fosters creative learning. Many teachers in clinical nursing seemed to have developed a compulsion for infalli-

ble performance, which led to intense anxiety during the performance and guilt feelings whenever it fell short of perfection; these same attitudes were reflected by student expectations. The time has come for us to examine realistically our rights and responsibilities. Do clinical teachers have a right to be wrong? If so, in what circumstances? Admittedly the process of providing a service to human beings in a clinical setting suggests that we do in fact have grave responsibilities for the preservation of life in every act of nursing. But provision of a learning environment that offers support and direction in helping students develop realistic sets of expectations about their performance may relieve the anxiety reactions created by the self-perpetuated doctrine of infallibility. More important, perhaps, than honestly admitting that error may accompany learning is discovering that an honest critique of errors can advance learning and understanding. The teacher, as a human being, has a better potential for becoming the role model of an expert clinician when expectations are realistic as opposed to threatening to individual integrity, which increases the possibilities of anxiety-laden, inferior performance.

The teacher who seeks to provide a creative learning environment for students must demonstrate clinical competence in the areas of (1) application of concepts and scientific principles to patient care situations, (2) performance of technical skills with a flexibility allowing for modifications to meet the immediate needs of the situation, (3) adequate assessment as a basis for making appropriate judgments, (4) planning, organizing, and directing various levels of personnel and disciplines in implementing learning experiences to meet the needs of the patients, and (5) establishment of effective communications and interpersonal relationships to provide the desired learning milieu. The competent teacher of clinical nursing relies on intellectual and motor skills in performing as a "live" example of clinical nursing performance. Although the teaching program is designed for the student, the example provided other nurses as the teacher functions in the clinical setting, coupled with effective interaction, improves the quality of nursing provided by the total staff in the given setting.

It is difficult to separate sharply the various competencies. With the basic assumption that the clinical nursing teacher has an adequate background of knowledge, technical skill, and the ability to establish interpersonal relationships and communication, the way in which the teacher uses these competencies in a given nursing situation reflects the creative ability. Clearly the teacher's clinical competence lies in the ability to use all skills in some form to provide the desired results; each used as a separate entity cannot suffice.

ESTABLISHING EFFECTIVE WORKING RELATIONSHIPS WITH OTHERS

Establishing effective working relationships with others provides the third dimension so necessary for the teacher of clinical nursing to be viewed as a creative individual. To paraphrase the adage, "one cannot give with a closed fist," the clinical nursing teacher cannot be a creative individual with a closed mind. The effectiveness of the total clinical nursing program is directly proportional to the kind of relationships the teacher establishes with students, peers, nursing service personnel, and representatives of related health and welfare disciplines.

Relationships with students

Contrary to the image of today's young adult perpetuated by the news media, studies done by educators, sociologists, nurses, and countless others have revealed a profile of the "new breed" of students that has profound implications for the total educational system, particularly nursing programs. Foshay has pointed out some of these changes as they are affecting curriculum patterns in nursing.[4] Many of today's students and certainly those of tomorrow have been exposed to educational systems that have provided them with ability to use problem-solving techniques; discuss crucial issues of our times; use learning innovations such as programmed instruction, independent study, and audiovisual devices; conduct group discussions; write clearly enough to communicate their views; pursue a project requiring extensive search of the literature; use the laboratory approach to solving a specific problem; and have an ability to base their understandings on concepts and principles and apply them in a variety of relationships. These students also are more emotionally and socially mature; they are willing to take responsibility for their own actions as adults. They seek help on occasion but in return expect to be able to enter into an adult relationship with the teacher in viewing various sides of the problem without having demands made on them that infringe on their rights and responsibilities. We no longer deal with just the late adolescent for whom we have elected to serve as parent surrogate. We now have a heterogeneous group of part-time and full-time students, some of whom are married, have children, and have had other careers. We must relinquish existing rules and regulations that tend to control the rights of students as individuals and that, in fact, do affect their educational development. Students of today seek opportunities to discuss their ideas with intellectually honest people; they have no respect for teachers who are unwilling to discuss issues and problems with them or who give answers leading them to dead-end learning situations. Thus a common bond of understanding regarding one's rights and responsibilities in an educational setting must exist between student and teacher before an effective student-teacher relationship can be established in the clinical nursing program.

It follows, then, that the provision of a learning environment fostering effective student-teacher relationships in the clinical nursing setting depends on the teacher's degree of self-acceptance and professional competence and the extent of recognition and acceptance of the knowledge, competencies, and personal characteristics that students bring to nursing from their total life experiences. The establishment of a learning environment in a clinical nursing setting involves both the personal characteristics necessary for creative teaching and the climate that has developed in each clinical nursing setting. The personal and professional behavior displayed by the teacher should provide an environment that stimulates and nourishes the students' zest for learning. Requisites to creativity in providing a favorable learning environment include the investment of self in the activities of teaching to the degree that reflects enjoyment of teaching and students but has no room for martyrdom; giving of self, reflecting warmth and friendliness, removing fear without destroying attitudes of mutual respect or expecting returns from students; possessing self-confidence in approach to the learning situation regardless of approaches used by others and showing confidence in students' ability to succeed; and possessing enough patience to allow students at different levels to grow at their own rate, learning by a process of self-discovery rather than by rote to meet the necessary goals within a prescribed time period.

Each setting used for clinical learning experiences has its own psychosocial climate that must be understood and interpreted to the students through positive examples set by the teacher. Teaching in any practice setting as if it were a laboratory in which one could attend only to the experiment or experience at hand can cut one off from important multiple learning possibilities. Students of nursing must learn how the interaction of those seeking health care, those producing it, and the organizations in which the two meet affect all involved and must gain some mastery of methods for dealing with the interactions. It is the *human factor* that is responsible for the success or failure of the student-teacher relationship, wherever it takes place. The teacher uses a problem-solving discussion to help students grow through situations they do not understand and for which they seek answers. Concern about

what the student is thinking and learning as well as the environmental problems motivates the teacher to continue to provide a clinical nursing environment conducive to learning, regardless of the obstacles. Creativity depends primarily on the teacher's courage to use his particular character assets flexibly and with spontaneity as such situations demand action.

Perhaps the greatest compliment the teacher affords students in clinical nursing is that of recognizing each as an individual in terms of goals to be pursued, approaches to solving nursing care problems, approaches to daily organization and planning for nursing care, and their individual beliefs regarding basic psychosocial issues and approaches to daily life situations. To consider individual differences in the attainment of goals, the clinical teacher must accept *all* students, have patience in helping each to reach his potential, allow freedom for each to progress in accord with his own learning ability, offer individual assistance to those seeking help, build curiosity into experiences for those who are ready to move ahead, provide source materials and new avenues of inquiry for those who question current ideas and practices, and provide opportunities for testing and evaluating new ideas. The blending of these facets of individualized learning is dependent on the clinical teacher's ability to provide the delicate balance between success and failure, enthusiasm and boredom in assisting individual students to progress toward the desired goals. Teachers who find mastery of knowledge and skills to be relatively easy cannot expect the students to be rubber-stamp images of their model; neither can teachers hold back those students who do, in fact, find it relatively easy to master the desired behaviors and then seek knowledge and experiences beyond that included in the teachers' original plans. Students requiring tutorial guidance and continued support should not be expected to reach the unattainable. If, after a reasonable expenditure of time and energy, the student is unable to meet the minimal goals, he should not be penalized by being allowed to continue in a program that affords marginal opportunities for self-fulfillment.

A part of individualizing the learning experience is that of communicating professional and ethical norms while honestly expressing personal values and preferences. A beginning student of any subject often searches for "right" answers to provide the security of rigid rules and minimize the risk of choices that might be in error. Although it is true that the new student may be confused by too broad a range of choices, it is also true that individual members of a profession must be capable of making ethical and professional judgments based not only on group norms but also on personal values. The instructor who exhibits rigid adherence to professional standards and is not honest about how these interact with, and sometimes conflict with, personal values will do students a disservice. The instructor who can share instances of such interaction and conflict and the eventual action decisions, will add a great deal to the development of students' abilities to function effectively as professionals.

The application of the concept of individual differences to the teaching of clinical nursing is not new. Rather, it is the *way* that it is used which is the crucial factor in planning clinical nursing experiences designed to release the individual student's potential for creative learning. Generally clinical teachers have relied heavily on consideration of individual differences in diagnosing learning problems encountered by students and helping them overcome these problems in the classroom or tutoring programs. The lack of consideration of individual differences in planning clinical nursing experiences is distressing, especially at a time when we have at our disposal resources for providing individualized learning, limited only by the teacher's ability to use them creatively. Ways must be found for selecting and planning clinical nursing experiences that recognize these individual student needs. By studying the

students' background and taking cues from their expressed needs, the creative teacher can identify multiple approaches to meet more nearly students' needs within the framework of the total course objectives. The example of such an approach described in Chapter 3* deserves further consideration if creative teachers truly believe in the concept of individual differences and are willing to risk themselves in providing an environment conducive to creative learning in which students are free to assess their own strengths and weaknesses and pursue learning experiences accordingly. This opportunity for self-discovery on an individual basis is accompanied by the teacher's guidance in helping students work through their problems, in seeing relationships from one experience to another, and in applying basic principles to each new experience. Another dimension in the consideration of individual differences in planning clinical nursing experiences utilizes some of the newer instructional technologies to help students proceed at their own rate. These are discussed in greater detail in Chapter 8.

Determining desirable student-faculty ratios for supervision of students in direct patient care experiences becomes less a problem of numbers and time allotments and more a matter of the clinical teacher's creative ability. The ability to lead from the background involves playing a supportive role in helping students focus on the appropriate actions needed to meet the desired goals. Creative clinical supervision of students involves a sensitivity to maintaining a situation that preserves the patients' physical and emotional safety but allows students the freedom to formulate a plan of action for accomplishing a given task. The suspended-judgment approach used by the clinical teacher offers students encouragement and confirmation of their ideas; the teacher's "silent partner" actions offer the students valuable learning cues

---

*Refer to Chapter 3, pp. 37 to 40.

for growing through difficult experiences while preserving their self-esteem. The clinical teacher who allows the student to describe their plan of work organization for the day and pursue it accordingly provides mutual student-teacher learning opportunities. If the student is allowed to pursue the plan, its success provides a learning experience for both teacher and student; if the student is unsuccessful, review and evaluation of the plan become a more meaningful and lasting learning experience because it was the student's idea, not that forced upon him by an authority figure. The teacher who uses creative approaches to the clinical supervision of students provides them with self-confidence, leading them to learn through self-discovery; they can function comfortably in the clinical situation with or without the presence of the teacher yet know that they can secure supportive assistance any time they need it.

Providing individual and group counseling demands a clinical teacher with an awareness of and sensitivity to others. There are those students who constantly seek teacher approval, but there are those who do not seek assistance, either because they are unaware of their problems or are unwilling to admit that they need assistance. Therefore the clinical teacher often identifies the need for individual or group counseling through a sense of timing in knowing when to offer guidance and when to allow students to manage their own affairs. The literature abounds with guidelines for counseling students. However, there is one rule that cuts across all problem areas in both individual and group counseling. *The creative teacher should project the image of never being too busy to discuss a problem with a student.* However, the student's self-image should be preserved by providing privacy for the counseling session, regardless of circumstances or time elements.

By our own admission, evaluation of clinical nursing performance suffers critically from a lack of established, reliable, valid criteria for use in analyzing results obtained through a variety of evaluation tools. At present the establishment of an effective teacher-student relationship for evaluating student progress is based on the clinical teacher's reinforcement of good performance by providing feedback regarding progress made during each successive clinical experience. The teacher's task involves being readily accessible to provide praise for successful performance, to provide needed support in redirecting the focus of learning, or to help students express or demonstrate ideas and action in an atmosphere fostering freedom of personal and professional growth. Immediacy of feedback is of particular importance to clinical nursing from two vantage points: (1) there is a need to preserve the patient's safety; and (2) there is a need to correct student misconceptions or gross errors in performance before proceeding. The teacher's approach in evaluating students' progress in clinical nursing must be consistent with approaches used to foster creative learning throughout the entire clinical nursing program. The teacher should accept the student's individual work pattern as satisfactory if it brings desired results and is compatible with the system in which the student is practicing, regardless of how it may differ from that of other students. Insofar as the process used reflects the self-actualization of the individual student, that student has succeeded, regardless of the teacher's preconceived goals. The teacher seeking to foster creative thinking and action in clinical nursing must recognize that the exact approach to the task and end results must be evaluated in a framework that includes student, patients, system, and instructor as well as course goals.

The creative teacher of clinical nursing knows that providing an atmosphere of freedom for learning and allowing students to recognize and accept their own failure is not enough. The teacher also assumes the responsibility for providing support to those who seek it and for setting standards of performance to be pursued. Periodically the teacher can assist students in determining their own progress and can help them clarify thinking regarding means of meeting their goals by raising thought-provoking questions and by suggesting various alternatives to be explored in resolving problems. Effective student-teacher relationships should be such an integral part of the total teaching-learning environment that there is no room for fear of the teacher, reluctance to express original ideas, or fear of ridicule from others. It means that the teacher can understand all sides of a problem and view each student in terms of individual potential. Such an approach helps students discover for themselves how far they have traveled toward self-fulfilled learning and provides them with a vision of how far they might go.

Relationships with faculty peers

The development of clinical specialization in nursing and the potential for parallel specialization within the curriculum, may lead to division within a school faculty. Current discussions in medical education, where specialization has had a longer, more direct impact, highlight the potential for problems. Newer curricular designs in nursing seem to be structured around courses that encourage collaboration across lines of specialization. In any school it is essential that faculty retain a commitment to the total educational goal as a focus of individual work.

When several clinical teachers are functioning within the same clinical area, every effort must be made to provide a learning milieu that represents unanimity of purpose without sacrificing the unique contributions of each clinical teacher. Extensive cooperative planning should be used to determine objectives to be met; methods of teaching and time allotments to be used; instructional materials to be secured, developed, and used at specified times; supervision of students by each faculty member; the role each teacher will play in teaching needed skills; use of other faculty members as resource persons; clinical facilities to be used; policies for students in providing patient care; and criteria for evaluation of student performance. The process of coordinating these activities demands an ability to share with others, changing the teaching environment to one in which freedom permeates the total teaching program. Teachers should feel free to communicate with one another regarding the sharing of learning experiences and should allow free interchange of students from one teacher to another. The habit of sharing information about individual student progress, patient progress, and other environmental factors in the clinical setting allows clinical teachers to expend their energies in constructive achievement of desired educational goals. Because students are constantly placed in an environment requiring them to work cooperatively with others, the clinical teachers must establish working relationships with one another to serve as role models for the students. An environment of unified faculty action and mutual respect is contagious. Students learn many valuable lessons by observing and experiencing interactions, especially those with other nurses and professionals. While cooperative planning is time consuming, its rewards outweigh its disadvantages in any experience where more than one teacher is involved.

Faculty members responsible for teaching in a given clinical nursing area know that the knowledge explosion makes it a major task for them to keep abreast of the current practices in their own area. Most faculty members are also aware of the need to remain cognizant of progress and problems related to nursing, health care, and the related disciplines. There is always the risk of becoming either too extended or too circumscribed in one's knowledge, though most faculty avoid either extreme. If faculty do no remain appropriately informed, students readily identify the problem, often through being subjected to either piecemeal or repetitious teaching that shows little relationship from one clinical area to another. There is a need for teachers from the various clinical nursing areas to meet together in an effort to coordinate the identification of new information and its inclusion in teaching, thus providing a unified approach that is greater than the sum of its individual clinical components. When colleagues can enter into this kind of cooperative planning, they also recognize the value of relying on each other to contribute their specialized knowledge and experience to appropriate aspects of various clinical areas. Communicating with one another regarding content and experiences taught in each clinical nursing area helps each teacher build on these experiences, prepare students for future experiences, and refer students seeking additional information to the clinical expert in another area. A professional respect for each clinical nursing teacher's ability and potential for contributing to the total nursing curriculum is an essential part of the sharing relationship that can be developed.

Just as the teaching of clinical nursing cannot be compartmentalized into neatly separated teaching programs for each clinical area, the total teaching of clinical nursing cannot be divorced from other professional courses or courses supporting the nursing major. Establishing cooperative working relationships with nonclinical faculty members offers teachers of clinical nursing the opportunity to know the content being taught and use it. The clinical teacher also has an opportunity to interpret students' learning needs and recommend course changes to facilitate application of basic knowledge to the most commonly encountered clinical nursing experiences. The nature of clinical nursing crosses all boundary lines in terms of kinds of learning experiences encountered because human beings have personal as well as medical and nursing needs. In this respect the clinical nursing teacher who establishes cooperative working relationships with nonclinical faculty members can rely on them as resource persons to sup-

plement background information needed to explain behavioral patterns, symptomatic manifestations, or new approaches to health care. The identification of the nurse/teacher as a member of a faculty will be divided between the roles of nurse and that of academician. A healthy balance is necessary; many younger nursing faculty are surprisingly delighted at the productivity and stimulation of exchange with college- or university-wide groups.

A plan of action for cooperative relationships with faculty peers both in nursing and non-nursing areas removes those blocks to communication and creativity all too often used as excuses for a clinical teacher's inability to provide a creative teaching-learning environment.

Relationships with nursing service agency personnel

The roles established by nursing service agencies and schools of nursing charge the clinical teacher with the responsibility for planning clinical nursing experiences for the students in conjunction with the agency; the ultimate goal of both the school of nursing and the nursing service agency is providing optimum patient care. The teacher of clinical nursing is in a strategic position to move either in the direction of providing clinical experiences completely divorced from the agency personnel or in the direction of providing clinical nursing experiences in an environment teeming with interactions of various levels of agency personnel and departments and school of nursing students and clinical teachers.

Nursing programs will not progress with teachers who provide clinical nursing experiences in a vacuum and who avoid suggestions of collaborating with nursing service agency personnel to make cooperative plans. The clinical nursing teacher who can discard the concept implied by "my students" is ready to explore with others the kinds of experiences and human resources that can contribute to the total desired learning outcomes, regardless of who makes the contribution. *The clinical nursing teacher remains in control of the total learning program but enters into a cooperative venture with various agency departments and personnel to the point where the students are commonly referred to as "our students."* The clinical teacher must enter into a cooperative relationship with an open mind and with the constant reminder that every contact with another human being offers one an opportunity to learn something new.

It has been said that Mahatma Gandhi's greatest asset was his fearlessness. In our society fearlessness is a rare commodity, perhaps because it requires an objective evaluation of one's self in order to establish mutually effective relationships with others. In the anxiety to accomplish necessary goals, our approach to a given situation may resemble that of a herd of elephants, leaving fear in its wake. That is, we can become so intent on planning and implementing a clinical nursing program in a nursing service agency that we do not take the time to explain the program, to seek collaboration with others, or to provide opportunities for the students and the personnel to establish mutually effective working relationships. As a result, nursing service personnel experience the fear of the unknown, which manifests itself in a variety of forms, depending on the situation and persons involved. Students, using practitioners as role models, may assume that avoidance and criticism mean that they are learning erroneous material or are becoming "bad" nurses. The clinical teacher, too, exhibits manifestations of fear of the unknown in not knowing exactly what to expect from the nursing personnel or how well an environment conducive to learning can be established. But the teacher of clinical nursing who enters into a partnership with the full range of nursing service personnel has little fear about the total program and helps to minimize fears and doubts on the part of the agency personnel. The teacher of clinical nursing seeks cooperative action in planning for student clinical experiences, providing orientation

programs, supervising students, evaluating student behavior and development, utilizing various persons as resource personnel, and collaborating with the nursing team and total health team in helping students use problem-solving approaches to patient care. This kind of cooperative approach to providing clinical nursing experience in an environment of support and acceptance does not add to the functions of the nursing service agency personnel nor remove these functions from the clinical nursing teacher. The gain in effective care provided by faculty and students adds to the care resources and should allow flexibility for the staff to share in education. The best cooperative efforts between agency personnel and school of nursing personnel are those fed by freedom and spontaneity, those that generate contributions without demanding them and give recognition and acceptance to each person making a worthwhile contribution. Initial explanations of the goals to be sought while students are in the agency help personnel to feel a part of the total program and to contribute useful ideas and information. Nursing personnel who know that the clinical teacher and students welcome their help and suggestions feel needed and accepted and are motivated to continue to make contributions and advance into areas not previously considered. The clinical teacher who takes the time to know and relate to the various nursing personnel also recognizes the potential many of these persons have for contributing to the educational program; a mere suggestion to them often sparks their particular talents, which may be used to enrich the clinical learning experiences for students. In the process of building these relationships, a reciprocal feeling often emanates within the nursing service agency whereby the teacher is sought for help of various kinds. The assistance may take various forms, including demonstration practice, consultation on specific care problems or issues, or participation in in-service and continuing education programs. This is an extremely healthy sign, indicating that the agency has accepted the clinical teacher as an individual of worth and is seeking ways and means of improving the educational environment for the students.

As the health and welfare needs of the nation shape the practice patterns of community agencies, schools of nursing should be seeking student clinical experiences from a wider range of health and welfare agencies or relying on personnel from these agencies as consultants in conferences and discussions. Here again the clinical teacher should seek a cooperative approach to the planning, supervision, and evaluation of clinical nursing experiences for students. The teacher must learn to communicate with those who have little orientation to nursing education. When time is not an immediate factor, the clinical teacher can establish an excellent give-and-take relationship with the desired agency in the same manner used with other nursing agencies. The specific content and framework of exchanges will be altered by the goals and programs of the agency involved. Working directly with personnel in such a situation allows the teacher to assess the agency in terms of the kinds of learning experiences and environment it can provide; the teacher can supply opportunities for the agency to learn about the objectives of the educational program and nursing as a profession and the goals to be realized by using the particular agency as a part of the total clinical nursing experience. When such a foundation has been established, the cooperative planning and implementation of a given program can come as a natural and integral part of the total experience.

The teacher of clinical nursing seeking to create a learning environment reflecting cooperative, coordinated actions between the school of nursing faculty and the service agency must proceed with courage and great patience in providing an atmosphere of education without fear. The establishment of these relationships comes about relatively slowly, but the teacher must recognize that each contribution by each individual, is a step in the direction that eventually leads to tangible evidence of cooperative relationships. When nursing service personnel know that they are not *required to* contribute to the program but experience the tangible results of having made a contribution, they are motivated to continue. Eventually the cooperative actions become a natural part of the daily activities. As this cooperative action grows and is reflected in the total learning experiences, the students, too, develop a sensitivity to the need for establishing cooperative relationships with agency personnel. When they see that they are wanted and are considered a necessary part of the total organization, they will turn to personnel for help, respect their judgment, and offer them assistance. But this fairy-tale ending becomes reality only when the nursing teacher and the nursing service personnel provide tangible evidence of these cooperative relationships as an integral part of the clinical learning experience.

The teacher of clinical nursing as a creative individual is a role model of many personal and professional qualities, it is the individual who establishes the creative act as an extension of the self. The true value of a given creative act must be established by the person, not by praise or criticism by others. It would seem trite to list characteristics of the creative teacher out of context; therefore, the foregoing discussion has attempted to provide a view of the creative teacher in relationship to self and others.

REFERENCES

1. Jersild, Arthur: When teachers face themselves, Nursing Forum 1:61-72, Fall, 1962.
2. Maslow, Abraham H.: Creativity in self-actualizing people. In Anderson, Harold, editor: Creativity and its cultivation, New York, 1959, Harper & Row, Publishers.
3. Quint, Jeanne C.: Hidden hazards for nurse teachers, Nursing Outlook 15:34-39, April, 1967.
4. Foshay, Arthur: Beware, your future students are learning to think! Nursing Outlook 13:47-49, Oct., 1965.

SUGGESTED READINGS

Batey, Marjorie: The two normative worlds of the university nursing faculty, Nursing Forum 8(1):4-16, 1969.

Dickoff, James, and James, Patricia: Power, American Journal of Nursing 68:2128-2132, Oct., 1968.

Hassenplug, Lulu W.: The good teacher, Nursing Outlook 13:24-27, Oct., 1965

Kiker, M.: Characteristics of the effective teacher, Nursing Outlook 21:721-723, Nov., 1973.

Kramer, Marlene: Reality shock: why nurses leave nursing, St. Louis, 1974, The C. V. Mosby Co.

Layton, Sister Mary M.: How instructors' attitudes affect students, Nursing Outlook 17:27-29, Jan., 1969.

Rauen, K. C.: The clinical instructor as role model . . . , Milwaukee Wisconsin, Journal of Nursing Education 13:33-40, Aug., 1974.

Williams, Frank E.: Intellectual creativity and the teacher, Journal of Creative Behavior 1:173-180. Spring, 1967.

Unit III Aspects of design for teaching programs in clinical nursing

We must think anew—and act anew.

6 Planning and selection of learning experiences for clinical nursing

Each school of nursing attempts to build a curriculum that will best meet the needs of those it seeks to serve. To this end educators frequently utilize Tyler's concept of curriculum development and instructional planning, which involves identifying the kinds of educational goals the school believes should be attained, determining the kind of educational experiences that are possible in attaining the goals, organizing the educational experiences to effectively achieve the goals, and evaluating the outcomes to determine how well the goals are attained.[1,2]

While the focus of this book is directed toward teaching in clinical nursing, such a program cannot be regarded as both a separate entity and the heart of the total curriculum plan. To determine meaningful objectives for the teaching program in clinical nursing, one must build on the philosophy and objectives of the total nursing program, so that each complements the other. The responsibility for translating the curriculum plan into action rests with the teacher. The responsibility for implementing a nursing curriculum that provides students with a base upon which to build a continuum of professional nursing practice rests with the teaching program in clinical nursing.

Just as the wise practitioner bases a diagnosis on a collection of relevant facts, the educator must rely on a variety of sources of information to provide a comprehensive basis for the selection of objectives for a given program in a school of nursing.

To clarify the relationship between the process of curriculum building for a total curriculum and the development of a clinical program in a particular subject area, a conceptual model is shown in Fig. 1. This model describes the process of curriculum planning that proceeds from the general to the specific. That is, the process becomes more specific at each hierarchical level, beginning with identifying students' needs, society's needs, and professional standards to formulate objectives. The objectives are screened so that they are in accord with the school's philosophy of education and its stated beliefs about the conditions for learning. This process gives a basis for formulating outcome or behavioral objectives first for the total curriculum, next for the specific subject areas, then for the clinical program for each subject area, and finally for the daily planning of clinical experiences. The hierarchy of objectives must be in harmony as each phase of the total curriculum is designed to bring about the desired behavioral outcomes of the students.

Once a thorough study of the sources of objectives has been made and the hierarchy of objectives has been established and screened, the clinical teacher determines the best ways of attaining those goals in the practice of nursing. The test of creativity lies in the teacher's ability to work with the students in determining individualized daily objectives for clinical learning and in planning satisfying and challenging experiences that are in accord with the total course and curriculum objectives.

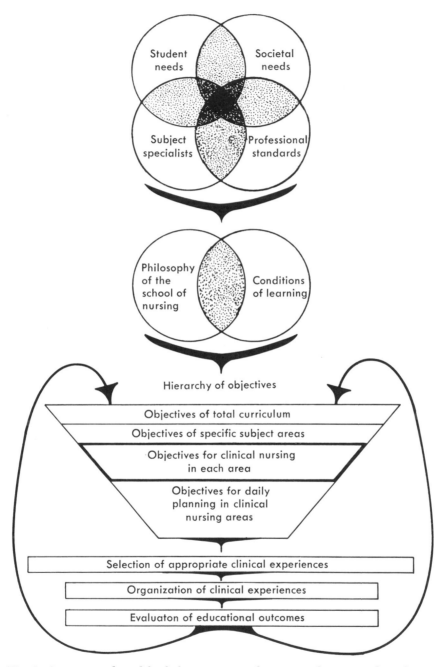

Fig. 1. A conceptual model of the processes inherent in planning and implementing teaching programs in clinical nursing. (Drawing revised by Howard F. Langhoff, Project Director for "Development and Evaluation of a System for Improving the Teaching-Learning Process in Nursing," Indiana University School of Nursing at Indiana University–Purdue University, Indianapolis, funded by PHS Grant No. NU 00244-01.)

SOURCES OF INFORMATION FOR DERIVING OBJECTIVES
Study of students' needs

Viewing nursing education as a continual process of changing students' behavioral patterns of thinking, feeling, and performing demands that the educational objectives sought by a given school of nursing reflect comparable kinds of behavioral changes. The frequent discovery of discrepancies between learning outcomes and desired objectives of a given learning experience is indicative of the difficulty of achieving an educational goal. In some cases, it may be necessary for educators to face the fact that the nature of the learner may be the key determinant of effectual outcomes of the teaching-learning process. Although educational objectives are dependent on the school's prevailing philosophy, the teachers' beliefs about the psychology of learning, and their commitment to the practice of those beliefs, we must also determine characteristics and needs of students and *use* this information in developing educational objectives.

The marked changes in the kinds of students enrolled in schools of nursing affect the way we relate to them in terms of understanding their attitudes and perceptions as well as their learning abilities. The most notable changes are the increasing variety in social and cultural backgrounds and the increasing knowledge expectations placed even on those newly recruited to nursing from so-called deprived backgrounds. We must also deal with a wide range of background of nursing experience; motivation for seeking nursing education; degree of productivity; response to environmental stimuli; need for authoritarian or permissive atmosphere; need for recognition, status, and acceptance; ability to make value judgments; rates and degrees of learning ability; ability to use problem-solving methods; and exposure to multimedia approaches to learning.

To study the needs of the student, a wide variety of methods can be employed, such as: examination of students' records, personal interviews with students and parents, or teacher observations of student behavior in both social and educational settings. A more sophisticated and reliable approach is that of utilizing testing devices yielding data that will meet the needs of the individual school and that can be used in a variety of ways in establishing objectives that enhance individuals' potentialities in accord with their assessed levels of abilities. There are any number of available standardized tests, such as: Edwards Personal Preference Schedule, Empathy Inventory, Nurse Attitudes Inventory, or Luther Hospital Sentence Completion Test. Most institutions of higher education have some type of internal research division that continually directs efforts toward gaining similar and additional data for use by all departments.

Analysis of whatever kind of data collected about the students constitutes a basis for considering the kinds of students' interests and needs in determining meaningful, relevant objectives for the educational program.

Study of society's needs

A second source for determining curriculum is the needs of contemporary society. The use of results of such information in proper perspective along with the other suggested sources of information is not only desirable but also necessary. The long-range effects of scientific and technological advancements, changing patterns of the socioeconomic condition of society, and changing patterns of health needs and resultant health care programs impose a need for careful observation and decision from those vitally concerned with total curriculum planning in schools of nursing. The exigencies brought about by our constantly changing contemporary life charge educators with the responsibility for curriculum planning that provides opportunities for students both to add to their current knowledge and to become prepared to discover new concepts. Time must be wisely spent by avoidance of teaching concepts that are possibly outdated or already known to most students, or striving to teach "everything" without regard for the rapidly changing social order.

Inferring school of nursing curriculum objectives from the needs of contemporary society generally involves the collection and analysis of data from epidemiological studies, population reports, public health surveys, morbidity and mortality statistics, longevity studies, birthrates, social problems related to health and disease, legislative programs related to health and welfare, socioeconomic health and welfare indices, geographic distribution and prevalence of various diseases, and health problems and needs resulting from natural and man-made disasters. This must include health needs related to social relationships and understanding human behavior. The significance of the key word—*contemporary*—in the study of this source of information cannot be overemphasized. One must be constantly looking at today's problems in order to be assured that nursing programs will be effectively planned to meet the problems and issues of society.

A variety of methods of investigating contemporary society can be utilized such as activity and job analysis, observation of behavior, sociological surveys, questionnaires and interviews to determine trends in thinking regarding social issues, community studies regarding particular problems, health surveys, analysis of contemporary literature about critical social issues, and statistical studies of social-economic-health problems. Fortunately for the nursing profession much of the information regarding health needs of society has already been compiled on international, national, state, and local levels and is ready for analysis leading to inference of the kind of educational objectives that will enable the nurse to practice in terms of the current needs of the consumers of nursing—society.

There are innumerable ways of analyzing contemporary society, as evidenced by the abundance of available studies. Regardless of the phase of life selected for study, the purpose remains that of securing data about the particular aspects of contemporary society most likely to have implications for the educational objectives of a particular curriculum. Here again, as in the case of determining student needs, data regarding the needs of society must be compared to norms and interpreted according to gaps in the present status before objectives can be inferred.

Study of subject matter suggested by specialists

If we say that each teacher responsible for planning a given course of study within the nursing curriculum presumably is an expert in the given subject matter, we automatically utilize the subject specialists as a third source of inferring educational objectives. Ideally this approach to determining suitable objectives for a total curriculum plan appears to have great merits. But the fallacy that often makes this approach unsound may be seen from two viewpoints: (1) too often those responsible for the course are not truly subject specialists and (2) legitimate subject specialists tend to pursue the course objectives in terms of highly technical or specialized information regarding the particular subject matter with no thought given to how the course contributes to broad general objectives permeating many areas of the curriculum.

There is available written material in general, professional, and nursing education that suggests ways in which specific areas of knowledge in the liberal arts and professional education could contribute to the enrichment of the general curriculum pattern and to the more specific functions of a particular subject area in its own right. An excellent example of the kinds of suggestions for objectives than can be obtained from a subject specialist in nursing is that described by Brodt,[3] who cites many examples of how various liberal arts courses contribute to the broad objectives regarding ability to use problem-solving techniques, communicate effectively and apply the understandings of the nature of man to the understanding of human behavior in nursing situations. She describes how nursing research activities can influence the curriculum planning regarding objectives that seek to provide quality nursing care for patients.

Interpretation of information presented by subject specialists for purposes of deriving educational objectives served by a given subject area is facilitated by seeking the answers to these two questions: (1) What major function can this subject serve? (2) What specific contribution can it make to the total curriculum pattern? Areas for contribution include the social, behavioral, and physical sciences, and those fields contributing to the ability to make value judgments and solve problems.

Study of professional standards

Those responsible for nursing education look to the needs expressed by students, contemporary society, and subject matter specialist in planning curriculum, but the responsibility for the development and maintenance of minimum standards for competent nursing practice and ethical behavior lies solely with the nursing profession. The state laws defining nursing practice provide a foundation for determining the kinds of experiences students need to meet the prescribed *minimum* standards of competence in nursing practice; and criteria set by various accrediting bodies provide the standards for measuring the quality of the total education program provided by a given school of nursing. With these minimal criteria in mind, the faculty as a school carry the individual and collective professional responsibility for determining the scope of nursing practice, the potential contribution of their graduates to that practice, and the level of expectations to be used as standards.

Since the time of Florence Nightingale, individual nurses and professional nursing groups have continued to attempt to define nursing. Research studies of nursing functions have been conducted and findings re-

ported; individual nursing leaders have expressed their views regarding the nature of nursing; and the American Nurses' Association's Board of Directors has made an official statement on the definition of nursing practice that was designed for use by the states for inclusion in their nurse practice acts.[4] New nurse practice acts in many states have contributed to the defining process. These provide guidance to schools of nursing in the preparation of nurses who are safe to practice nursing in society, but allow individual schools of nursing to experiment with curriculum by virtue of the minimum requirements set by the act. Additionally, more academic definitions have come from the nursing theorists, including Johnson, Peplau, Rogers, and Roy. These statements provide models, not only for definition but also for practice, teaching, and research.

Accrediting bodies seek to improve the quality of total education programs offered by colleges or universities and the professional components such as schools of nursing through the standards set by the educational group making up the particular accrediting body. Such accrediting bodies serve a necessary and useful purpose as incentives to the continuous improvement of programs offered by a school of nursing while allowing for attainment of the objectives of the school. When they allow little regard for the achievement of the school's objectives, they cease to be useful. Schools of nursing reveal much evidence of the accreditation processes of the National League for Nursing, some of which have fostered creative development. In some schools, however, they have been accepted as rigid rules and used to limit rather than to support growth.

Information regarding the standards expected of graduates of nursing as well as the total educational program a school establishes to provide a competent nurse has implications for the kinds of objectives a school seeks to achieve. The key to the successful use of this information lies in the recognition by nurse educators that the responsibility of the profession is the assurance of standards but in no way implies that there should be a standardization of curriculum for schools of nursing.

RELATIONSHIPS BETWEEN SCHOOL OF NURSING PHILOSOPHY AND OBJECTIVES

The process of studying needs of students, needs of contemporary society, suggestions from subject matter specialists, and professional standards produces a heterogeneous collection of objectives that are too unwieldy to utilize in curriculum planning. At this point the school of nursing faculty must take a long, hard look at the collection of objectives in terms of compatibility with the school's philosophy, compatibility with one another, ability to accomplish all of the objectives within the prescribed time limits, and ability to measure the objectives in terms of desired behavioral outcomes.

The first criterion for screening these objectives is a clearly stated philosophy of the school of nursing. The list of objectives can be compared with the basic philosophical beliefs of the school; those objectives that most readily agree with the philosophy can be assigned a high priority, whereas those not in agreement can be eliminated.

Each philosophy reflects the viewpoints of those charged with the responsibility for planning and implementing the curriculum. Detailed discussion of various philosophical viewpoints is left to other textbooks and references dealing specifically with such issues. However, today's students tend to view higher education with a seriousness of purpose that seeks to improve the existing social order. This reality-oriented philosophy of life requires that basic philosophical approaches to nursing be reexamined to consider a more humanistic approach to problem-solving, which would deal with identification and acceptance of basic human needs as expressed in a variety of life styles existing in a wide range of community settings. The school of nursing then uses this knowledge to determine the kinds of values, ideals, and practices that constitute the philosophy underlying the kinds of behavioral patterns to be represented by the objectives of the total curriculum and each definitive portion of the program.

RELATIONSHIPS BETWEEN CONDITIONS FOR LEARNING AND OBJECTIVES ESTABLISHED BY SCHOOL OF NURSING

A second screening device for clarifying and organizing the statement of objectives for the total curriculum is that of determining the basic beliefs of a given school of nursing regarding the conditions that are most conducive to learning. Since the educational objectives represent the results achieved by learning, it is obvious that the stated objectives must be in accord with the stated conditions for learning as perceived by the faculty. A study of various conditions for learning as described by educational psychology expects can be used as the basis for formulating a statement of beliefs regarding the learning process that seems reasonable and applicable to the given situation.

In general, such a statement would attempt to explain how learning occurs, under what conditions, and by what sorts of mechanisms. Those committed to the concept of fostering a learning environment conducive to creative thinking and action will want to address themselves to the conditions for learning that foster creativity. This implies an examination of some of the emerging concepts of education and teaching. With the teaching-learning process focused on creativity, there is a need to consider an existential approach to learning that addresses itself to the active involvement of the student in dealing with a changing social order. A discussion by Frank[5] regarding the application of the concept of teaching without learning to nursing education poses some provocative thoughts that should be studied in depth by those seeking to provide a creative learning environment for students.

The newer dimensions of curriculum development alluded to in Chapter 1 might well be considered in terms of taking a new look at the relationships between the current and projected needs of the learner and the teaching innovations being used to implement the curricula of schools of nursing. In his commentary concerning changes in his position regarding curriculum development, Tyler[2] suggests that those concerned with curriculum development reevaluate their current thinking regarding the following:

1. Consider the delicate balance between providing learning experiences that foster conformity and those in which complete control is held by the learner. The latter approach implies a belief in the learner as an active, purposeful human being, which predicates the provision of learning experiences to help the individual recognize his rights and responsibilities for learning—that is, present in every learning situation are some things that the learner can manipulate for meeting his personal objectives and some things for which an adjustment must be made in order to meet the teacher's objectives.

2. Consider the learner's role in developing and using knowledge. Before formulating objectives for a particular area of study, it would be well to investigate the structure of the discipline and nature of the knowledge it involves. Using this information, along with the concept that one learns by discovery, allows one to formulate objectives that will enable the learner to treat knowledge as a growing product of man's effort to understand.

3. Consider the relationship between learning conditions that draw on the use of specific stimulus-response learning and learning resulting from generalizations. There may be a point at which both kinds of learning enter into the accomplishment of the objective in that the level of generality to be expected by the student can be stated, while at the same time the student can recognize how the generalization applies to a number of specifics and vice versa.

DEFINING THE HIERARCHY OF OBJECTIVES

Regardless of the hierarchical level, a statement of objectives describes the expected changes in student behavior as determined by the faculty of a given school of nursing. The stated objectives then serve as criteria for guiding those activities that contribute to curriculum planning, implementation, and evaluation. Specifically, objectives function as guides to definition of the desired behavioral outcomes, selection of content, selection and organization of desirable learning activities, selection of the teaching techniques best suited to meet the desired outcomes, and measurement of the effectiveness of the selected teaching-learning activities.

To be used efficiently, objectives should be expressed in two-dimensional terms: (1) the behavioral aspect to be developed in the students and (2) the content aspect, which specifies the particular kinds of situations with which the behavioral aspects may be identified.

The behavioral aspects are often classified as follows in terms of the mental functions involved in the achievement of the desired behaviors:

1. *Cognitive (knowledge)*. This refers to objectives concerned with the acquisition and application of knowledge and the development of intellectual abilities and skills involving remembering, reasoning, problem-solving, concept formation and application, ability to see relationships, understanding of principles, creative thinking, and making value judgments.

2. *Affective (attitudes)*. This refers to objectives concerned with personal ad-

justment, social sensitivity, professional responsibilities, establishment of habits of conduct, changes in interests, attitudes, and values, and development of appreciations.

3. *Conative (skills).* This refers to objectives concerned with developing specific motor abilities and general adaptive abilities that may be mental or motor, with consideration given to the degree of skill desired as related to the level of experience.[6,7]

The content aspect relates to each of the behavioral aspects, either in general subject matter areas or areas related to patients, society, and the student as an individual. This provides a clear-cut picture of how the specific behavioral changes apply to particular subject areas, ideas, or kinds of clinical nursing situations.

After considering the sources of information for deriving objectives and using the school's stated philosophy and theories of learning as screening devices, clearly stated objectives should emerge. If we accept the premise that the purpose of objectives is to indicate the desired changes in students' behavior as related to specific content, it follows that objectives should concern that behavior rather than describe either the school's or the teacher's functions.

The hierarchy of objectives described in Fig. 1 attempts to show the interrelationship between the various levels of objectives for curriculum planning, ranging from the general to the specific and vice versa. Such a diagram can be of assistance to the curriculum planner in testing the objectives formulated for the various levels. Proceeding from the general to the specific, the *first level of hierarchy* defines those objectives related to the total curriculum pattern for the school of nursing. They are designed to reflect the basic ingredients of the institution of which the school is a part, the philosophy of nursing and nursing education, and the conditions for learning accepted by the school of nursing. The objectives are general in nature, applying to the total curriculum pattern for the school; they serve as guides for determining more specific objectives for each succeeding level of the curriculum plan.

The *second level of hierarchy* defines the objectives for specific subject areas. At this level the objectives usually refer to a core of related courses established according to the particular curriculum pattern of the school. This could refer to a broad fields grouping of courses related to an integrated curriculum, or a grouping of liberal arts courses and a grouping of professional courses, or a series of separate courses. Many other combinations are within the realm of possibility. Regardless of the approach used to establish courses or groups of courses, the objectives at this level are derived from the basic beliefs expressed in the objectives of the first hierarchical level but now relate specifically to each course or group of courses at this second level.

The core of the total curriculum pattern appears at the *third level of hierarchy,* in which the objectives of nursing are established according to the specific learning needs for the clinical areas. Here again, objectives are tailored to meet those learning needs identified as characteristic for each nursing specialty area or general clinical nursing area in accord with the basic beliefs expressed in the objectives for the two preceding hierarchical levels. It is this strategic level of objectives that sets the stage for the successful accomplishment of the objectives sought by a school of nursing. The exact division of nursing content into areas may be done using a variety of models. Common are medical subdivisions, age and development groups, and divisions derived from a specific nursing theory. Each may work if used with care; selection should have occurred at the level of stating the school's philosophy and objectives.

This third level is also important in setting the stage for the *fourth level of hierarchy* in which objectives must be planned to meet daily clinical learning activities within the framework of the broad scope of the clinical areas and the total program.

OBJECTIVES FOR SPECIFIC AREAS OF TEACHING IN CLINICAL NURSING

For teachers in clinical nursing, the availability of clinical resources including the latest electronic devices, of research scientists providing the latest in treatments, and of patients seeking health care in diversified settings ranging from primary care to hospital and extended care facilities may produce an overwhelming confusion. It is not enough for the teacher to believe that a teaching program in clinical nursing needs only the proper modern facilities in order to provide an educationally sound program! Regardless of available resources, the essence of a sound educational program at the clinical level lies in the careful selection and planning of experiences that fulfil those objectives specifically stated for the needs of the particular clinical nursing area in accord with the total curriculum objectives.

At the clinical nursing level the teacher must determine the specific objectives to be met in a particular area using the following guidelines:

1. Objectives for a given clinical experience should contribute to the total development of the students by including the cognitive, conative, and affective aspects of desired behavioral changes.

2. Acceptance of the concept that the primary purpose of education is to bring about behavioral changes in the students charges one with the responsibility for stating objectives in terms of the kinds of changes *expected of students.*

3. Each objective should be so stated that it contains a behavioral and a content component. Clinical nursing objectives should express those kinds of behavioral changes expected of students that are related to the particular clinical situation.

4. Objectives must be stated in terms that clearly define the desired specific behavioral changes. To accomplish this task successfully, it is extremely help-

ful to analyze each stated objective by asking, "How can I measure this clinical behavior to determine the degree to which the student attains this objective?" When the list of behavioral outcomes used to describe a given objective *can be measured clinically* in terms of degree of attainment by students, the objective in all probability is clearly stated.

5. The desired changes in behavior reflected by the objectives for learning in the clinical nursing areas should be consistent with the objectives for the specific subject areas, the total curriculum, the conditions for learning, and educational philosophy adopted by the school of nursing and the college or university.

6. Objectives must be attainable within the prescribed time available for a given clinical nursing program. The need for adequate time and available clinical experiences to accommodate the growing number of students has altered the traditional pattern of clinical learning. The rapid growth in the utilization of various electronic devices and visual aids makes it possible for students to learn certain skills on an independent study basis according to their own levels of ability. Upon completion of the clinical nursing program in a given area, the specific objectives are attained, although the time pattern and methods utilized vary widely among individual students. Such an approach allows for the flexibility necessary for creativity in the utilization of the concept of totality in determining objectives to be attained within a given clinical nursing program.

7. Objectives should be flexible enough to provide for planning clinical nursing experiences that allow for progression according to the ability levels of individual students.

8. The teacher should understand the objectives and assume responsibility for interpreting them to the students. A

cooperative student-teacher discussion of objectives serves as a motivating force in guiding the teaching-learning process.

9. Objectives provide the structural framework for the direction to be taken in planning clinical learning experiences, but the extent to which provision is made for creative learning activities for students rests with the teacher who recognizes the need for using creative approaches in meeting the prescribed objectives rather than considering objectives as limiting factors in planning clinical nursing programs.

Objectives for the clinical nursing aspect of the curriculum too commonly are equated with the refinement of nursing skills. However, clinical nursing involves such kinds of skill learning as application of basic science and nursing theory to clinical nursing situations; development of a wide range of specific kinds of observation and assessment skills; development of skill in establishing interpersonal relationships ranging from self-understanding to relationships with peers, patients and their families, nursing personnel, health team members, and school of nursing personnel; skill in making judgments regarding many facets of planning and implementing patient care; application of scientific principles to the development of motor skills; and the ability to master motor skills concomitantly with providing patient-centered nursing care. (Detailed discussion of these learning skills will be found in Chapter 7.) However, a careful examination of those objectives related to skill development would reveal that the cognitive and affective behavioral aspects are interrelated with the conative aspects. For example, to apply basic science and nursing theory to clinical nursing situations requires objectives from the realm of cognitive behavior whereby knowledge must be learned if it is to be applied; skills in relating to others involve a knowledge and understanding about one's self, and human behavior and a development of attitudes that assist in accepting behavior as it exists. The

learning of a particular motor skill involves intellectual mastery of the principles underlying the skill and an appreciation and understanding of the existing variables in order to simultaneously meet the patient's needs and acquire the motor skill.

The use of these guidelines in determining the most desirable objectives for a given clinical nursing program provides the teacher with a clearly defined set of criteria for selecting content, planning learning activities, selecting teaching techniques, and evaluating the effectiveness of the learning experiences.

USE OF SURVEY IN SELECTION OF LEARNING EXPERIENCES FOR CLINICAL NURSING

The establishment of meaningful, measurable objectives for a teaching program in clinical nursing leads to the selection and organization of those kinds of experiences needed for the attainment of the desired behavioral changes. The survey to determine the availability of appropriate resources has long been utilized by educators in the initial planning for all levels of curriculum development. Periodic reevaluation of facilities are equally important in determining the availability of the kinds of facilities needed to produce curriculum changes that best meet the changing needs of students and society. (If a faculty is actively engaged in the practice of professional nursing, and acting on the professional responsibility for community involvement, it will remain abreast of changes in available facilities, and less often need to resort to research-model surveys.)

In nursing education, surveys have been used to identify students' needs, goals, characteristics, motivation for entering nursing, family relationships, social relationships, and educational background; descriptions of facilities in which nursing care is given; kind and amount of supplies and equipment used in providing nursing care; administrative and organizational patterns for the provision of patient care; data describing health care needs of the community and community services available to meet these health care needs; and availability of resource consultants from related community health and welfare agencies. The question of who should conduct the survey to determine the kinds of desirable clinical facilities available must be resolved by the given faculty. There is also a growing trend toward engaging consultants to collect information and to make recommendations according to their findings. This kind of approach can be attempted by a relatively short but intensive consultation visit by an expert or team of experts who study the particular problem and make recommendations regarding the findings or by the development of a long-range experimental research design to pursue a descriptive survey of facilities in terms of meeting both broad and specific needs. For example, the use of an experimental design for the assessment of quality of patient care could, when properly validated, provide reliable criteria for assessing clinical facilities in a given situation.

Survey data collected by direct observation, interviews, questionnaires, and critical incidence can be interpreted by comparing them with reliable criteria determined by other surveys, established professional standards, and standards recommended by the investigating institution. The resultant analysis of these data should reveal a descriptive list of existing background information regarding the learners, the educational setting, the clinical facilities, and the community resources. These data then serve as a ready source of information in the selection and organization of those learning experiences needed to meet the desired objectives for clinical nursing.

Information about students

Information gained about the students in a given school of nursing provides the teachers with a wealth of knowledge about existing backgrounds of the students for purposes of comparison with the desired behavioral changes defined by the course objectives. Such information about the student's background assists the teacher in planning clin-

ical learning experiences that reinforce and build on previous clinical experiences and allow for recognition and growth of the individual's potential creative abilities. For example, knowledge about the student's pattern of interpersonal relationships, when used constructively, can greatly enhance the establishment of mutually acceptable teacher-student relationships in determining meaningful, relevant clinical nursing experiences.

Information about clinical facilities and educational unit

To make the best use of a variety of available facilities, each teacher must assume responsibility for continual review to select desirable learning experiences in clinical nursing. With the growing number of students enrolling in collegiate schools of nursing, it is entirely possible that a number of hospitals and community health centers having related facilities may need to be utilized to meet common goals for clinical nursing experiences. The geographic location of facilities must be considered so that a reasonable travel time to desirable facilities can be provided without seriously interfering with time allotted for clinical nursing experience.

Of particular concern to the clinical teacher is information that reveals the kind of educational environment provided in the clinical setting. Therefore study items should include the following: administrative philosophy regarding measures for providing continuous quality patient care, inservice programs to upgrade professional nurses, provision of an environment reflecting acceptance of students as assets, number and kinds of physical facilities, kinds and numbers of patients available, number and kinds of other students using the same patient-care facilities, degree of freedom and responsibility involved in planning for the use of facilities by various levels of students, and provision for legal responsibilities of students assigned to a given institution. Information about the educational unit is needed to clarify for the teacher such items as the educational philosophy, administrative control and regulation of policies, and budgetary policies affecting the kinds and amount of needed equipment. The clinical teacher must have a well-grounded understanding of the relationships between the administrative officers of the educational unit and those in the participating hospitals or agencies in order to select and organize clinical nursing experiences that can be implemented to satisfactorily meet the objectives.

Information about the community

The survey of the community provides the teacher of clinical nursing with two distinct kinds of data: (1) data about prevailing population factors, socioeconomic problems, and patterns of health within the community and (2) information about existing health, education, and welfare agencies regarding the services offered to the public, the kinds of facilities that could be utilized for clinical nursing experiences, and the availability of specialized consultants as resource persons.

A sample of a categorical list that can be used as a guide in making a survey to assist in the provision of clinical nursing experiences needed to meet the objectives of the clinical nursing program is shown in the following outline.

Guide for survey of resources to be used in selection of learning experiences for clinical nursing

I. Survey of students
  A. General information
    1. Number of students in the school
    2. Number of students in each class
    3. Number of students in particular courses
    4. Age, sex, and background of students
  B. Selection of career and school of nursing
    1. Reason for choosing nursing as a career
    2. Source of information regarding the school of choice
    3. Reason for selecting the particular school and particular type of school
    4. Previous experience in other schools of nursing
    5. Expectations from the school
    6. Future plans in nursing
    7. Familiarity with the geographic location of the school
  C. Home background and family relationships
    1. Parents (living or dead): religion, education, occupations, nationality, and birthplace
    2. Siblings
    3. Location of home before entering school of nursing; type and size of community
    4. Health history of family and student
    5. Attitude of parents and/or spouse toward student's educational adventure
    6. Family-student relationships and responsibilities
  D. Education and experience
    1. High school size and location; scholastic ratings; curriculum
    2. Other schools or courses attended
    3. Type of occupation before admission to the school of nursing
    4. Scholastic and professional rating in the school of nursing
    5. Courses in school of nursing completed prior to current courses
    6. Clinical experience prior to current clinical course
    7. Student evaluation of self; successes and failures
    8. Participation in extracurricular activities; extent and kinds of activities
    9. Relationships between scholastic achievement, health, work, and home responsibilities
II. Survey of the educational unit
  A. History of the school of nursing
    1. Historical development
    2. Contributions of the school and its graduates to nursing and to the community
    3. Community attitude toward the school
    4. Recent developments of the school
    5. Accreditation status
    6. Current enrolment of students; number and kinds of other students assigned to the school
  B. Organization and administration of the school of nursing
    1. Administrative control
    2. Philosophy, aims, and objectives of the school
    3. Unity of organization, lines of administration, and responsibilities delegated in terms of functions
    4. Faculty organization and activities
    5. Record system
    6. Amount and kind of educational research being done
  C. Finance
    1. Sources of finance
    2. Administration of the budget

D. Facilities
1. Classrooms: number, adequacy, equipment, arrangement, upkeep, and location relative to clinical areas
2. Laboratories: number, kinds, adequacy, equipment, arrangement, and upkeep
3. Library: extent, organization, maintenance, equipment, and materials
4. School health program
5. Equipment and supplies: maintenance, method of obtaining, and method of selection
6. Living conditions
7. Guidance services available

E. Personnel
1. Number of personnel; student-personnel ratio; frequency of change
2. Qualifications; education; experience; personal qualities
3. Morale of faculty
4. Practice, research, and continuing education activities

F. Curriculum
1. Committee or persons responsible for overall planning of curriculum
2. Extent of participation by faculty members
3. Philosophy and aims of school curriculum
4. Plan for clinical assignments
5. Affiliations with other schools or agencies
6. Review of standards
   a. Nursing school standards related to the curriculum
   b. Admission standards
   c. Graduation standards
7. Number of hours of instruction and distribution
8. Determination of course content
9. Placement of courses in relation to established curricular pattern
10. Courses of study
    a. Content; determination of points and extent of overlapping with other subjects; needed emphasis
    b. Distribution of hours
    c. Teaching personnel

III. Survey of clinical facilities (primary care facilities, hospitals, extended care facilities)
A. Kinds of patients
1. Sex and age
2. Stage and length of health problems
3. Nursing diagnoses presented by patients
4. Range of socioeconomic-cultural background

B. Physical facilities
1. Arrangement of units
2. Availability of supporting departmental services
3. Quality of nursing and health care given to patients
4. Degree of continuity of hospital-home care
5. Method of patient care assignment; use of nursing care plans
6. Instructional facilities
   a. Conference rooms adjacent to patient service area
   b. Office space provided for clinical teachers in patient service area
   c. Closed circuit television systems available for teaching students
   d. Interdisciplinary teaching activites available to nursing students
   e. Library facilities in patient service area
7. Record system

C. Administrative aspects
1. Administrative control
2. Lines of communications and delegation of responsibilities
3. Relationships between supervisors, head nurses, and staff and reciprocal relationships between agency personnel and school of nursing personnel
4. Accreditation status of the hospital or agency
5. Philosophy of the hospital or agency regarding patient care
6. Philosophy regarding interdisciplinary team approach to patient care
7. Amount and kind of clinical research being done
8. Degree of influence exerted by various professions in policies
9. Number and levels of professional and nonprofessional personnel assigned to each unit
10. Degree to which unit personnel adhere to hospital and school policies

D. Human resources
1. Availability of experts in specialized fields for use as consultants
2. Availability of personnel who could serve as resource persons by virtue of their particular health problem
3. Availability of voluntary members of community health and welfare agencies who could serve as resource consultants
4. Availability of other faculty members who could make a contribution to the particular clinical program

IV. Survey of the community
A. Distribution of population by age, race, sex, and cultural background

B. Political structure of community
  1. Governmental organization
  2. Political party affiliations
  3. Power and pressure groups
  4. Community goals and problems
C. Major industries contributing to the economy and welfare of the community
D. Trends in the health picture
  1. Birthrate
  2. Major causes of death
  3. Mortality and death rates
  4. Major causes of disability and disability rate
  5. Distribution and frequency of major health problems in terms of age, sex, economic, and social factors
  6. Number and types of health facilities available
  7. Kinds of regional health centers available
  8. Services offered by the state health department and local health departments
  9. Types of voluntary health and welfare organizations available and services offered
  10. Clubs, service groups, and others interested in health and welfare
  11. Available professional personnel
E. Social and welfare agencies
  1. Types
  2. Services offered and how they are available
  3. Personnel available for use as resource persons and consultants
  4. Literature available to promote health and social welfare
  5. Governmental agencies providing socioeconomic welfare
F. Educational facilities
  1. Colleges and universities; junior colleges
  2. Vocational schools or programs
  3. Adult education programs
  4. Elementary and secondary schools
  5. Day nurseries and other day care facilities
  6. Governmental agency educational programs
  7. Church-supported educational programs

Data revealed by such a survey can provide valuable information for use in the selection of those clinical nursing experiences that clearly relate to the desired objectives. The extent to which the information is used effectively is dependent in part on the teacher's ability to provide a total learning environment that fosters freedom for self-expression and creative activity. Tyler's principles for planning learning experiences include ten conditions necessary for effective learning.[2] These conditions suggest that the teacher's responsibility lies in the setting of conditions that allow the learner to practice the behavior implied by the objectives through the process of self-actualization. Given the guidance needed to learn a new skill, sufficient materials with which to work, time to refine the skill, and opportunities for sequential application of the newly learned skill and immediate knowledge of progress, the learner should be motivated to become involved in trying new ways of learning, setting standards that require greater performance levels than previously attained and beyond those set by the teacher, and ultimately should derive satisfaction from the particular learning experience.

ORGANIZATION OF LEARNING EXPERIENCES FOR CLINICAL NURSING

Selection of appropriate experiences requires the judicious organization of clinical learning experiences in order to establish relationships with other activities that will produce a combined cumulative effect in attaining the objectives of the total clinical nursing program. Complexities in the curriculum pattern for a school of nursing validate the need for using several approaches to the organization of learning experiences. Approaches would vary according to basic beliefs of a given faculty and to the kind of objectives being sought for a given clinical nursing course in a particular area at a given time.

Curriculum experts have substantiated the effects of organizing learning experiences to produce the desired elements of vertical and horizontal relationships for establishing a pattern of learning experiences. Traditionally, the criteria generally accepted as guides for the effective organization of learning experiences are *continuity, sequence,* and *integration;* however this pattern is beginning to undergo alterations as we move into more flexible and creative approaches to teaching.

Continuity is the organization of learning experiences providing for a vertical relationship between different levels of the same subject matter or skills. It provides sustained and recurrent opportunities for skills to be practiced or concepts and skills to be developed from small beginning ideas into major meaningful concepts and abilities.

Sequence is the organization of learning experiences providing for progressive development of knowledge and skills. It provides opportunities for building a relationship between previous learning experiences and each successive learning experience on a higher level of understanding, with a broader and deeper extension of the application of knowledge and skills.

Integration is the organization of learning experiences providing for horizontal relationships between various elements in the total curriculum. This kind of organization provides opportunities for students to analyze various aspects of the total experience until they become a meaningful whole, resulting in unified behavior in dealing with various elements of the learning situation.

Application of criteria to organization of clinical nursing experience

Determination of the individual student's level of understanding and ability to achieve the desired behavioral outcomes furnishes the clinical teacher with guidelines on which to build the progression of learning experiences. To show how the clinical teacher meets the criteria for organizing selected learning experiences in a given clinical nursing situation, a sample objective has been developed in terms of organizing clinical experiences meeting the criteria of *continuity*, *sequence*, and *integration*. The objective considered is: to interpret by use of developmental theory behavior patterns of patients having long-term illnesses.

Continuity and *sequence* are provided as the teacher assists students to observe patients for behaviors and to determine the commonalities of behaviors in reactions of patients toward specific experiences. Some of these experiences might be terminal diagnosis, admission to the hospital, referral to a clinic, acute illness, pain, separation from family, dietary restrictions or requirements, kind of therapy prescribed, socioeconomic effects of illness, and cultural and religious beliefs and their effects on illness. These behavioral reactions should be observed repeatedly in varying combinations. In the beginning the teacher assists the student in recognizing these behavioral responses; but as they begin to take on meaning, the student is able to apply earlier observations of a singular nature to those of a more intricate and complex nature. Early experiences would attempt to provide readily observable, simple behavioral patterns of patients. As the student progresses to more complex learning situations, the combination of new and previously learned behavioral patterns takes on new meaning. For example, it would seem relatively simple to recognize the behavior associated with daily treatment of a chronically ill patient. But nursing experiences in the complete care of this patient involve multiple problems that must be considered in studying the patient's responses. Each experience in the nursing care of the chronically ill patient in the various clinical areas builds on the previous learning and leads to higher and broadened levels of learning.

Integration is planned by providing opportunities for students to integrate various learning experiences into an understanding of the total care situation. As the behavioral problems of the patient are observed and identified, the student needs the opportunity to apply previously learned principles from psychology, sociology, philosophy, anthropology, literature, history, biological and physical sciences, and other professional courses in seeking understanding of the behavior. As the student learns to use the concepts and principles learned in courses to explain the observed behaviors of patients, integrated learning takes place. This integration grows to more sophisticated levels as the student continues to use previously learned theoretical and clinical knowledge in new relationships that serve as useful tools in implementing solutions to nursing care problems.

For students to *experience* growth in the reorganization and unification of previous learning experiences in light of new perspectives, the creative clinical teacher plays a crucial role in planning and selecting appropriate experiences. Effectively planned clinical nursing programs are built on the philosophy and objectives of the total nursing program, are operationally defined in terms of specific expected behavioral outcomes, are planned in accord with changing needs of students and society, make efficient use of available facilities and allow students to assume responsibility for learning how to examine issues critically as a basis for developing judgments in problem-solving situations.

Such carefully laid plans as described in this chapter may eventually fall short of their mark because we cannot currently identify the kinds of clinical nursing skills that will be needed during the next decade. Unless clinical teachers are willing to face the challenges of the unfamiliar, creative planning will perish. Every teacher in clinical nursing is charged with the responsibility of providing experiences that develop skills in learning how to find information, how to utilize opportunities to learn, how to assume responsibility for self-learning, how to solve problems, and how to apply learned knowledge and skills to new situations.

The startling realization that we can no longer teach *everything* (if in fact we ever could) to equip students to practice in a society that is in truth unknown to us has led to an unprecedented increase in curriculum study by schools of nursing. The resultant experimentation in planning clinical nursing experiences is opening new avenues of teaching, calling for teachers with vision and courage to use creative approaches to the planning and organization of clinical nursing experiences that allow students to integrate them into meaningful relationships.

REFERENCES

1. Tyler, Ralph W.: Basic principles of curriculum and instruction, Chicago, 1950, University of Chicago Press.
2. Tyler, Ralph W.: New dimensions in curriculum development, Phi Delta Kappan **68:** 25-28, Sept., 1966.
3. Brodt, Dagmar E.: Education today for nursing service tomorrow, Journal of Nursing Education **5:**7-13, Jan., 1966.
4. Auxiliary personnel in nursing service, American Journal of Nursing **62:**72, July, 1962.
5. Frank, Edwina D.: Teaching without learning? Nursing Forum **9**(2):131-145, 1970.
6. Bloom, Benjamin, editor: Taxonomy of educational objectives. Handbook I. Cognitive domain, New York, 1956, David McKay Co., Inc.
7. Bloom, Benjamin, and others: Taxonomy of educational objectives. Handbook II. Affective domain, New York, 1964, David McKay Co., Inc.

SUGGESTED READINGS

Brunclik, Helen, and others: The empathy inventory, Nursing Outlook **15:**42-42, June, 1967.
deTornay, Rheba: Strategies for teaching nursing, New York, 1971, John Wiley & Sons, Inc.
Gagné, Robert M.: The conditions of learning, New York, 1965, Holt, Rinehart and Winston, Inc.
Geissler, E. M.: Matching course objectives to course content, Nursing Outlook **22:**579-582, Sept., 1974.
Hayter, Jean: Guidelines for selecting learning experiences, Nursing Outlook **15:**63-65, Dec., 1967.
Henderson, Virginia: The nature of nursing, New York, 1966, Macmillan, Inc.
Kramer, M.: The concept of modelling as a teaching strategy, Nursing Forum **11**(1):48-70, 1972.
Kramer, M., and others: Self actualization and role adaptation of baccalaureate degree nurses, Nursing Research **21:**111-123, March/April, 1972.
Langhoff, H. F.: Instructional development in nursing, Audiovisual Guide, **51:**9-12, Oct., 1972.
Little, D., and others: Complexities of teaching in the clinical laboratory, Journal of Nursing Education **11:**15-22, Jan., 1972.
Mager, Robert F.: Preparing objectives for programmed instruction, Belmont, Calif., 1962, Fearon Publishers.
McAttee, Patricia: The human side of curriculum development, Nursing Forum **8**(2):144-150, 1969.
Rauen, K., and others: The teaching contract, Nursing Outlook **20:**594-596, Sept., 1972.

Rogers, Carl R.: Freedom to learn, Columbus, Ohio, 1969, Charles E. Merrill Publishing Co.

Rosenauer, J. A., and others: Teaching strategies for interdisciplinary education, Nursing Outlook **21**:159-162, March, 1973.

Skinner, B. F.: Beyond freedom and dignity, New York, 1971, Alfred A. Knopf, Inc.

Werley, H. H.: Research in nursing as input to educational programs, Journal of Nursing Education **11**:29-38, Nov., 1972.

Whitehead, Alfred N.: The aims of education, New York, 1963, Macmillan, Inc.

Wilson, Christopher: The effect of cloisterization on students of nursing, American Journal of Nursing **70**:1726-1729, Aug., 1970.

7 Creativity in planning and providing patient-centered clinical nursing experiences

The teacher of clinical nursing is constantly faced with finding ways of planning and providing patient-centered clinical nursing experiences for students. While the basic purpose of this book is to show how the teacher functions creatively in clinical nursing as an integral part of the total program of the school of nursing, the tasks related to the teaching of patient-centered clinical nursing are isolated for purposes of discussion. Clinical nursing experiences are examined in terms of the broad concept of skill learning in its relationship to any clinical nursing setting. The teacher who seeks ways of using creative approaches to the teaching of patient-centered clinical nursing must employ the concepts of (1) cooperative student-teaching planning and selection of clinical learning experiences, (2) planning clinical nursing experiences in accord with individual student's levels of ability and expressed needs, and (3) fostering student self-actualization in providing patient-centered nursing care. Many of the ideas discussed do not answer questions; rather, they pose questions that, hopefully, will stimulate thinking about past and present practices in terms of discovering new ways of providing patient-centered clinical nursing experiences clearly relating to individual learning needs of students.

SKILL LEARNING NEEDED FOR PATIENT-CENTERED CLINICAL NURSING EXPERIENCES

A skill is a learned response to a given situation, which will be used depending on judgments regarding sequence of actions, and appropriate adaptations depending on a wide range of variables. Although skills are primarily considered psychomotor, the practice of nursing involves a number of interactive, psychosocial skills as well.

CREATIVITY IN PLANNING PATIENT-CENTERED CLINICAL NURSING EXPERIENCES

Patient-centered learning activities involve the use and development of skills as a complex act that is an integral part of a whole. Creative teaching in clinical nursing demands that we first consider the kind of nursing practitioner we want to prepare rather than the tasks the nursing practitioner must be able to perform. What is needed is a clinical teaching approach that promotes inquiry and acquisition of knowledge on the universality and temporality of human beings; this knowledge can be used in assisting learners to perform motor responses that are performed as a unified act while coping with change, encounter, and involvement.

Skill learning should take place in a context that includes consideration of factors selected from universal experience, which influence one's efforts to cope with health and illness. Such an approach assists the learner in understanding the total situation and the relationships between principles and their application to individual patients.

Learners need opportunities to explore and experiment, to ask questions, to study diagrams, and to observe skilled performances by others before applying any skills in a direct patient care situation. There should follow various opportunities for students to develop given skills in a variety of settings utilizing a wide range of patient care experiences. It must be remembered that ability to perform skills varies from person to person, from time to time with the same person, and from situation to situation. Thus, the degree to which a particular skill is developed is related to the individual's ability to move through the process of gradual refinement into a unified, wholistic approach to patient care.

Currently the development of skills related to patient-centered clinical nursing is the subject of much discussion in many schools of nursing. Chapter 8 further describes a variety of means that could be used by the creative teacher in these situations.

KINDS OF SKILL LEARNING NEEDED FOR PATIENT-CENTERED CLINICAL NURSING EXPERIENCES

Regardless of how one proceeds to differentiate kinds of learning needed in a given situation, the processes of learning should be organized to produce a unified whole. In setting objectives for learning in patient-centered situations, it is clear that various kinds of needed skills form a pattern of interrelationships. While the following discussion is largely concerned with a wide variety of skill learning, inherent in every clinical situation is opportunity for the learning of new knowledge and attitudes and their application to the learning of skills. To illustrate the kinds of skill learning needed, the following skills have been arbitrarily separated for discussion purposes.

Skills in the application of concepts and scientific principles to clinical nursing situations

The total process of learning involves the acquisition of knowledge, enabling one to form concepts, see relationships, and derive generalizations as a basis for taking action in a given situation. The teaching of nursing involves the use of intellectual skills in the identification of scientific principles and concepts plus judgment in determining how they apply to any given patient care situation. Thus, it becomes a matter of providing a framework of knowledge from the various physical, biological, and social sciences and from the nursing theory on which to build

quality nursing care practices through direct patient care experiences. Development of skill in the utilization of this background information is an essential ingredient for the learning of clinical nursing. However, it would be unrealistic to assume that students automatically remember to apply concepts and principles in the given clinical situation. The clinical teacher should provide a role model for the use of concepts related to such aspects of patient care as for example, behavioral patterns indicating physiological, psychological, or sociological stress and resultant effects on the patient's state of health or equilibrium. With the instructor, students can utilize this information for making judgments regarding the assessment of patient's needs and for creative decision-making relative to setting priorities for nursing care goals and evaluating outcomes of the plan of action. As a role model, the instructor not only shares conclusions but should discuss the intellectual process utilized. In subsequent interactions students will more readily utilize the theory to reach decisions and also begin to master the process.

Observation skills

While the clinical nursing setting provides unlimited opportunities for observation, this does not automatically assure one's ability to become skilled in making selective observations. Development of this skill is indispensable to the determination of appropriate nursing actions in providing expert patient care. To make meaningful observations requires the use of all one's sensory perceptions—sight, hearing, touch, taste, and smell—and the discovery of what each conveys in providing a total picture of significant characteristics from which to make judgments leading to nursing action. Selective perception is developed as a skill through practice in analyzing that which each sensory experience conveys, in looking for patterns of relationships, and in focusing attention on the details until they reveal significant data related to the total observations. Observation is subjective, conditioned by one's system of thought patterns. Observations become more skillful as the mind becomes conditioned to a new framework for selective response. Once one has developed skill in observations, the cycle of learning must be completed by understanding the observable phenomena and using the information to provide skilled nursing care. In the process of developing skill in observation one must guard against being more concerned about accomplishing one's personal goals than in seeking ways of helping the patient to learn about himself. When the goals of observation are related to collection of data regarding the physiological, psychological, or sociological nature of the patient, the nurse will learn a great deal of valuable information. The next step is learning how best to use the information in a way that will help the patient to help himself. When the goal relates to performing a specific nursing care task, the task itself can overshadow the nurse's ability to observe the patient's verbal or nonverbal responses. Through the use of the various senses one learns to observe the patient's facial expressions, body movements, and posture, to hear how a patient speaks—his tone of voice, choice of words, relevance of subject—and to become aware of inconsistencies between verbal and nonverbal communications.

Historically, nurses have made observation from a distance, leaving the closer observations of palpation, percussion, and auscultation to the physician. Changing role perceptions and care-giving practices of the last decade have led to marked changes. Many undergraduate nursing students now begin developing skills in use of hands, eyes, ears, stethoscope, oto-opthalmoscope, and other tools to discover more precisely a patient's state of health or illness. Only time will tell if those additional skills are truly useful in gathering sufficient data to make nursing diagnoses and monitor the progress of interventions, or if they merely allow nurses to poorly mimic physicians without functioning as professionals themselves.

Inherent in the development of these observation skills is the ability to develop selective perception, interpret, and make judgments leading to positive action involving the following aspects of clinical nursing: physiological manifestations of health and illnesses and related conditions of patients; behavioral patterns displayed by patients; patterns of interpersonal relationships that have effects on the problems of the patient or the ability of the nurse to function; and changes in patient behavior patterns, progress, or interpersonal relationships.

Interpersonal relationship skills

In nursing practice the development of interpersonal relationships becomes an extension of one's ability to make meaningful observations; the ensuing interaction is the product of the nurse's interpretation of the observable patient behavior. The degree to which the nurse may or may not interpret the observations in accord with the patient's point of view necessitates efforts to develop mutually satisfying nurse-patient relationships. Every contact students have with patients and their families, various members of the nursing team, the total health team, and school of nursing personnel responsible for clinical nursing teaching programs will be improved by working knowledge of interpersonal relationships.

The development of interpersonal relationship skills as an integral component of the total learning skills needed for participation in direct patient care involves (1) understanding one's own feelings, abilities, limitations, and degree of self-acceptance regarding these factors; (2) developing one's own potentials through multiple processes; (3) understanding behaviors of patients and families and acknowledging their assets in helping them reach their greatest potential through their own process of self-actualization; (4) establishing a therapeutic environment for nurse-patient interaction; (5) establishing effective liaison relationships among the patient's family, the patient, the physician, and others contributing to his welfare as a patient and an individual; and (6) establishing effective interpersonal relationships with nursing personnel and other health team members. Each clinical nursing experience is unique, but inherent in each situation is a need for a combination of all available interpersonal skills.

Skill in making judgments

Levine reminds us that service in medicine and nursing is built on the concept of the capacity of the human being to respond in particular ways to the usual variations of the environment and to those unusual situations activating the defense potential. Many of these responses are common to many people, yet one must also look for the unique way in which each individual activates his own defense mechanisms.[1]

Nurses are increasingly aware that the initial judgment of a nurse after evaluating a person presenting himself for care is a diagnosis. While in many instances the nurse may provide care based on the medical diagnosis, the principal reason for the professional nurse remaining involved in a treatment situation should be to treat diagnosed health problems that fall within the realm of nursing.[2] Having made a nursing diagnosis, one then makes judgments regarding the specific interventions to be attempted and the variations in response that can be expected.

Judgments leading to decisions regarding nursing intervention are based on one's observations of the individual patient's behavior and relevant data measured against scientific principles describing requirements of all patients.

The development of skill in making judgments based on scientific clinical knowledge involves (1) recognizing signs and symptoms of altered health states; (2) analyzing these states to arrive at a nursing diagnosis; (3) developing and implementing appropriate nursing action; (4) assessing effectiveness of the care, making necessary adjustments to meet the changing needs of patients or changes in judgments concerning the nursing care problems; (5) interpreting and reporting observations and judgments with accuracy; (6) coordinating services of team members as needed to assist patients through various stages of illness; and (7) teaching patients information in accord with their changing daily needs and ability to assimilate information.

Motor skills

Regardless of the approaches taken to provide a curriculum built on the concepts of patient-centered nursing care (such as that advanced by Abdellah and associates[3]), one cannot deny that certain motor skills must be developed by students in order to provide safe, therapeutic nursing care measures for patients. Direct patient care experiences provide opportunities for students to develop various motor skills, but there is a crucial need for teachers of clinical nursing to view the development of these motor skills in their proper perspective. That is, the clinical nursing program must provide for prerequisite understanding of a wide range of scientific principles in a three-dimensional application: (1) to the development of specific motor skills, (2) to the understanding of electronic or mechanical devices and the interpretation of their results, and (3) to the modification of motor skills in order to meet the needs of the patient in a given situation. Students having the opportunities to develop motor skills based on understanding of how various scientific principles apply to the given situation readily adopt a concept of patient-centered goals of nursing practice as opposed to task-centered goals.

PROVIDING CLINICAL EXPERIENCES TO MEET VARIOUS LEVELS OF ACHIEVEMENT

Educational literature over the last decade abounds with the indictments of elementary and secondary education for wasting the vast reservoir of students with high potential for intellectual and creative achievements. Professional schools in higher education become both the recipients of these students and the perpetuators of some of the same practices of ineffective utilization of students' intellectual abilities and creative talents. What do we do in schools of nursing to provide learning experiences commensurate with individual levels of abilities when we continue to have students who "go through" a program without making an identifiable contribution, without challenge, without individual attention, and often with unresolved negative feelings regarding their learning experience? There is, in truth, an enormous reservoir of the population who have a high potential for intellectual and creative achievement, whom we ignore for mere inability to find suitable ways of identifying them. To face this educational dilemma realistically we must consider students of all levels of achievement and ability. Having joined forces with other social and educational institutions in the fight to maintain and promote an improved society, we must find ways of helping a wide range of students without lowering our standards of achievement. To offer graduates from our schools of nursing to society we have a responsibility for ensuring a level of achievement that we can be sure is not only minimally safe but adequate to contribute to meeting the health needs of society. It is unrealistic to expect that we will ever find a single measure of determining individual potential for achievement; therefore it is incumbent on each school of nursing to give careful consideration to ways of determining valid criteria to use in measuring levels of achievement according to the individual student's potential ability for growth and the desired outcomes of each experience.

The idea of identifying levels of ability from cognitive functioning to abilities to apply knowledge and to develop skills considered necessary is not new, but it remains largely unapplied for want of integrated, comparable measurements of implementation. As a result, even in those schools recognizing the need to identify and deal with individual learning problems of students, progress seems to halt as faculty members raise questions regarding implementation of changes. The following

very real issues are often expressed: How does one identify differences in backgrounds that students bring with them to the clinical nursing setting? How do we know where to set minimum and maximum limits of performance? How much practice or experience in the learning of a given skill is enough? How can we identify those students having varying levels of ability in order to provide them with the kind of help they most need? What do we do with students who appear to be overachievers? How do we know when to advance a student to new learning? What happens to students when they are grouped according to abilities? How do we establish standards for placing students in ability groupings? How do we determine standardized grading systems for students if we establish a plan of allowing them to proceed at their own rate of learning? How do we build in flexible scheduling of classes and clinical nursing experiences to allow for individualized study?

These are only a few of the unanswered questions that have posed barriers to teachers of clinical nursing who have considered the need for providing more meaningful learning experiences for students of differing abilities. There are schools of nursing in which faculty members have proceeded to work out a program to accomplish these tasks and answer many of these questions. Some schools have attempted to reorganize the total curriculum pattern to meet these needs. Others have selected one area as a pilot study from which to develop a sound approach. Still other schools have utilized the honors program existing with the university to provide students with opportunities to advance at their own rate in the nonnursing areas and have developed their own nursing honors program. The state of flux apparent in this vital area of learning prompts the following general suggestions. These approaches do not constitute an absolute and do not purport to answer the issues raised; they are offered because there is a need for creative clinical teachers to devise ways of developing nursing programs based on these concepts and with the hope that they will give careful consideration to the total problem and undertake projects that will contribute to the development of clinical nursing programs designed to allow each student to reach maximal potential.

General approach to development of clinical nursing programs designed to meet individual levels of ability

The practice of presenting clinical nursing experiences and related nursing theory as an integrated whole necessitates the provision of both creative clinical nursing experiences and well-presented nursing theory. The creative teacher of clinical nursing is concerned with developing a total program of clinical nursing aimed at providing the level of content, speed of learning, and methodology commensurate with the individual learning needs of students. Such a program requires three essential elements: (1) teachers who devise objective ways of diagnosing and measuring individual student learning needs and abilities as the student assumes responsibility for mastery of the various kinds of clinical nursing skills, (2) students who assume responsibility for their learning in order to move toward their particular needs and interests, and (3) a modification of the traditional clinical teacher's role in helping students direct their own learning activities as a cooperative venture. Such an approach requires (1) continual diagnosis of learning progress; (2) initiation of avenues of learning to be pursued; (3) coordination of the overall pattern of activities of learning; (4) consultation, individually and in groups, with students as needed; and (5) allowing students to proceed at their own rate, assuming responsibility for seeking advice or approval regarding achievement of a given task. This kind of approach may be used, but does not necessitate the grouping of students, not in terms of academic ability but in terms of particular kinds of experiences to meet students' needs at a given time.

At first glance it would appear that these three elements could provide a reasonable approach to the establishment of clinical learning experiences designed to meet individual levels of ability. However, each element carries its built-in barriers to the effective establishment of such a program; it is these barriers with which one must deal in order to break the lockstep of rigidly set patterns of clinical nursing experiences for students. The most obvious barriers to be overcome are those of helping the teacher recognize the need for objective criteria for measuring individual achievement rather than relying on intuitive judgments regarding individual student progress; recognizing that students are not only willing but also capable of assuming responsibility for their own learning; helping students recognize and accept the teacher's sincerity of purpose in allowing them to pursue learning experiences in accord with their needs and abilities, accepting concepts of flexible scheduling, and applying the newly developed teaching innovations to clinical nursing skills in order to provide for individualized learning opportunities that will not jeopardize the patient's safety.

One approach to the development of a clinical nursing program designed to meet individual levels of abilities of students would be following the process of curriculum building as described in Chapter 6. As previously stated, the objectives must be in harmony as each phase of the curriculum is designed in order to allow the desired outcomes for the students. A review of the previously stated guidelines for establishing objectives for clinical nursing programs serves as the basis of discussion in establishing measurable behavioral changes as the criteria for determining individual attainment of desired levels of skill development in clinical nursing.

A first condition for the development of clinical nursing programs is that of determining measurable competencies for each level of progression to be met by each objective for the total learning experience.

This implies that within the total time period in a given clinical nursing area these specific levels of competencies should be met in order to accomplish the total objectives. It further implies that each student is provided with a framework of total time allotted for learning specific kinds of skills but that the rate at which these are pursued and learned depends on the individual student.

A second condition necessary for planning this kind of clinical learning experience is that of knowing about the student's background of knowledge, experience, interests, attitudes, and previous behavioral patterns regarding his approach to learning. This means more than ascertaining the student's scores made on standardized tests. It means establishing a working knowledge of the achievement already attained by the student, the kinds of activities the student envisions in the present situation as extensions of projects pursued in previous clinical settings, new ideas the student expects to pursue in the current setting, the student's general attitude regarding the kinds of life situations to be dealt with in this particular clinical experience, and current personal and professional problems the student may be facing that could affect his motivational pattern or rate of learning. Some of this information is available from the student's record and could be obtained by interviewing and observing the student. Another means of determining the student's readiness for a given learning situation is that of using comprehensive, validated placement examinations. These should be based on the previously defined specific outcomes prior to assignment to a clinical area to determine readiness for the experience and the strengths and weaknesses to be considered in helping each student progress according to his abilities. This same test could be given either totally or in part, as a means of determining when the student is ready to move on to a new realm of learning. Although patient-centered clinical learning experience may be more difficult to test, we are at a point in time when we can no longer rely on personal judgments to make such decisions. The newer educational technologies have concentrated great effort on various skill developments and their measurement through diverse programming techniques. If we truly expect to bridge the gap between health care needs and the supply of capable, professional nurses, now is the time to look at every possibility to utilize our students' capacities to the fullest extent.

A third condition is that of providing flexible scheduling conditions. If we plan a clinical nursing program in terms of meeting individual students' levels of abilities, we must plan for flexibility conducive to individualized instruction. This approach involves (1) altering the size and type of class situations to allow for small seminar groups, independent study, large assembly classes, individual conferences, or other means best suited to accomplishing the goals in accord with the individual student's needs; (2) altering requirements in terms of time required for mastery as opposed to arbitrarily set time patterns as part of a daily routine; (3) keeping student assignments on the clinical nursing units flexible enough to allow each to accomplish his goals rather than requiring all to be present x number of hours on x days of the week; (4) providing students with freedom to seek needed experiences wherever they are to be found; and (5) providing teachers with opportunities to contribute to various aspects of the learning situation in accord with that which each is best equipped to handle. Flexible scheduling is an approach to the teaching-learning process based on the teacher's professional judgment and the student's responsibility for assuming his own learning, whether he be considered superior, average, or slow, interested, or disinterested. Furthermore, one of its greatest assets in terms of clinical nursing is that it approaches each day's learning activities according to that which presents itself rather than an orderly schedule of time for each activity in a given time limit. Much depends on the particular requirements of each kind of assignment in determining both the size of a particular group to be taught and the time needed for accomplishing the purposes.

Quite apart from making actual time schedules from day to day, the greatest problems lie in interpreting the concept of such a framework to the students, the teachers, and nursing service personnel. Even after the concept of flexible scheduling has been throughly discussed and explained with all levels of personnel and the students themselves, certain barriers may affect the implementation of the program. Teachers and administrators must work constantly to remove these obstacles. For example, the length of time and number of times per week a class or conference is scheduled to meet or the number of times a student is required to perform a particular skill must be decided on the basis of mastery by students rather than by dividing clock hours and calendar days into equal parts for each experience. The excuse that nursing accrediting agencies are unwilling to accept new concepts in accrediting a school is often used as a crutch for those who are unwilling to accept change; often a change needs only a written proposal along with a rationale submitted to the accrediting agency for approval. Educators make up the accrediting agencies and they do seek educational change; if the proposal is well conceived and justified, there should be little problem regarding its approval for use in a school of nursing. Change often means increased cost; however, the plan of flexible scheduling is not necessarily more expensive. It utilizes personnel and facilities in different combinations, often without requiring additional personnel or facilities. Frequently it is difficult for teachers and nursing service personnel to accept change. Close examination of these attitudes, however, usually reveals that these people have been asked to move from a traditional plan to a plan about which they know very little. Before being asked to participate in such a program, they should understand its rationale, know what the outcomes for such a program should be, know why the change is needed, and understand how they personally fit into the plan.

Change in learning behavior takes time and effort on the part of both student and teacher. Students entering a program in which this concept of individualized instruction is being utilized need a thorough orientation to the concepts on which it is based, its purposes, and how the school expects the students to function as a part of the system. Change of this nature may take a great deal of time for students entering from schools with traditional learning backgrounds. Often the students are suspicious regarding the teacher's motives or do not accept responsibility for their own learning. However, students do begin to see its values and to settle into the pattern. Before one hastily evaluates students' responses to such an approach, it is well to remember that not all students contributed satisfactorily to the traditional methods of teaching, either.

For students, personnel, and teachers, the various facets of individualized instruction make up a complex teaching-learning environment beyond the provision of time, small groups, independent study, and adequate learning resources. It means that teachers of clinical nursing must stretch their creative potentials to the greatest extent in helping students become self-directive, purposeful learners, in guiding them to become effective thinkers, and in supervising them in the development of patient-centered clinical nursing skills without wasting time in repetitive, nonproductive tasks. In addition, each teacher must develop criteria for assessing an individual student's ability to function effectively in the patient care situation. This aspect of the problem is discussed more fully in Chapter 9.

Regardless of the kind of flexible schedule teachers of clinical nursing devise, thought must be given to how to provide those experiences needed by individual students in helping them reach their maximum potential. Some suggestions might include the following: (1) providing flexible interchange of students from one clinical area to another as needed from day to day; (2) providing ample opportunity for independent study laboratories designed to promote mastery of skills before or during the actual patient care experiences, the only requirement being that a given level of skill be developed within the total time period for that particular clinical nursing area; (3) providing opportunities for students who have an ability to master skills very quickly either to move on to more complex related activities or to pursue an independent study project that is of particular interest and is designed to contribute additional knowledge and understanding of the given situation but is not required as a part of the objectives of the clinical nursing experience; and (4) allowing the individual student to progress from one clinical area to another on successful completion of the necessary behavioral objectives. This practice creates administrative problems within the total school curriculum and may sacrifice depth and breadth of learning for quantitative learning in shortened time periods. It is a variation of the old practice in elementary education of allowing students to skip a grade, and it carries all the problems of that practice. On the other hand, if students are proficient, are we doing them and society a disservice by not letting them contribute as fully and quickly as possible as professional nurses?

In whatever way a teacher of clinical nursing elects to devise and implement a program in which students are allowed to develop the necessary nursing skills according to their own rate, needs, and abilities, the crucial factors for succeeding with such a program lie in (1) defining the specific outcomes to be achieved at each level of performance for each objective and (2) preparing and utilizing evaluation tools to provide objective means of determining the student's readiness to proceed to new learning experiences.

GUIDELINES FOR PLANNING AND SELECTING CLINICAL LEARNING EXPERIENCES

Because the process of planning and selecting clinical learning experiences in accord with the philosophy and objectives of a clinical course is a many-faceted task, the following problems deserve careful consideration: Finding sufficient learning experiences for the increased number of students, limited faculty time, changing patterns of health care and health needs of patients, limitations of time for functioning in the clinical nursing situations, diverse patterns of integrated clinical nursing courses, and increasing frequency with which students are expressing their desires to participate in the selection of their clinical nursing experiences. The selection of clinical nursing experiences should be based on a concept of the total learning process, leading to integrated learning of knowledge and skills in accord with the individual student's ability. To help the clinical teacher in planning and selecting clinical nursing learning experiences designed to accomplish the desired behavioral outcomes, the following guidelines are suggested.

Providing essential learning experiences for all students. The teacher of clinical nursing who has developed a carefully determined set of objectives indicating desired competencies for a given clinical area is well equipped to proceed with the total process of planning, selecting, implementing, and evaluating clinical nursing experiences. The carefully planned, specific, desired behavioral outcomes are the determinants of the kinds of learning experiences considered essential for students within a given clinical area. But it is the *way* in which the creative teacher of clinical nursing *uses* the desired specific behavioral outcomes that provides the delicate balance between sterotyped and individualized clinical nursing assignments for students. If, indeed, the teacher of clinical nursing seeks to provide *individualized* essential learning experiences for each student, the following factors must become an integral part of the total plan:

1. The accomplishment of the desired behavioral outcomes should be in terms of the *total time allotment* for the clinical nursing course as opposed to arbitrarily set time limits as the measure of attainment to be met equally by all students.
2. Students should have opportunities to practice and participate in the kinds of clinical learning experiences defined by the objectives.
3. Students must be allowed to advance at their own rate and level of attainment of the desired skills by moving on to new learning according to their own readiness, ultimately meeting the desired goals.
4. The desired skills can be met in several ways; flexibility allows the teacher to plan various kinds of clinical nursing experiences as they are available, ultimately meeting the same desired behavioral outcomes for all students.

Consideration of principles of learning in meeting students' needs and abilities. The successful development of the various kinds of skills needed in clinical nursing is dependent on the teacher's recognition of the many variables in any given situation that can affect the individual's desire to learn and ability to master the needed skills; clinical nursing assignments must be tailored to meet these needs and abilities of individual students. Clinical experiences must provide meaning for the student according to the particular background of knowledge and skill each brings to the clinical situation. Thus, there is a learning continuum that moves from the simple to the complex and allows for maximal development of individual growth. This concept recognizes each student as an individual in interests, needs, knowledge, abilities, genetic endowment, and sociocultural backgrounds, and respects each as an individual of worth and dignity, regardless of the teacher's expectations and goals. Similarly, motivation patterns underlying clinical performance are highly individualized; students tend to be more highly motivated when they can see a direct relationship between the learning activity and their own learning needs. The creative teacher of clinical nursing must be aware of these variations by considering the underlying factors on an individual basis in planning clinical experiences to meet satisfactorily the range of motivation.

The presence of a wide spectrum of variables producing positive and negative forms of reinforcement has the potential for enhancing or destroying learning. Awareness of the subtle and complex negative and positive responses to students by personnel in the clinical settings helps the clinical teacher identify the kinds of responses that generate the positive reinforcement needed for optimal learning conditions.

There are great variations in the abilities needed to master the skills in clinical nursing. Some skills are readily perfected with a minimum of manipulative ability; many others require simultaneous complex physical manipulation and coordination and use of mental and social processes; still others require only a high degree of use of mental and social processes. Performance leading to the desired mastery of these skills presents wide variations of achievement among individual students within the same range and among different groups considered by age or previous experience. Therefore, the creative teacher of clinical nursing must plan and adapt learning experiences that meet the individual student's mode of learning, allowing each to progress in terms of readiness. The clinical teacher should plan length and amount of practice periods for each student in terms of the ease each experiences in developing competence in the wide range of skills.

Cooperative student-teacher planning and selection of clinical learning experiences. For years eminent educational psychologists have advocated the concept of cooperative student-teacher action to determine the learning goals and the kinds of daily learning experiences needed to accomplish these goals. Many educators, and particularly nursing educators, have ignored this approach to learning by rationalizing that students are not in a position to know what they need in order to meet the course objectives. More often than not the real problem lies in the teacher's inability to use the course objectives as the framework for providing opportunities for students to seek experiences commensurate with their ability. If clinical teachers do, indeed, believe in planning and selecting clinical nursing experiences in accord with students' individual differences of needs, abilities, and goals, cooperative student-teacher planning must become an integral part of the design for teaching. Whatever the program offered by a school of nursing, it does, in fact, exist for the primary purpose of educating the student. The total teaching-learning situation is a cooperative venture, involving student-teacher interaction in the planning, implementation, and evaluation of an educational program that meets the individual learning needs of students while seeking to accomplish the long-term goals set for the curriculum. To plan and select clinical nursing experiences that are at once challenging and commensurate with the individual's level of development, teachers need to build in new experiences and opportunities for applying basic concepts and principles in new and meaningful combinations and to reinforce previously learned experiences. Evidences of experimentation in the direction of cooperative student-teacher planning of clinical experiences along with flexibility in providing desired experiences are in the nursing literature. For those who view this concept with skepticism, the following two basic tenets must be understood:

1. Joint student-teacher planning of clinical nursing experiences implies that the teacher represents a recognized authority in the given clinical nursing area and, as such, assumes responsibility for identifying the desired goals and contributing to the attainment of the total curriculum goals regardless of the methods used to involve the learner.

2. Changes taking place in elementary and secondary education are providing schools of nursing with students who possess a greater degree of maturity of judgment, ability to think, and ability to function effectively in using many of the technological innovations now in many schools of nursing.

Foshay's description of some of these changes provides new perspectives regarding the quality of students entering schools of nursing.[4] The particular way in which cooperative student-teacher planning and selecting of clinical nursing experiences are accomplished depends on the ability of the individual teacher of clinical nursing. However, the following elements should be considered:

1. The degree of student involvement should be commensurate with levels of ability, progressing on a continuum from dependent, short-term goals to independent, long-term goals.

2. Group conferences should be provided to acquaint students with the desired objectives that serve as the framework for the development of their related goals and desired experiences.

3. Individual conferences should be used frequently to determine specific student needs and offer necessary guidance in focusing on meaningful goals and experiences.

4. Terms used by students regarding desired experiences should be clarified, since students tend to use global terms having specific meaning to them but quite different meaning to others; that is, the term *complex nursing care* has distinct meanings for each student as well as the teacher.

5. Students should be helped to understand the value of some repetitive learning experiences in developing needed skills.

6. Students should be helped to recognize the need for and ultimate value in setting long-term goals involving

continuity of experiences as opposed to only short-term goals providing little continuity or sequence of learning experiences.

7. A variety of means should be provided for helping students meet their goals.*

This early involvement of learners in planning and selecting clinical nursing experiences places the focus of learning on them and serves as a motivating force in assuming responsibility for continuously seeking new avenues of inquiry. It exerts long-term effects in helping them to plan nursing care for individual patients and to participate in numerous kinds of planning activities expected of the graduate nurse. The creative teacher of clinical nursing utilizes every opportunity—planned or incidental, formal or informal—to involve students in selecting their learning experiences.

Flexibility in selecting available resources for clinical experience assignments. A necessary adjunct to the implementation of cooperative student-teacher planning of clinical nursing experiences is that of flexibility in the use of available clinical nursing resources to provide needed learning opportunities. The familar practice of confining student experiences to a particular pattern of clinical rotation in various kinds of settings places arbitrary restrictions on students' learning experiences and in no way guarantees that desired experiences are available on the assigned unit. Initiating a clinical nursing program utilizing cooperative student-teacher planning and selection of experiences underlines the need to develop flexible clinical assignments for students, with clinical teachers having the freedom to select experiences according to need rather than by stereotyped design. To bring desired learning experiences into focus with nursing theory courses challenges the creative abilities of clinical teach-

ers. But an educational program providing for flexibility of student clinical assignments enhances the opportunities for successfully meeting the challenge. A report by Schumann describes how the University of Washington School of Nursing provided flexible clinical nursing assignments for students in medical-surgical nursing.[5]

Because many patients have multiple medical and nursing problems, it is easier to recognize that the particular organizational setting is of minor importance as compared to the experiences provided by specific patient situations. Freedom to select clinical nursing experiences from a wide variety of settings within the total community increases the opportunities for providing all students with the desired experience at the time needed. An even greater advantage to the use of the flexible assignment concept is that it enables instructors to plan sequential, meaningful experiences according to individual student needs and ability levels instead of repetitive experiences that can occur in the circumscribed clinical block rotation.

In addition to planning clinical nursing experiences through the use of flexible assignments, cooperative planning with all nursing faculty and nursing service personnel is essential. Flexible scheduling of clinical nursing assignments is dependent on the ability of the clinical nursing faculty members to work cooperatively, with a common bond of understanding and willingness to share available experiences with one another. There is little room for clinical nursing teachers who are either unwilling to seek those learning opportunities needed to meet the individual needs of students or unwilling to share knowledge about available resources with other faculty members.

Another barrier in the use of flexible clinical nursing assignments is that related to maintaining an environment of acceptance by nursing service personnel. While teachers of clinical nursing control the assignments for students, they hold the responsibility for establishing a cooperative

---

*Consider various approaches to learning discussed in Chapter 8.

working relationship with nursing service personnel. In using a flexible scheduling approach to clinical nursing assignments, the clinical teacher must make every effort to include nursing service personnel in the planning by (1) orienting nursing service personnel to the total plan, its purposes, and expected outcomes; (2) planning clinical nursing experiences in a manner that avoids disruption of patient care; (3) seeking assistance from nursing service personnel in determining desirable experiences available; and (4) soliciting information regarding areas of assistance needed by students.

Individualized clinical experiences do not mean that students necessarily can or should change clinical assignments on a daily basis. Great care must be taken to keep students with each patient and setting long enough for gain on the part of both student and others, yet not beyond the time when learning is occurring. Too frequent change in all spheres is a hazard of modern life[6]; we should take care not to add unnecessarily to the stress.

While it may appear that with such flexibility not all of the desired learning experiences will be covered, a single problem situation can be used to bring out a wide range of problems in caring for a patient. Clinical conference discussions frequently serve as the springboard for action in related problem areas as a discussion of one set of problems precipitates interest in another set of problems. This approach embraces the concept of utilizing many ways to meet a given objective. It is obviously unsound to advocate uniform adoption of flexible clinical nursing assignments. What *is* needed is study to determine how this method of student assignment can be utilized to the best advantage and how to overcome the barriers in order to use it in appropriate clinical learning situations.

Maximum utilization of clinical resources. Nursing encompasses a broad spectrum of life situations and health care within the hospital, the patient's home

environment, and various community settings, such as rehabilitation centers, schools, physicians' offices, public health agencies, various voluntary health and social agencies, regional health agencies, and neighborhood health clinics. To prepare the professional nurse to function in such a variety of settings demands that clinical nursing experiences provide opportunities for developing skills in various health care situations. It is incumbent on each teacher to stretch the limits of the nursing experiences to include these different settings as an integral part of the clinical experiences. For too long clinical nursing experiences have been planned on a model of medical, surgical, maternity, pediatric, psychiatric, and public health nursing, each for a given time period. We must broaden the scope of facilities used to include a wide range of settings in which the student can learn to apply the desired knowledge and skills. Nursing educators are, in fact, opening the doors to these widened horizons of learning. Such an approach was needed yesterday, is needed today, and is the foundation for the future in preparing nurses to fulfill their responsibilities as professional practitioners.

Selection of desirable time periods for clinical nursing experiences. Many teachers of clinical nursing are constantly faced with the problem of providing sufficient clinical nursing experiences in a limited setting for increased numbers of students, without a comparable increase in the number of available patients. Some teachers view the traditional 24-hour segments of the days, evenings, and nights as offering vastly different kinds of learning experiences for students; still others believe that students do not learn sufficient new knowledge to warrant the provision of clinical nursing experiences on the evening and night shifts. The basic issue here lies in seeking answers to the following three questions:

1. Can behavioral outcomes be developed for use in assigning students to clinical nursing experiences at var-

ious time periods throughout the 24 hours?

2. Can some of the same behavioral outcomes be satisfactorily achieved throughout the 24-hour time period, or is it necessary to expand the total course objectives to provide for those experiences that differ from one another during given time periods?

3. Can students be provided with appropriate clinical supervision on an around-the-clock basis?

Serious consideration of these questions by a faculty should be taken in accord with the basic philosophy and objectives of the curriculum. Depending on evidence relative to these questions, nursing experiences can be planned for any or all of the time periods. An interim rule of thumb may be helpful in determining timing for planning and supervising clinical nursing experiences: *Clinical nursing experiences should be provided whenever and wherever there are available those experiences needed to meet both the stated objectives and the individual needs and abilities of the students.*

Utilization of vicarious learning experiences. A basic premise on which clinical nursing is built is that students best develop when they have direct contact with real or "live" situations. Unfortunately there are occasions in which adequate clinical nursing experiences are not available to meet the desired objectives. The individual teacher's first line of defense is to seek these desired experiences in other areas of the hospital or community agencies and alter the clinical assignment accordingly. When it is impossible to manipulate assignments in order to provide these desired experiences, the creative ability of the teacher of clinical nursing must be utilized to provide vicarious teaching material that is appropriate to the nature of the desired experience rather than relying on the chance that the student may have the opportunity for the experience later. Through the use of teaching methods such as role-playing, case history analysis, pro-grammed instructional materials, and the teacher's accurate description of the situation, conceptual learning can result. Examination and study of the materials described in Chapter 8 may prove helpful in devising ways and means of providing such meaningful learning experiences.

The prevailing theme of this discussion has been that of relying on the creative abilities of teachers of clinical nursing to implement changes in providing meaningful, satisfying, and stimulating clinical nursing experiences commensurate with the individual needs, abilities, and objectives of the students. In providing these experiences it is essential that the teacher possess a mastery of nursing knowledge in the given field and be well acquainted with the health needs of patients in order to meet the learning needs of each student.

GUIDING STUDENT EXPERIENCES IN PATIENT-CENTERED CLINICAL NURSING

Having defined the objectives for the clinical experiences, determined individual student learning needs, and planned the desired clinical nursing experiences, the teacher faces the equally demanding, complex, and rewarding task of supervising students in their nursing practice. To function in this capacity requires special knowledge of clinical nursing, an ability to function as an expert nursing practitioner, and an ability to recognize individual needs of students in terms of stress situations as well as mastery of skills. In addition the teacher must have developed a compassionate understanding of how to accept and cope with daily nursing situations involving personal commitment not only to patients but also to students, nursing service personnel, and allied health team members.

The teacher of clinical nursing functions as a guide for the students, playing a helping, supportive role while giving students responsibilities for active participation in the planned activities within the realm of safe nursing care practices. Regardless of the approach used in providing clinical nursing experiences, the teacher-student ratio, or the size and type of physical facilities, the teacher of clinical nursing must (1) establish a rapport with students that fosters a feeling of freedom to seek help; (2) be readily available to students when they seek assistance; (3) circulate among students for the purposes of assessing performance at various stages leading to the finished task; (4) allow enough time for all students, avoiding helping a few at the expense of the total group; (5) allow time for unanticipated events; and (6) manipulate the individual student's learning opportunities in a way that moves him from dependent action to increasingly greater independence of action and ultimately to assume full responsibility for pursuing learning opportunities. Small wonder that the teacher is so frequently exhausted at the end of the day! The need for supportive resources for the teacher should be obvious after studying such a list.

The clinical teacher assumes responsibility for guiding the students in those planned experiences designed to meet the desired outcomes for the given course. The following examples are not intended to be exhaustive but to show how the creative teacher of clinical nursing functions in supervising clinical experiences based on the previously described skills in providing patient care experiences.

Assisting students in planning and organizing daily assignments. From the time students begin to function within the clinical nursing units they need to learn to plan their daily approach to assignments, considering economical use of time, materials, and energy expenditure as they ultimately affect the patient. The teacher has a dual responsibility in helping students plan and organize their daily assignments: (1) establishing a sequence for accomplishing tasks in terms of patient needs, discriminating between essentials and nonessentials, and preserving time, energy, and equipment; and (2) adjusting plans to meet conditions in the clinical setting and patient needs, revising ineffective plans, or

pursuing additional experiences to meet the learning needs best. Planning for clinical nursing experiences on a continuum from the simple to the complex requires comparable clinical supervision. The teacher of clinical nursing needs to provide sustained guidence; from the very beginning students and teachers should share in decisions. Often this can be done effectively by using reflective questions to help students analyze the situation and suggest approaches; the clinical teacher *guides* the student but does not *take over* or finish an assignment for a student. As students progress in their individual abilities to plan and implement effective nursing care, the teacher of clinical nursing should provide guidance in gradually diminishing amounts, offering students opportunities to assume increased responsibility for planning their daily learning experiences, along with the freedom to seek approval or guidance as necessary.

When the recognition of individual differences pervades the total clinical nursing program, the creative teacher guides students in a manner that allows them to express their own creative talents to cope with daily planning problems through increasingly independent actions. There is nothing wrong in allowing students to implement a plan of action that is within the realm of safe nursing practice although it appears illogical or awkward and certainly not the way you, the teacher, would plan it. Only two effects can result, each of which serves as a learning experience: (1) the student learns the plan is unsatisfactory and must be revised in order to accomplish the desired goals; or (2) the plan is successfully implemented, and the teacher identifies a new approach to accomplish the same goals. Students learn far more by recognizing *their own* mistakes than from simply being told by the clinical teacher that the plan will not work. Individualized guidance in planning and organizing daily assignments by students does not mean that the teacher abdicates supervising students. It means that daily conferences, either group, individual, or both, are held for the purpose of discussing each student's plans for the day and for providing initial guidance in needed areas. Throughout the experience the teacher confers individually with students to guide them in implementing the plan of action, revising it where needed, and evaluating the total effects on completion of the assignment.

In the guidance of students the teacher must be able to relate to students sufficiently to be considered as helper and supporter; sufficiently open-minded enough to allow students to proceed in a manner conducive to developing their own creative approaches to nursing; sufficiently aware of patients' needs to guide students in making effective nursing care plans; sufficiently flexible to allow for changes in planning of care or approaches used as necessitated by a given situation at a given time; and sufficiently aware of learning needs and problems of individual students to help them analyze their strengths and weaknesses and plan and organize their learning experiences accordingly.

Assisting students in application of concepts and principles to clinical nursing situation. While much of this chapter is given to the discussion of a wide range of skills to be developed by students as a result of their clinical nursing experiences, integrated learning involving the application of theoretical knowledge to the development of nursing skills is also necessary. To acquire integrated clinical knowledge and skills, students need learning experiences that provide opportunities for sequential practice of broader, more complex elements of skill development, drawing repeatedly on basic concepts and scientific principles in new and more complex combinations in their application to the given situation. Learning is most effective when teachers consistently ask students *why* patients react as they do, why certain symptoms are indicative of certain physiological manifestation, why certain drugs are used for vastly differing kinds of symptomatic treat-

ment, why certain nursing measures are needed in the care of various patients, and why nurses must exercise judgment and proper timing in their interpersonal communications. Just as clinical nursing teachers habitually seek these answers in helping students identify the relationships between theoretical knowledge and clinical experiences, so the students develop this habit of inquiry. The teacher guides students in recognizing and analyzing the concepts and scientific principles to determine why and how they apply to each in new and different relationships. An inquiring mind begets an inquiring attitude of mind; as the teacher of clinical nursing poses questions and problems to show the application of concepts to the daily nursing situations, the students are motivated to keep pace with the teacher, frequently moving into individual study in related areas. This approach to guiding student experiences in clinical nursing is basic to the entire program because it helps students to understand the relationships between theoretical knowledge and clinical experiences as they discover how concepts and principles can be used in unlimited combinations to provide knowledgeable nursing care for patients. For example, Levine's discussion regarding the application of four conservative principles to patient care, while limited in scope, describes how nursing care can be based on the nurse's knowledge of scientific principles.[7]

Assisting students in development of observation skills. Providing clinical learning experiences designed to assist students in developing observation skills goes beyond the historic purpose of observing to secure data for records. It is information perceived through the use of the combined sensory organs which is understood and leads to sound action, which places the powers of observation among the desired and necessary skills in providing direct patient care. The development of the ability to organize a wide range of observations into an integrated, meaningful whole serves dual purposes in providing effective patient care:

(1) to enable the nurse to accurately diagnose health conditions and plan care accordingly, and (2) to reflect on observations in providing responses that best help patients become aware of themselves. Here again the teacher should guide the students in the development of observation skills on a progressive basis starting with carefully planned activities from the earliest clinical nursing experiences, with each successive activity becoming more complex, and moving from teacher-directed to student-initiated activities.

To provide meaningful guidance in the development of observation skills according to students' individual needs and abilities, it is wise to begin by assigning specific observations to be made, focusing at first on a singular objective and asking students to describe their observations in a given situation such as a classroom, a social setting, or a selected experience in a clinical setting. Each subsequent experience should be so designed as to provide increasingly complex observations, broadening to include those that include participant observation and instrumentation. Each experience should provide opportunities for new and different kinds of observations, while the amount of assistance provided by the teacher regarding clues to observations decreases.

In addition to providing guidance in terms of *what to observe,* the teacher of clinical nursing has the responsibility for helping students to interpret their findings and plan nursing care accordingly. The use of group and individual conferences is essential to determine the extent and kind of observations students make as they progress from simple to multisensory observations in a variety of nursing situations. Students should be given the opportunity to discuss their own interpretations of their observations while being guided by the clinical teacher in understanding the meanings of their observations.

Faculty should be capable of teaching students the difference between description and designation, and designation and diagnosis (as discussed by Feinstein[8]). Mastery should lead to a decrease in mistaken early interpretation of findings and associated ineffective actions.

Follow-up discussions regarding resultant action from the student's observations are essential to complete the learning cycle, for it is one thing to be able to observe and interpret the findings accurately but it is another to be able to initiate appropriate action. As the students progress, they should become increasingly skilled in observing multiple details and in responding to patients effectively.

Assisting students in development of interpersonal relationship skills. Helping students to develop observation and communications skills necessary for establishing satisfying interpersonal relationships is difficult, even when taught as an integrating thread permeating the total curriculum. A report of one school of nursing described how instructors utilized a non-nursing course on the dynamics of communication for preparing students to be able to communicate more effectively in clinical nursing settings. Because the course focused on laboratory activities that forced students to identify communication behaviors and find ways of coping with them, the stage was set for individual development of awareness of the effects of people on one another.[9] A course of this type, offered prior to clinical nursing experience, could prove extremely helpful as a basic foundation for developing the kind of facilitative communication techniques that foster therapeutic interpersonal relationships. The teaching of interpersonal relationship skills can then be continued in an integrated manner in all clinical nursing experiences throughout the total nursing program. Johnson, Dunham, and Culver have described an approach to teaching these skills in an integrated manner by building concepts and developing skills from the simple to the complex.[10,11] Of particular signicance was their approach to the early development of beginning skills in interpersonal relationships based on the underlying concept of the effect one's individual behavior has on another. Use of such an approach allows those concepts to be learned, repeated, and applied over an extended time period, contributing to the total understanding of human behavior in the variety of ways needed to meet the unique psychosocial and physical needs of patients in all clinical nursing areas.

In addition to having a workable understanding of various theories of human behavior, the development of satisfying and satisfactory interpersonal relationships involves empathy and compassion. To provide care for patients, nurses should develop self-understanding that will sustain the high level of personal commitment and involvement necessary to practice nursing. Given the nature of nursing as a caring art, it is the person of the nurse that is often the therapeutic tool. For this tool to be useful, the nurse must have self-awareness and self-acceptance. Nursing literature reflects a growing evidence that these factors are of real concern to professional nurses and deserve further consideration by teachers in planning clinical nursing experiences.

The University of Vermont School of Nursing serves as an example of one school that devised an approach to understanding and helping students develop their own self-awareness. Using the FEL technique they offer a nongraded group session laboratory for purposes of improving interpersonal relationships through self-understanding.[12]

Teachers of clinical nursing must possess the self-awareness needed to cope with their own feelings in care situations so they can assist students seeking to learn from similar events. Teachers with self-awareness can offer students the necessary support and guidance in helping them recognize their feelings and the reasons for them and in learning ways of responding to them creatively.

The clinical teacher can be of assistance in helping the nursing service personnel, since the way in which they react to situations in the clinical setting directly affects the way in which the students react. There are often occasions when students seek help from nursing service personnel; therefore, the learning environment should allow the students freedom to express anxieties and receive needed support in reaching an adjustment for functioning effectively in providing compassionate, supportive nursing care for patients.

Otto suggests that nurse educators consider taking a periodic inventory of students' personality assets to help them identify and develop their unique potentials as human beings through the process of self-actualization. The same suggested inventory process can also be used to assess the patients' potentials so that the nurse can better assist patients by helping them actualize their own potentials.[13] Guiding students in the development of the interpersonal relationship skills appropriate to a given situation demands that the clinical nursing teacher know the total patient situation, recognize the presenting problems, provide a learning environment, and use counseling techniques in helping students analyze their strengths and weaknesses in their progressive development of any or all of the needed interpersonal relationship skills each time students enter into a patient care situation. Creative teachers of clinical nursing set the example by their role-model of self-understanding, of understanding behavior patterns of patients, and of nonverbal and verbal communication conveying the attitude of acceptance, support, and basic belief in the patient's potential for restoration of health and well-being.

Assisting students in development of skill in making judgments. Use of the nursing process of assessment, diagnosis, goal setting, intervention, and evaluation is an orderly and effective means of providing patient-centered nursing care. This systematic approach to planning patient care based on a scientific foundation provides many avenues for solving the problems presented by patients. But one of the keys to its success is that of *developing skill in making sound judgments.* The development of skill in using judgment to plan and implement quality nursing care comprises the core of the clinical nursing program.

Nurses have recognized that jumping from observation or assessment to care without making explicit the intervening stages of diagnosis and goal setting makes it more difficult for the student to learn and more difficult to evaluate the efficacy of the care given. Just as the student physician is evaluated, not only for skill in performing a cholecystectomy but also for accuracy in identifying gall bladder disease, the student nurse must be evaluated for skill in both applying comfort measures *and* accuracy in diagnosing the presence of pain. The nursing diagnoses made and the goals set for overcoming or adapting to the diagnoses should be clearly documented in patient records and in student papers.

The use of the nursing process usually involves formulating a written nursing care plan or nursing orders. This plan serves as a useful tool in implementing care designed to meet the assessed needs of the patient. To prepare and implement such a plan calls for making skilled judgments so that the plan is based on diagnosis—specific, realistic, and achievable. There is need to provide for individual patient differences by using common or master plans flexibly to help students plan effective nursing care. Careful consideration should be given to where and how students share their care plans. While practicing nurses often do not need before them all the detail required of the student, the students and practitioners both gain if documentation is on the regular record rather than only turned in to teachers.

Assisting students in development of motor skills. It has been found that motor skills learned in an isolated laboratory setting tend to degenerate when they are not soon followed by transferred learning experiences in a "live" situation. Therefore the various clinical nursing settings provide ideal conditions for the development

of specific desired motor skills. The teacher of clinical nursing has a dual role in helping students develop motor skills: (1) to provide opportunities to use a given learned motor skill in the natural clinical setting soon after having perfected it in the classroom setting and (2) to continue to guide the student until he has fully transferred the learning, bringing the level of performance of the skill with patients up to that previously achieved in the classroom laboratory. The teacher should continue to provide opportunities for application of the learned skills in similar or new combinations or in modifications to various kinds of patients, helping students maintain their level of performance and as a foundation for the mastery of more complicated skills. If, in fact, motor skills are learned in terms of general steps to be followed, based on sound scientific principles, flexibility must become a built-in feature in their effective development. Such flexibility allows for the performance of motor skills that not only safeguard the patient but also meet the demands and limitations imposed by the setting in which the task is being done. Students must not only be taught basic principles but must also be shown how these apply in a number of similar patterns, according to the available equipment and supplies, the physical environment, or the patient's condition.

When provided with a flexible learning environment, students can approach each performance of a skill with a relaxed feeling of being able to satisfy the patient by adjusting the procedure without anxiety about the outcome and its ultimate effect on the performance record. As students grow toward mastery of motor skills in an environment of this nature, they quickly learn to teach procedures to patients in accord with their level of learning, adapting them to fit their particular resources, equipment, and abilities. A third dimension of adaptation occurs in the changes that take place in the clinical nursing setting when new equipment or new methods are introduced. Having learned to develop motor skills based on scientific principles and flexibility of use, students readily adapt to these measures and become reliable resource persons for teaching others.

The creative teacher of clinical nursing is responsible for guiding the student's development of motor skills by: (1) helping students identify a sequence of action needed to develop form based on identifiable principles; (2) guiding students in making beginning movements until they sense the body movements needed to coordinate the action; (3) keeping attention focused on the objectives, allowing for flexibility in manipulation according to the students' learning needs; (4) evaluating strengths and weaknesses to help students correct errors as they are learning the skill rather than after they have learned it haphazardly; (5) allowing sufficient amounts of rest and activity periods to avoid fatigue yet continue development of the skill; (6) providing for application of the same principles in a wide range of settings and adaptations; (7) requiring students to explain their motions or actions in terms of the existing circumstances as they relate to principles; (8) helping students feel sufficiently secure so that they can make modifications according to the demands of the situation while remaining within the realm of safe practice; and (9) using communications to indicate needed change of action during a procedure in a manner that students can exemplify as a role model.

Creativity in the planning and guiding of student experiences involving patient-centered clinical nursing activities requires a clinical teacher who can provide an environment conducive to the student's ability to develop skills into functioning ability in accord with the desired competencies of the program.

The cycle is completed when the teacher of clinical nursing assumes responsibility for making continuous observations of student progress and performance relative to (1) ability to plan and organize work assignments; (2) degree of use of initiative and self-direction; (3) application of scientific principles to the patient care situation; (4) development of observation skills; (5) development of interpersonal relationship skills; (6) ability to communicate effectively with patients and others; (7) ability to express oneself adequately in writing and reporting; (8) ability to assess patients, make a nursing diagnosis, establish a goal-directed plan of care, assess the effectiveness of the plan, and make necessary adjustments; (9) ability to use sound judgment in responses to patients and others; (10) ability to initiate appropriate action in communicating with others; (11) ability to use scientific principles in adapting nursing procedures to meet individual patient's needs or the demands of the situation; (12) ability to perform procedures flexibly within the realm of safe practices; (13) ability to organize work; and (14) ability to teach patients and others effectively. To be of value, these observations must be recorded and interpreted through the use of various tools and techniques designed to provide objective, evaluative measures. These are described in more detail in Chapter 9.

As students learn to integrate various kinds of skill learning, so, too, the creative teacher of clinical nursing guides the students' desired learning activities by integrating the functions of (1) determining the specific, expected levels of competencies in accord with the objectives of the given program; (2) planning and selecting clinical learning experiences with the students in accord with their various learning needs and abilities; (3) guiding student experiences in direct patient care; and (4) observing student progress and performance in the integrated development of skills needed to provide patient-centered nursing care.

REFERENCES

1. Levine, Myra: Adaptation and assessment, a rationale for nursing intervention, American Journal of Nursing 66:2452, Nov., 1966.
2. Gebbie, Kristine, and Lavin, Mary Ann: Classification of nursing diagnoses, St. Louis, 1975, The C. V. Mosby Co.

3. Abdellah, Faye G., and others: Patient-centered approaches to nursing, New York, 1960, Macmillan, Inc.
4. Foshay, Arthur: Beware, your future students are learning to think! Nursing Outlook **13**: 47-49, Oct., 1965.
5. Schumann, Delores M.: Improved method of making clinical assignments, Nursing Outlook **15**:52-55, April, 1967.
6. Toffler, Alvin: Future shock, New York, 1970, Random House, Inc.
7. Levine, Myra: The four conservation principles of nursing, Nuring Forum **6**(1):45-59, 1967.
8. Feinstein, Allan: Clinical judgement, Baltimore, 1967, The Williams & Wilkins Co.
9. Hanson, Rachel, Minor, Gene, and Wirick, Elizabeth: Tuning in on tuning out, Nursing Outlook **16**:40-42, May, 1968.
10. Johnson, Betty S., Dunham, Frances, and Culver, Charles: Teaching interpersonal skills to nursing students, Nursing Outlook **2**(1): 79-85, 1963.
11. Culver, Charles, Dunham, Frances, and Johnson, Betty S.: A first course in interpersonal relations, Nursing Forum **2**(1):79-85, 1963.
12. Chase, Phillip H., Farnham, Beverly, and Magee, Frances: FEL—a process for teaching interpersonal relationships, American Journal of Nursing **70**:524-528, March, 1970.
13. Otto, Herbert A.: The human potentialities of nurses and patients, Nursing Outlook **13**: 32-35, Aug., 1965.

SUGGESTED READINGS

Brodie, Barbara: Reexamination of reinforcement in the learning process, Journal of Nursing Education **8**:27-32, April, 1969.
Durand, Mary, and Prince, Rosemary: Nursing diagnosis; process and decision, Nursing Forum **5**(4):50-64, 1966.
Folta, Jeannete R., and Deck, Edith S.: A sociological framework for patient care, New York, 1966, John Wiley & Sons, Inc.
Fuhr, Mary T.: Clinical experience: record and nursing care planning, St. Louis, 1972, The C. V. Mosby Co.
Gezi, Kalil, and Hadley, Florence: Strategies for developing critical thinking, Journal of Nursing Education **9**:9-14, April, 1970.
Gragg, Shirley, and Rees, Olive M.: Scientific principles in nursing, St. Louis, 1974, The C. V. Mosby Co.
Kron, Thora: Communication in nursing, Philadelphia, 1972, W. B. Saunders Co.
Lewis, Lucile: This I believe about the nursing process—key to care, Nursing Outlook **16**:26-29, May, 1968.
Little, Dolores, and Carnevali, Doris: Nursing care plans: let's be practical about them, Nursing Forum **6**(1):61-76, 1967.
Manlove, Donald C., and Beggs, David W., III: Flexible scheduling: bold new venture, Bloomington, Ind., 1965, Indiana University Press.
Martucci, Elizabeth: Students view faculty roles in the learning process, Nursing Outlook **16**:22-23, Nov., 1968.
McAttee, Patricia: The human side of curriculum development, Nursing Forum **8**(2):144-150, 1969.
Olsen, James: Should we group ability? Journal of Teacher Education **18**:201-205, Summer, 1967.
Ortelt, Judith, and Glichman, Carole: An undergraduate honors program in nursing, Nursing Outlook **15**:66-68, July, 1967.
Ramphal, Marjorie M.: A rationale for assignments, American Journal of Nursing **67**:1630-1633, Aug., 1967.
Schwalb, Roberta B., and Clark, Emily A.: The obstetrician's office as a clinical field, Nursing Outlook **16**:32-33, March, 1968.
Searight, Mary: A planning laboratory, Nursing Outlook **15**:58-59, Dec., 1967.
Sorensen, Gladys: An honors program in nursing, Nursing Outlook **16**:59-61, May, 1968.
Wagner, Berniece: Care plans: right, reasonable, and reachable, American Journal of Nursing **69**: 986-990, May, 1969.
Walsh, Joan E., and Monat, Cecelia A.: Expected competencies as a basis for selecting content in psychiatric nursing, Nursing Outlook **15**:58-62, July, 1967.
White, Marjorie A.: Teaching the superior nursing student, Journal of Nursing Education **4**:9-14, April, 1965.
Zimmerman, Donna, and Gohrke, Carol: The goal-directed nursing approach: it does work, American Journal of Nursing **70**:306-310, Feb., 1970.

8 Teaching methods and devices adaptable to the creative teaching of clinical nursing

Vast amounts of research have given little substantiating evidence to suggest that certain teaching methods or devices automatically produce better results than others. The current movement is toward the development of theoretical research designs for the study of the processes of teaching and learning and their ultimate effects on self-appropriated learning. Teachers must rely on currently available information and their own resourcefulness in the selection, adaptation, and evaluation of effective teaching-learning methods and devices.

Educators continue to seek ways of having personal and close contact with master teachers who inspire through their ability to communicate their knowledge of the subject field and their understanding of the student as an individual. Although there is no substitute for intimate contact with the expert teacher, it must be remembered that one cannot guarantee that small groups of students with a teacher offer the best educational opportunities. The very nature of this environment would, in some instances, merely perpetuate mediocrity; it is possible for a given student or group of students to learn more by being exposed to expert knowledge through one or several modes of education. Utilization of a wide variety of communications media as an integral part of the total teaching-learning process may lead the way to creativity by offering students opportunities to pursue individual inquiry along with tutorial assistance from truly expert teachers who do not impose their views and attitudes on the students. Just as we recognize that a single learning theory does not describe the di-

versity of ways in which individuals learn, neither can we identify one teaching theory that describes the range of activities and devices used by teachers. Creative learning is dependent on some underlying scheme leading to self-discovered learning; thus, teaching processes cannot always be readily identified. They exist in a variety of shapes and forms and are comprised of a variety of operations providing for learner involvement in the acquisition of knowledge and skill. We are now at a point for teachers to reexamine their teaching approaches, identifying those methods and instructional strategies that provide for more flexibility in the use of processes leading to creative learning in the clinical nursing situation.

The procedural aspects of the teaching-learning process in nursing consist of a system of communications involving teachers and others familiar with the use of teaching methods and audiovisual media. This chapter is limited to the discussion of those teaching methods and devices that, presumably, the creative teacher can adapt for use in the clinical nursing situation. Although the teaching of clinical nursing can involve a wide range of methods, educational communication media, and multimedia approaches in a variety of combinations, each broad category is described separately so that the reader can gain information about the use of specific teaching approaches and devices.

Teaching methods refer to any kind of an orderly, logical course of action taken to accomplish a particular educational goal. A wide range of methods of teaching has been devised and used in a variety of combinations depending on the objectives to be accomplished, the students, and the ability of the teacher. Creativity in the use of these methods is reflected by the individual teacher's distinctive manner of performance in a given situation.

GUIDELINES FOR SELECTION OF METHODS ADAPTED FOR USE IN CLINICAL TEACHING

A creative teaching-learning milieu provides the freedom for discovery so vital to learning professional responsibilities. In an article Mereness describes six freedoms and responsibilities she believes should be provided by any educational institution.[1] The clinical teacher who provides opportunities for learning through discovery and makes teaching selections based on the democratic concept that *for every right granted an individual there is an equal responsibility* should experience the joy of self-fulfilment. This broad concept offers clinical teachers the opportunity to increase their potential for fostering creativity through their ability to purposefully select and adapt a wide range of teaching methods to the clinical setting. The following guidelines can be used in the selection of methods of teaching appropriate for use in the clinical setting.

Selection of method must be appropriate to objectives and desired behavioral changes. There may be any number of methods that could be used to meet the specific objectives, but there are instances in which certain methods could not accomplish the objective. For example, to learn some of the skills described in the preceding chapter, some type of learning experience involving practice of the skills is needed in addition to the use of the lecture method. A clinical conference could also be utilized to meet the behavioral outcomes by helping students discuss the problems inherent in the nursing situation and see relationships between the theoretical background of knowledge and its application to patient care situations.

Creativity in the selection of methods best suited to the objectives can be accom-plished through a cooperative venture whereby students suggest ways of learning within the framework defined by the teacher. The teacher holds the responsibility for interpreting the educational goals, society's needs, and patients' needs; the student holds the responsibility for determining learning experiences that are in accord with these stated needs and goals, and with their individual needs. In this era of technological advancement and knowledge explosion the student population is becoming increasingly sophisticated and aware that there seldom exists one perfect, correct solution to a problem. Students need a learning environment that allows them to pursue educational goals by proposing and experimenting with "new" or "different" methods of solving problems related to clinical nursing. Freedom to learn in this dimension invokes the student's responsibility for defining the problem and describing the purpose and expected outcomes for the selected approach. The teacher is responsible for allowing spontaneity that fosters creativity and for providing the necessary support needed by the student regardless of success or failure.

Selection of method must be in accord with principles of learning. Success or failure in the use of selected teaching methods is also dependent on the teacher's ability to organize materials, ideas, and people within the social context of the learning environment. The teacher must have a basic understanding of how people learn, variations of individual learning rates, reinforcement techniques, interpersonal relationships affecting motivation, and active as opposed to passive student involvement in the learning process. A more detailed pattern of the application of psychological principles of learning to the teaching process was described in Chapter 6.

Today's world demands that people learn how to think deeply regarding actions to be taken and the potential consequences of the actions. Individuals who learn how to discover knowledge, how to inquire and examine all issues, and how to arrive at their own decisions readily learn how to assume responsibility for their own actions and how to evaluate the results. The selection of teaching methods fostering this kind of learning is largely dependent on the teacher's ability to consider the significance these learning principles have for the individual learner and to translate these concepts into meaningful approaches to teaching.

The creative teacher in clinical nursing has the responsibility of selecting methods of teaching that offer freedom to explore unusual concepts, examine many sides of an issue, and express individual ideas. To learn in an environment fostering this individual freedom of expression, students assume the responsibility for inquiry that assists them in identifying the philosophical and intellectual basis for making value judgments. Helping students to understand *why* certain action is taken and to question the consequence of actions in terms of patients' responses should become a part of the routine pattern of professional thought.

Selection of method must be in accord with capacity of student. Know your students! The acknowledgment that individual differences are far greater than similarities underlines the need to develop a greater concern for the individual student. Each new group of students must be studied carefully to determine individual variations in intellectual maturity, emotional development, social or environmental orientation to learning, and previous experience with various kinds of teaching methods. The selection of teaching methods in accord with this basic information suggests the need to employ a flexible plan with a wide variety of methods that can offer the individual student a feeling of security, accomplishment, and self-fulfillment. Inherent in this concept is the need for teachers to recognize that they must provide ways of avoiding premature and unreasonable demands on students while seeking to develop them as competent nurse practitioners.

The teacher should select those methods that provide an atmosphere of security to assist the learner in gaining mastery of a

technical skill, the establishment of satisfying relationships with others, the application of previously learned material to a new setting, or the solving of a complex care problem. The teacher holds the responsibility for assisting students to reach their potential by fostering curiosity, being encouraging of novel or different responses, and being open-minded toward those who do not follow the prescribed patterns. The student is responsible for pursuing learning activities that make wise use of time and self and for developing a conceptual framework for understanding and validating the chosen plan of action in patient care.

Selection of method must be in accord with availability of resources. Effectiveness of selected teaching methods is dependent on the availability of the necessary resources. Teaching innovations are being tried, tested, and reported at a rate faster than one dares to imagine, providing teachers with encouragement to vary facilities and methods. The teacher's responsibility lies in carefully evaluating new techniques and devices for practicality in a given situation, making the best use of the available materials to meet the objectives of the program, becoming familiar with the use of new devices, making advance preparations and plans, and preparing the students for their use. Where newer methods and devices are currently not in use, it is imperative that planning for their future use take place, even as the readily available resources are being used in the current teaching program. Students have the opportunity to stretch their minds by learning with new teaching techniques and devices. Their responsibility lies in their willingness to accept change, by becoming involved in working with the new processes and devices and evaluating their effectiveness in contributing to the total learning situation.

Selection of method must be in accord with teacher's ability to use it effectively and creatively. Know yourself! As early as 1910 research related to teacher effectiveness gained popularity, and it has continued to gather momentum. Even in the face of this expansive evidence regarding the method or combination of methods the teacher should use in order to facilitate creative, effective learning, it remains difficult to determine the precise degree of change in student behavior that can be attributed directly to the teacher. Research studies have provided a long list of desirable traits for successful teachers. The very act of teaching involves the individual teacher's feelings, beliefs, interests, psychological reactions, sociocultural orientation, background of knowledge and experience, knowledge of subject matter, and use of teaching methods.

It remains for each teacher to adopt and develop that style of teaching that best suits the individual's particular abilities and is appropriate to the given situation. The road to creativity is characterized by a combination of the individual's self-awareness of aptitudes and the courage to experiment with ideas and innovations that could be adapted effectively to the teaching of clinical nursing.

Students need the freedom to experience relationships in which the teacher serves as a role model in teaching and as a vital, caring human being. The teacher who is not limited by excessive self-interest or anxieties but can share much of the self in daily relationships with others will experience the joy of helping students feel a freedom for creative expression. Teachers who search for ways of realizing the potentials that lie within each person and find freedom *for* a creative giving of the self will foster student responsibility for the development of comparable attitudes in an environment of mutual respect and concern.

TEACHING METHODS ADAPTABLE TO CREATIVE TEACHING OF CLINICAL NURSING

The methods a given teacher selects for teaching clinical nursing do not guarantee the student's automatic changes. For teaching that is *authoritative* rather than *authoritarian* we need creative clinical teachers who use imagination, ability, knowledge, and courage in the selection and use of teaching methods. The discussion of teaching methods is limited to a representative group of those appearing to be the most adaptable for teaching clinical nursing.

Laboratory method

According to Webster's *New Collegiate Dictionary* the laboratory method had its beginnings in the teaching of chemistry, whereby students went to a workroom for purposes of experimental study involving testing, analyzing, and preparing chemical substances. This concept of experimental problem-solving became an integral part of the study of a variety of the science components of nursing curricula. Soon the nursing components of the curricula became a natural media for the use of the laboratory method by providing opportunities for students to use a problem-solving approach to the development of techniques in a controlled learning environment. In undergraduate study the early laboratory experiences are usually performances of well-known actions that, when followed correctly, allow the student to share in reaching a known goal. At graduate levels the laboratory is the site for exploration and discovery of new knowledge.

Explicitly the laboratory method of teaching utilizes a problem-solving approach to learning that offers students opportunities for supervised, individualized, direct experiences in the testing and application of previously learned theory and principles and the refinement of specific skills or complex abilities. The learning experiences are planned so that the theory and laboratory experiences complement each other. This concept has been expanded to include the clinical setting in the hospital, the home, and community health agencies in providing students with opportunities for using problem-solving techniques to study patients with varying degrees and kinds of nursing and health problems. Unlike chemical laboratories, patient care settings can rarely be sufficiently controlled so that the instructor can guarantee the details of the student's findings. Even the beginning undergraduate student must be prepared to discover something new about human experience with health and illness.

Many schools of nursing have expanded the use of the laboratory method to include prolonged observational studies within the clinical and community setting. This technique has proved particularly successful in the study of growth and development patterns and of interpersonal relationships to gain an understanding of behavioral patterns of children and adults. A recent experimental study in the use of prolonged observations of hospitalized children as a teaching technique for nursing students is described by Schulman and co-workers.[2]

As schools of nursing modernize their teaching facilities, they are providing laboratories equipped with one-way viewing devices for observation studies by small groups of students. The objectives for the observational study vary according to the subject, such as (1) parent-child interactions; (2) growth and development patterns of various age groups; (3) demonstrations of group therapy; (4) nurse-patient interaction; and (5) counseling and interviewing patients with specific problems such as long-term illness, death and dying, drug dependency, unwed parents, or other family crisis situations. The purpose for using this technique and its variations is to build observation skills by allowing the interaction to occur in a more natural way than if the observer is seen, and to allow interaction among observers during the event. Alternating observations of specific situations with participation in these settings and later student/teacher interaction can be very effective.

A demonstration of this kind necessitates ethical consideration of the rights of the subjects being viewed. Prior to the observation session the persons working directly with the patients should clearly explain the purpose of the demonstration, describe the viewing audience, and provide sufficient explanation to the subjects to allow each to make an intelligent decision about his willingness to participate in the observation study. Situations involving patients must be evaluated on an individualized basis to determine whether the demonstration will help or hinder their progress.

The demonstration-observation requires careful planning and should be conducted by an expert in the given subject matter who already has established a rapport with the subjects. For a productive learning situation, observations should be (1) conducted at frequent intervals over a sufficient period of time, (2) evaluated by students in accord with their objectives and their theoretical insights, and (3) followed by teacher-observer conferences to validate findings, develop new insights regarding observed responses of patients, discuss observer reactions to the problem, and explore ways that will lead to better patient understanding.

Variations of this device are frequently used in medicine. One excellent example is described by Marschak and Call in observations of parental influence on disturbed children.[3] In another, Kübler-Ross interviewed dying patients to determine their feelings about death and dying, followed by a seminar with the observers representing a wide range of professional disciplines to help them understand their own feelings about the patient and provide the support and understanding needed.[4] Careful study of these techniques furnishes the creative teacher with numerous ideas regarding ways of adapting this method to selected areas of clinical nursing.

While both teacher and student have definite responsibilities for the effective use of the laboratory method, its creative use is dependent on the teacher-student milieu. The extent to which the teacher fosters self-direction through cooperative planning, action, and validation of results is directly proportional to the degree of creative action expressed by the student. Table 1 is intended for use as a quick reference of the

Table 1. Technique for the laboratory method

Teacher responsibilities	Student responsibilities
1. Specify objectives for laboratory experience and make them known to students.	1. Study necessary background material in accord with outlined objectives.
2. Outline general plan of activities in accord with objectives; provide for correlation of activities with theory courses.	2. Formulate own objectives for pursuing assignments.
3. Arrange for needed facilities in advance—*know* patients and projected area of study.	3. Outline plan of investigation, using own objectives, teacher objectives, background knowledge, and prepared instructions; be prepared to justify plan of action.
4. Provide necessary equipment; check for availability and working condition.	4. Pursue plan of action, using teacher as resource for guidance in completing plan.
5. Prepare instructions—verbal, written, taped, or in manual form—but avoid excessive detail in order to provide for creative thinking.	5. Make needs known to teacher; seek assistance in validation of data.
6. Plan for sequential learning experiences; allow progression according to individual abilities.	6. Seek additional theoretical information by reading and further study in order to understand and work through presenting problem.
7. Supervise students through questions and example; timing of guidance must be strategically planned—know when to act, when to withhold action.	7. Validate actions with classmates, nursing service personnel, and other health team members.
8. Provide reinforcement at regular intervals; keep records of daily progress.	8. Summarize data frequently to keep goals clearly in focus.
9. Make self available for group or individual help.	9. Report findings to group, reviewing problem, plan of action, significant data, findings, conclusions, and recommendations.
10. Summarize through discussions and individual conferences, data collection, organization of findings, methods of solving problems, common problems encountered, individual accomplishments, and implications for use in solving other nursing problems.	10. Evaluate self regarding progress made, areas of strengths and weaknesses, and needed areas of help to ensure future growth. (Use originally established objectives as means of self-evaluation.)
11. Report results of progress to individual students and use information as basis for planning future learning experiences.	

responsibilities of teacher and student in the use of the laboratory method; but its application to actual practice depends on its translation into cooperative teacher-student action, as described in Chapter 7.

In clinical nursing the use of the laboratory method becomes procedure for providing students with well-planned, supervised experiences in translating principles of nursing into active, problem-solving for nursing problems. The laboratory method serves as the foundation for building in those combinations of teaching methods best suited for establishing a structural framework to bridge the gap between the theoretical study of nursing and the study of patients. Therefore, the following methods of teaching can be viewed both in

terms of their singular uses or their integral contribution to the total laboratory method.

Demonstration method

In clinical nursing the demonstration method can be both indirect and direct. Of the indirect routes, the most obvious are those of nursing acts performed by learned members of the health team and witnessed by students during the normal daily assignments. It therefore behooves educators to seek those clinical settings offering reasonable opportunities for finding health team members who can and do serve as favorable role models for students to follow.

A more direct version of the demonstration method is a carefully prepared, expertly presented replication of how to perform a given task. Through the simultaneous use of several senses it seeks to show how the underlying principles apply to the given process. When the objective is to present information in a lifelike situation or to illustrate relationships between theory and practice, a return demonstration may not be required. If the goal of the demonstration is to assist students to develop greater skills, the demonstration must include opportunities for supervised practice of desired skills followed by return demonstrations.

Within the clinical nursing setting the demonstration method provides a natural and readily adaptable means of teaching, particularly in combination with the laboratory method. Most commonly it is used (1) to teach new procedures either at the bedside or in the ward-teaching center, (2) to illustrate modifications of basic procedures to meet the immediate nursing situation, (3) to make application of the knowledge of underlying scientific principles to nursing care situations, (4) to teach the use and care of new equipment, (5) to teach application of observation techniques and skills to nursing situations, (6) to teach ways of establishing effective nurse-patient communications and interpersonal relationships, and (7) to teach health maintenance and preventive health care measures to patients and families.

A variation of the demonstration method is described by Brown[5] as Nursing Rounds. This method utilizes the patient's bedside as a "live" teaching field for single concept demonstrations of a variety of nursing care situations. The central purpose is to provide direct, purposeful experiences aimed at improving selected clinical nursing abilities. Therefore, selection of concepts for demonstration is usually made from particular nursing care situations encountered in the clinical setting. This method can be used to advantage in selected situations involving a limited number of students.

Regardless of the type of demonstration or the objectives for using it, the funda-

mental responsibilities of the teacher and student listed in Table 2 contribute in large measure to its successful use as a teaching method in clinical nursing. While the demonstration has classically been used in nursing to teach psychomotor techniques such as catheterization, it is valid for teaching other skills such as the patient interview to obtain health history.

Traditional use of the demonstration method to teach procedures has perpetrated such practices as (1) requiring repetitive practice of a given procedure until it can be repeated correctly step to step by the student, regardless of how well it is understood and (2) requiring every student to practice a given procedure for a designated number of times prior to being considered "safe" to administer it to patients without supervision. Students need opportunities to exercise and develop their intellectual abilities in the direction of curiosity, resourcefulness, inventiveness, and discovery while learning the various skills needed for the practice of nursing. Opportunities for productive thinking add new dimensions to the learning of skills by bringing out each student's potential ability to view the activities in a new light, to create something new, and to be ready for new ideas developed by others.

Although it must be recognized that the development of mechanical nursing skills requires a disciplined kind of teaching-learning situation, the key to the development of such skills lies in one's ability to practice *safe* nursing care with a minimum of time and effort expenditure on the part of the nurse and the patient through the economic utilization of available equipment. Herein lie the opportunities for creative teaching-learning experiences. The following suggestions are meant as stimulants to the consideration of ways of fostering creativity in the use of the demonstration method to teach skills for nursing.

1. Prior to the demonstration of specific procedures the clinical teacher should provide an orientation period to demonstrate

Table 2. Technique for the demonstration method

Teacher responsibilities	Student responsibilities
1. Time demonstration in accord with students' background of knowledge and readiness for practice of new knowledge.	1. Familiarize self with objectives for demonstration.
2. Arrange for demonstration to be as much like actual situation as possible.	2. Study written material and suggested references.
3. Select patient or other person to serve as model requiring nursing activity to be demonstrated; explain purpose of demonstration and obtain necessary legal clearance prior to demonstration.	3. Observe patients and equipment in use as examples for planned demonstration.
4. Obtain necessary equipment, duplicating that being used and including variations in other available types; test to make certain it is in proper working order.	4. Follow steps being demonstrated along with written information.
5. Study directions and practice demonstration *exactly* as it would be performed before observers.	5. Contribute to follow-up discussion by the following:
6. Provide students with advance information regarding activity to be demonstrated. (For on-the-spot demonstrations provide reference materials for follow-up information.)	a. Identify basic principles underlying activity.
7. Arrange physical setting for demonstration so that all observers are comfortably located to hear and see; repeated demonstrations may be needed to accommodate a large group.	b. Identify how activity can be modified to meet individual needs of patients.
8. Explain purpose of activity, results desired, equipment to be used.	c. Ask for clarification of points not understood.
9. Proceed with each step of activity in logical sequence but pace so that motions can be clearly identified and interpreted.	6. Translate observation of demonstration into return performance.
10. Coordinate each step with running comments, explaining exactly what is being done:	7. Seek opportunities to practice activity until needed skill is reached.
a. Make clear, definite, complete sentences.	8. Evaluate self regarding growth and areas of help needed to perfect desired skill.
b. Introduce statements with verbs.	9. Seek opportunities to build on newly gained knowledge and skill in making application to other areas.
c. Use positive terms describing *only that which is to be done.*	10. Demonstrate learned activities to others needing assistance.
d. State pertinent scientific principles underlying steps of activity.	11. Recognize patient's needs for learning procedure and proceed with necessary arrangements for a demonstration.
11. Show how various aspects of activity could be modified to meet immediate needs of patients.	12. Request demonstrations of unfamiliar procedures or equipment.
12. Provide discussion period immediately after demonstration; repeat portions needing clarification.	
13. Provide opportunities for prompt, supervised practice periods in accord with objectives of demonstration and needs of individual students.	
14. Evaluate individual student progress in accord with expected levels of ability in development of desired skill.	
15. Plan follow-up experiences needed to assist students in learning activity and in applying it to other situations.	

those activities basic to *all* procedures, such as securing and organizing equipment, preparation of the patient, modifications for meeting patients' needs, teaching opportunities, aftercare of the patient, aftercare of equipment, and record keeping. Once these activities are conceptualized as the scientific basis for the practice of *all* procedures, it becomes the student's responsibility to practice them as an integral part of each procedure. Responsibility is centered in the student, with the teacher acting as the catalyst by providing a wide range of freedom along with thought-provoking questions.

2. In presenting the demonstration the clinical teacher should eliminate detailed steps that seem so obvious as to insult the intelligence of the student. In demonstrating a procedural technique such terms as place, carry, pick up, unwrap might well be eliminated with the assumption that anyone would automatically make those movements in order to proceed with the task.

3. The clinical teacher should use scientific principles to explain the key steps of the demonstrated skill. This is a basic ingredient for fostering creativity when students are given the freedom to perform later in terms of their own perceptions based on defensible scientific principles.

4. Creativity in the use of the demonstration method is dependent on the teacher's effective use of self in the art of inquiry. Vesting the student with the responsibility for learning charges the teacher with the responsibility for determining student progress through inquiry. The teacher must be prepared to raise thought-provoking questions and be equally prepared to allow sufficient opportunity for students to explore the questions and conceptualize answers. For example, the performance of procedures in accord with the student's self-perceived ideas can be tested by the teacher who asks questions that identify the basic scientific principles the student used in the performance. This contributes to creative learning (a) when it is used to help students think and to move them from one simple thought to a variety of thoughts and (b) when students feel that their thoughts, questions, and comments will be considered and used for growth rather than criticized. Free discussion periods are of value in helping students conceptualize application of the activity to meet the needs of the patient. There need not always be a right or wrong answer—the concepts considered in discussions may be of more lasting value in the transfer of learning than any pat answer that the teacher could supply.

Another dimension of the "art of inquiry" relates to the teacher's ability to allow students to question. Teachers who are comfortable enough to allow students to ask and pursue questions, regardless of whether or not they can be answered at the time, do more toward fostering creative ideas for the present and the future than those who stifle questions or those who have ready-made answers for all questions. Time pressures on the curriculum become the scapegoat for teachers who prefer to *give* information to be received, stored, and hopefully used at some point in time. Creativity is fostered by those who allow time to be spent in exploring ideas and raising questions and issues.

5. Students need the opportunity to perfect their skills at their own rate of learning. Mastery of a given skill loses its creativity when it is measured in terms of speed of accomplishment rather than in terms of quality. Within a reasonable time period all students need to know that they have an opportunity to achieve; the difference in the rate of learning lies in the variation of breadth and depth each student acquires.

Students should be thoroughly acquainted with the established criteria for achievement in a situation. Provisions should then be made for students to work at their own rate and be kept informed of their progress. Students mastering the material with relatively few practice periods should be provided with opportunities for new avenues of inquiry and mastery; students who initiate a new approach to a procedure need opportunities to pursue it. Additional experiences and practice periods along with individual assistance should be provided according to each student's individual learning pattern. Once the "feeling tone" is established, learners having difficulties may undergo a metamorphosis and perform along with more able students.

6. Joint teacher-student conferences regarding performance achievement should be a continuous process. The teacher can foster creative learning by being a good listener while students analyze their strengths and weaknesses to gain insight into their problems without losing face by having the teacher "point a finger" at them. On the other hand students may not be able to diagnose their difficulties or determine action to be taken without the guidance of the teacher. Students need realistic goals to work toward and confidence to build on in reaching them. The creative teacher must provide guidance that fosters the motivation needed to reach these goals. This involves careful consideration of such variables as the following: whether or not the students can attain the goals they set, the point at which the teacher intervenes, the effect the teacher's intervention will have on the student, and the results if the teacher does not intervene.

The creative teacher knows how to use the demonstration method to modify concepts and skills and to maximize the possibilities for transfer of learning so that the students can use previously acquired knowledge in new contexts. As more skills are developed, new kinds of knowledge also develop, leading to the creation of new ideas.

Group discussion methods

A cursory review of stated objectives for educational programs in schools of nursing reveals a unanimity of purpose in seeking to develop professional nurses who can function effectively in a complex, dynamic society. More specifically, professional nurses are usually expected to make accurate assessments of patients' needs; use problem-solving techniques; make judgments; seek assistance in meeting patients' needs; establish mutually effective interpersonal relationships with patients, peers, and others; and develop a sense of social responsibility. Such objectives suggest that a large portion of the professional nurse's learning opportunities should be directed toward the development of those skills and understandings necessary for effective, productive group work. It therefore seems appropriate to provide opportunities for the group discussion method in teaching clinical nursing.

For the purposes of this book the group discussion method is defined as consisting of two or more persons having a shared interest in a common problem who meet together, either formally or informally, in a working relationship under the guidance of a leader for the purpose of constructive discussion of the problem, leading to a decision regarding its solution or conclusion. This definition specifies that effective group discussions are dependent on the presence of the following conditions:

1. A group of two or more persons having similar backgrounds and a shared interest in a common problem.
2. Recognition of a desire to meet together, either formally or informally, for cooperative action in attacking a problem.
3. Cooperative problem-solving action leading to individual acceptance of responsibilities as well as rights along with respect for and acceptance of individual group members' opinions and actions.
4. Individual participation involving active listening, thinking, and cooperative discussion of the cause and effect relationships of the shared information leading to the solution of a common problem.
5. The accomplishment of purposeful

group discussion with the effective use of knowledgeable leadership.

Some contend that the process of group-centered problem-solving necessarily involves consensus, and that this destroys creative thinking. However, consensus may indeed be arrival at a creative solution. Alternately, the final decision of a creative group may be decided by majority vote or by allowing the acknowledged leader of the subsequent action to select from the options presented. Group discussions foster critical analysis of problems by providing opportunities for the formation of new patterns of insight not previously identified. As group members contribute their thoughts to the discussion, the process opens new avenues of thought and new ways of responding to the problem.

Others decry the use of group activities because of their own personal unrewarding, frustrating experiences. While there may be a real justification for such a response, the answer to the dilemma lies not in bypassing those teaching methods but in discovering the underlying causes and seeking a remedy. There is no magic formula for the successful use of group discussion methods in teaching clinical nursing, but there are certain prerequisites that will greatly enhance the effectiveness of these methods. Of prime importance is that the teacher must be well grounded in the dynamics of group behavior and in their application to the learning situation. While today's students have had previous experiences in learning through the use of group processes, we cannot leave to chance the supposition that *all* students are ready for this kind of learning. Prior to the use of any group discussion method, the teacher should orient the students to the processes involved in group dynamics, the role the leader will assume, and the roles the group members are expected to play, in addition to the goals to be accomplished. The teacher should be certain that the problem for study lends itself to the chosen discussion method. Detailed directions for the effective use of group discussion methods have been prepared by many experts in this particular field; for further assistance in handling specific problems, refer to the References.[6-13]

The group discussion method and its variations have diverse purposes, such as:

1. Developing self-directive learning habits through active participation in group activity.

2. Developing attitudes of esprit de corps in arriving at group solutions to problem-solving situations.

3. Exploring and determining a plan of action in solving a professional problem common to the group.

4. Acquiring new knowledge about a given subject.

5. Developing the art of self-expression by face-to-face interaction with the group members.

6. Developing the ability to make personal and social adjustments by learning to accept the ideas and actions of others as contributing members of the group.

7. Discussing and examining varying viewpoints of an issue—positive, negative, new or speculative, accepting, rejecting—whatever the decision.

8. Sharpening critical thinking ability by analyzing contributions of others and reexamining one's own concepts in light of the newly examined information.

9. Sharpening powers of observation and subsequent validation of observed phenomena in terms of group findings and analysis.

10. Evaluating and validating one's beliefs in order to clarify values that may be in conflict with the fulfilment of the professional responsibilities.

11. Helping the teacher identify student strengths and weaknesses, background knowledge, ability to solve problems and see relationships, ability to establish effective interpersonal relationships, and degree of

Table 3. Techniques for group discussion

Teacher or leader responsibilities	Student responsibilities

1. Have knowledge and skill in use of group dynamics.
  a. Recognize differences between authoritarian, democratic, and laissez-faire leadership and know when each is appropriate.
  b. Understand group behavior.
2. Know how to adapt principles of group discussion techniques to a variety of kinds of learning situations.
3. Acquaint students with requisite skills of group discussion before attempting it in a teaching-learning situation.
  a. Distinguish between "talking" and discussion with a purpose.
  b. Help students recognize and accept differences in values as each contributes to discussion.
  c. Help students recognize barriers to effective group action and discuss ways and means of handling these situations.
  d. Demonstrate various roles students must learn to play in the group discussion process and provide opportunities for them to function in these roles.
4. Provide informal atmosphere allowing for freedom of expression without criticism or ridicule.
5. Provide physical arrangements so that all students have face-to-face contact with each other and the teacher, everyone can hear, and seating is comfortable yet fosters discussion.
6. Provide for adequate introductions.
7. Be familiar with students in order to draw on their knowledge and experiences in assisting them to contribute to discussion.
8. Be well informed about subject matter or provide someone who is an authority on subject; consider use of a consultant in a specialized area as a resource person during discussion.
9. Begin discussion by the following:
  a. Have the problem well defined prior to group meeting.
  b. Assist students to define particular problem they seek to discuss.
10. Help students identify goals and procedure to follow to apply problem-solving techniques to situation.
11. Keep goals before group.
  a. Create discussion by asking "how" or "why" questions.
  b. Pose questions that remind students of their own mental processes and those of others in group.
	1. Accept responsibility for learning how to function effectively as a group participant.
	2. Be prepared with necessary background information pertinent to discussion when topic is assigned prior to group conference; or seek necessary information when needed to solve immediate problems.
	3. Approach discussion with an open mind, allowing free discussion of ideas by others.
	4. *Share* mutual responsibility for defining problem, setting goals, discussing course of action, making recommendations, and evaluating outcomes of the discussion.
	5. Maintain welfare of entire group by the following:
	  a. *Listen* to contributions of others as each views various issues.
	  b. Attempt to understand other person's point of view, regardless of personal beliefs.
	  c. Present own point of view without forcing acceptance.
	  d. Help each other in free expression of ideas.
	  e. Ask questions of one another to clarify various issues or to help reticent participants express themselves.
	  f. Prevent discussion from being dominated by a few persons.
	  g. Support and be responsive to others and their ideas.
	  h. Promote solution to problem.
	  i. Share information about particular situation or other sources of obtaining information.
	  j. Maintain physical arrangements needed to provide opportunities for each member to make contribution and function as unified group.
	6. Clarify points of discussion at frequent intervals in order to maintain understanding of problem, agreement regarding goals, and ways of accomplishing them through systematic problem-solving process.
	7. Diagnose problem areas that are barriers to effective group discussion and seek necessary assistance in resolving them.
	8. Allow time for self-evaluation of group effectiveness at close of conference.
	9. Seek assistance from teacher regarding progress made in solution of problem.
	10. Offer feedback information regarding outcome of action taken as recommended by consensus of group.

Table 3. Techniques for group discussion—cont'd

Teacher or leader responsibilities	Student responsibilities
c. Refrain from answering question; use comments and question to serve as guides in directing inquiry into avenue of learning; follow with relevant questions designed to help students express themselves more clearly.	11. Offer feedback information to teacher regarding value of conference in promoting learning.
12. Maintain atmosphere of group sharing without allowing two-way conversation or argument to dominate discussion.	
13. Remain flexible as discussion proceeds.	
14. Maintain leadership role by leading, knowing when to intervene to clarify issues, using problem-solving techniques or introducing new source materials to solve problem.	
15. Summarize discussion at intervals as necessary to keep goals clarified and to terminate discussion.	
16. Admit own limitations of knowledge when asked questions you cannot answer; refer students to sources or resource persons who can supply needed information.	
17. Encourage group evaluation of progress made through discussion:	
a. Allow students to discuss problems arising from interpersonal relationships in terms of evaluating reasons for behavior and possible solutions to problem.	
b. Ask group to summarize progress made toward solution of problem at intervals during discussion.	
c. Consider follow-up discussions as necessary to provide feedback regarding kind of results obtained through implementation of recommendations by group.	
d. Request follow-up evaluation from students to furnish feedback regarding progress made in learning.	

progress made during the total experience.

Table 3 lists the responsibilities of the teacher and the student and serves as a guide in the adaptation of the group discussion method to a variety of ways of teaching clinical nursing.

The group discussion method lends itself to a variety of adaptations in the teaching of clinical nursing in direct proportion to the teacher's creative ability to make the adaptation. Group discussion methods have been used successfully for a long time in dealing with psychiatric patients and are overly identified with the mental health field. All too often those on the psychiatric nursing faculty are the only ones who understand and utilize group techniques effectively. This can promote the idea that any time one participates in a group, one is in danger of being "therapized," rather than having an opportunity to become open to growing and learning.

The following discussion is centered on ways of applying group methods to the teaching of clinical nursing in many settings.

Team teaching conferences

The concept of team teaching refers to the use of two or more teachers, each having special competencies and knowledge in the cooperative planning, teaching, supervision, and evaluation of a given group of students. This approach has many variations in the utilization of teaching personnel, according to the objectives to be achieved. It involves cooperative planning by the team teachers in terms of material to be taught to the total group of students; which teacher can best teach each aspect of content; material to be taught by group discussion within the clinical setting; kinds of clinical experiences needed to apply the theoretical information; and evaluation of the students' progress in class, clinical learning, and group discussion. This team approach implies a sharing of knowledge among faculty as well as students. All members of the teaching team work as a group by attending all formal class sessions.

The team teaching conference utilizes each team teacher as a leader of a group discussion, offering students the opportunity to discuss the implications of the theoretical information for application to selected clinical nursing experiences and subsequent evaluation of clinical performance. This approach is the most effective when it is kept flexible enough to provide the students with the teacher or teachers who can make the most valuable contribution to the particular group discussion session. Thus, consideration should be given to the utilization of those faculty members or related personnel who could make the best contribution rather than rigidly adhering to the use of faculty within the confines of a given clinical area or group.

When individual faculty members recognize the contribution a given faculty member can make to the presenting problem, regardless of the clinical specialty, an environment fostering freedom to learn, to seek new knowledge, and to develop imaginative ideas is established. This climate fosters faculty cohesiveness, enabling it to function effectively. The clinical teacher who assumes responsibility as coordinator of the teaching team must possess those qualities desirable of any group leader, and each team teacher must assume those responsibilities desirable for making cooperative contributions to the team. The success of the team teaching conference depends on the degree to which the team can function as a dynamic, cohesive group that serves as a model for students in the conduct of their group discussions.

Nursing care conference

The clinical nursing conference has come to be recognized as a pivotal component of the total teaching plan in clinical nursing. The nursing care conference consists of a group discussion using problem-solving techniques* to determine ways of providing care for patients to whom students are assigned as a part of their clinical nursing experience. The use of problem-solving techniques constitutes the core of the nursing care conference, with each new patient situation calling for a solution.

Problem-solving discussions arise from three sources: (1) the objectives of the clinical nursing program, (2) the patients, and (3) the students. The teacher and the students are responsible for knowing the objectives to be accomplished for a given situation, and to this end they plan for appropriate learning experiences. A danger of this lies in its application to the learning situation to the extent that the patients' needs and often the students' needs are lost in the course objectives. There is evidence o show that the clinical nursing conferences have been used to serve many masters. Some of these practices must be modified if we truly seek to educate today's students beyond the point of perpetuating the past—to be open-minded enough to accept new ideas and develop-

---

*Problem-solving in this instance refers to the practice of the same steps of problem-solving used in other kinds of learning situations: identifying, defining, and analyzing a problem; collecting data; stating and testing possible solutions; and making conclusions and recommendations.

ments activating their own creative potentials for coping with today's problems and for understanding the future.

It is time to recognize that dynamic, creative clinical nursing experiences have no room for such practices as the use of a master plan of arbitrarily set numbers of scheduled nursing care conferences per week covering predetermined nursing care subject areas or the use of the clinical nursing conference time to continue formal theory classes in order to "cover" all of the content. Although the care conference for students is also touted as preliminary to such conferences in practice, teachers should also be honest: in many settings truly creative, problem-solving conferences of nursing staff are rare. Students may be encouraged to identify the causes of this and to anticipate how they will receive collegial assistance in solving problems once in practice.

There is need for *spontaneity* in terms of the presenting problems, which are reality to the patient and to the student and must be dealt with as such before learning can occur. Students need opportunities to learn to cope with and *work through* the "now problems" as they perceive or are confronted with them in their daily nursing experiences. Such an approach can be accomplished effectively through the use of on-the-spot, problem-solving nursing care conferences. For example, if the current unit of study and clinical nursing experience is related to the nursing care of patients with chronic respiratory diseases, the clinical nursing conferences are determined by the problems as they present themselves, either through needs expressed by patients or perceived by students. The same techniques for discussion and problem-solving are used, but the timing of the conferences and the subject of the discussions arise from the spontaneity of the situation rather than from a fixed sequence of topics during a specific course. The nursing care conference will contribute to the total objectives, but the problems for the discussion arise from the learning situation itself, with action based on the learner's abilities at the given time.

These on-the-spot clinical nursing conferences must be in an environment of informality and permissiveness fostering student involvement in problem-solving discussions. The teacher must be flexible enough to allow spontaneity, yet know how and when to channel the discussion by helping students to examine their contributions, apply previous learning to the current situation, determine how current information may lead to other areas to be explored, and see relationships between their findings and how they contribute to the immediate problem and to the long-range objectives of the total learning experience. Through the teacher's ability to lead the group discussion from the background the objectives are met, but the students have had the opportunity to be actively involved in discussions of nursing care problems as they perceived them. This ability is characterized by the teacher who is constantly aware of presenting problems and willingly adjusts the teaching plans accordingly; raises questions, poses ideas for discussion, and suggests related readings; recalls previously learned concepts as they relate to the problem under discussion; utilizes the potential contribution of each student in the most favorable light; and summarizes the problem in terms of its immediate effect on the patient and its total learning contribution.

While the nursing care conference should be patterned in accord with the basic principles of group discussion techniques and problem-solving processes, it should also be aimed at helping students use information in creative ways. The nursing care conference viewed as a creative act provides a learning environment that fosters opportunities for students to *think through* challenging and worthwhile problems, allowing for their completion and evaluation while simultaneously learning new subject matter. The extent to which the clinical nursing conference contributes to the development of the student's creative potential is dependent on the teacher's ability to set the stage for each learning situation. This freedom to explore problems and seek their solution with imaginative ideas carries with it the responsibility for evaluating them in terms of their effectiveness and safety in reaching the desired goals. One example of such an approach is that described by Heller who initiated and developed her own discussion group by asking a group of handicapped patients to meet together to discuss their common concerns and needs while gaining understanding and emotional support from one another.[14]

Nursing team conference

Application of the basic concept of the clinical nursing conference and the principles of group dynamics is extended to the clinical setting as students pursue clinical nursing experiences within the framework of the nursing team and participate in the nursing team conferences.

Regardless of the structural organization of the nursing team in a given setting, the nursing team conference is used to plan for the daily continuity of nursing care that best meets the patients' needs. The team leader reviews the patients in terms of current objectives of nursing care and ways of altering the nursing care plan to meet the changing needs of the patients. Team members, professional and nonprofessional, discuss their observations and findings regarding the patients and their responses to treatment and nursing care. Problems are identified by the group, and modifications in the nursing care plan are suggested in an attempt to solve the problems. Resource persons from other disciplines are often utilized in arriving at a satisfactory plan of action.

Where these conferences occur in practice settings, students will be expected to participate as team members and team leaders. If students have been provided with opportunities to become active, creative participants in clinical nursing conferences, transfer of learning should assist them in participation in the nursing team conferences. An article by Melody and Clark described a variation of the team conference as "walking-planning rounds."[15] Another article by Hall and Little described how a group of students representing several clinical areas worked as a team to systemically evaluate patient care through the use of group dynamics.[16] Creative clinical teachers concerned with the teaching of basic concepts of team nursing to upper division students could pursue these approaches and modify them to meet their particular situation.

The nursing team conference as a teaching tool offers valuable opportunities for learning. The ability to observe, report, and analyze significant findings is put to its greatest test as students are confronted with this daily responsibility. Concomitant values gained by this type of experience are related to the ability to share knowledge of patients' needs and to work cooperatively with other members of the nursing team and total health team. Such experiences inevitably lead to the improved performance of nursing care activities in the clinical nursing setting.

Nursing clinic

The nursing clinic or patient presentation utilizes the presence of a selected patient as its focus for group discussion. It affords a direct experience in the discussion of principles and practices of nursing care relative to a given patient. The purpose is the improvement of nursing care. Students have the opportunity to sharpen their observation and interviewing skills while simultaneously developing increased ability to see relationships between the patient's concept of his health and nursing problems and his resources for coping with the total problem and the nurse's concept of the patient's problem and how it might be solved.

The most effective nursing clinics are those that are planned, which involves (1) determining the purpose; (2) selecting a patient for whom students have given nursing care; (3) securing the patient's consent and proper legal clearance; (4) selecting the setting to be used—the patient's bedside or a conference room visited by the patient; and (5) providing advance preparation of the student in terms of the name of the patient, the purpose, place, date and time, and any specific instructions regarding preparation for the discussion.

The group discussion generally consists of three phases: (1) the introduction, (2) the patient-centered discussion, and (3) the evaluation discussion; the patient is present only during phase two. The introductory phase serves to acquaint the students with the patient's background, presenting nursing care situation, the purpose of the discussion, significant observations, types of questions to be asked, and needed information. During the patient-centered discussion, a few simply asked questions directed to the patient are usually sufficient for obtaining the needed information. Ample opportunities should be allowed for patients to verbalize their needs and how they see their particular problem. Sometimes demonstrating a particular nursing care measure or allowing the patient to do so is sufficient for meeting the purpose. When the patient appears unresponsive or tired, it is wise to close the discussion, even though the purpose may not have been accomplished. The evaluation discussion offers an excellent opportunity for students to evaluate the patient's behavior, ability to solve his own problems, and various other aspects. The students can be evaluated in terms of their observations and ability to use problem-solving techniques. The discussion should be summarized in terms of application of background knowledge to the given nursing care problem and goals accomplished, with provisions made for follow-up on comparisons between the students' views of the patient's problems and the patient's views of his problems. Such an approach opens the door to many other ways of developing the student's ability to respond to the expressed needs of a variety of patients.

This same basic pattern can be adapted easily for use in planning and implementing interdisciplinary patient-centered clinics. The modification would be in terms of identify-ing kinds of input needed from each team member and seeking appropriate contributions from each.

Nursing care study

Closely aligned with the nursing care conference and nursing clinic is the nursing care study. Although the nursing care study is generally viewed as an individual learning activity rather than a group project, the nursing care conference and clinic serve as vehicles for the development, study, evaluation, and implementation of the nursing care study as presented by the student. In addition, the clinical teacher and the student work on a tutorial basis in the development of the study and preparation of the report. Thus, it is a group technique in that the student and teacher are a group of two during its development, and it is frequently presented, formally or informally, to other students in a group meeting.

The nursing care study is a problem solving activity whereby the student undertakes the comprehensive assessment of a particular patient's nursing problems leading to the planning, implementing, and evaluating of appropriate nursing care measures. It provides opportunities for the application of previously learned knowledge and skills to a patient for whom the student is providing daily nursing care. Development of a nursing care study presupposes that the student gives consideration to the physical, emotional, and social factors affecting the nursing care needs of the patients, and it includes services of other health team members in planning for adequate continuity of health care.

The range of possibilities for problem-solving and making judgments regarding nursing care and health maintenance is as simple or as complex as the particular patient selected for study. Thus, the patient must be within the realm of comprehension and abilities of the individual student. The student must have sufficient background information to cope with the problems yet have an opportunity to channel previous learning into new avenues of thought with each successive study. Students also need sufficient library facilities and time to pursue the comprehensive study *while actually giving nursing care to the patient.*

Although the use of the nursing care study continues to flourish as a method of teaching in clinical nursing, creativity in its use is long overdue. Suggestions for fostering the creative use of this tool follow:

1. When students are exposed to a total program of clinical nursing that builds on a problem-solving, patient-centered nursing care approach, the concept becomes an integral part of the pattern of learning they pursue. We do not require *x* number of clinical conferences, seminars, or clinics for each student in each clinical area; therefore the nursing care study should be viewed within this same context of flexibility in the use of methods in the teaching of clinical nursing.

2. As a natural corollary, the nursing care study should be used when the need exists at a particular time for a particular student, because it is the *best method* to use in accomplishing the objective. If used flexibly, students might apply this teaching method in each clinical area, in some clinical areas, or in none at all.

3. Students who experience the prevailing philosophy of flexibility in the use of teaching methods will not resist or question the use or lack of it any more than any other method, and perhaps less than those who are required to submit a quota of *x* number of nursing care studies.

4. Flexible use of nursing care studies necessitates preparing and presenting the study as an integral part of the clinical experience.

5. Guidelines for preparing nursing care studies should be limited to the basic directions regarding the format of the written report, leaving opportunities for the students to organize their materials and approaches to problem-solving according to their own abilities.

For example, Hepler describes a nursing care study written in free verse by a student who was willing to use a creative approach to a written assignment.[17]

6. A written nursing care study offers opportunities for students to learn to organize their thinking and writing in logical order and acceptable form; meaningful relationships between theory and its application to actual patient problems are perceived when the student presents the care study orally to the group members.

7. The nursing care conference and clinic serve as useful media for the discussion of the nursing care study from the early identification of the problem through periodic progress reports and final evaluation and follow-up reports. Within this framework the discussion takes on new meanings for the individual student and for the group conference members.

8. Further investigation should be directed toward creating new combinations or new approaches to the use of the nursing care study or toward determining ways of combining the use of the nursing care study with other methods of teaching such as case analysis or role-playing.

The effective use of the nursing care study will flourish in the hands of those who use it creatively; it will perish in the hands of those who cling to it as an end in itself.

Process record

Like the nursing care study the process record usually is considered an individual learning technique, but functionally it can be considered an effective adjunct to the written nursing care study and to the group discussion of specific patients during the nursing care conference.

The process record consists of the verbal and nonverbal communications between two individuals, along with observations on their meaning, for the purpose of assessing the interactions to improve understandings and interpersonal relationships. Within the context of clinical nursing, the process record can be used to study nurse interaction with patients, patients' families, other health team members, and other nurses. Some schools of nursing are using the concepts of the process record in requiring students to develop clinical diaries.

Use of the process record in clinical nursing as a tool for developing skills of nurse-patient relationships should follow a logical pattern of (1) teacher-student collaboration in defining the specific objectives to be accomplished through the use of the tool; (2) discussion of the relationship between the use of the process record and the accomplishment of the established goals; (3) careful, detailed explanation of the total observation, interviewing, and recording process; (4) preparation of the patient for the experience; (5) the student's reporting of the interaction soon after its occurrence, including the student's feelings, actions, and interpretations of feelings and actions communicated by the patient; (6) the student's analysis of recordings to serve as clues to self-understanding and understanding of the patient's needs; (7) individual student-teacher conferences for purposes of providing immediate feedback regarding the student's growth in self-understanding and understanding of the patients; and (8) the use of clinical nursing conferences for discussion of significant findings by students who are willing to share their experiences with others.

While this pattern for using the process record may seem relatively simple, its purpose implies the necessity for certain learning conditions. First and foremost, the teacher must have an understanding of the dynamics of human behavior, be highly skilled in the use of the technique, and know how to *guide* students through learning to analyze and evaluate communications and improve skills in interpersonal relationships. The purpose of using process recordings varies with the objectives for learning in a given clinical setting and with the level of ability of the students; therefore, each teacher must determine the exact purposes

that can be accomplished realistically. For beginning students the focus should be on *one* purpose, such as dealing with verbal communications as they relate to the student's self-understanding and understanding of the patient. Subsequent achievement of each purpose is a building process ultimately leading to the achievement of related purposes requiring integrated understanding of the total process of interpersonal relationships. The degree to which the technique effectively meets the intended purposes is in direct proportion to the degree to which the total use of the process record is understood by the teacher and the student.

The teacher should also consider such timing variables as the total length of time available for accomplishing the desired purposes in using the process record, the student-faculty ratio relative to the amount of individual supervision needed for each student, and the provision of time for making recordings immediately after interaction experiences. During the total course of the process recording, students must experience a learning milieu that fosters freedom of expression in a supportive manner while learning to build satisfying interpersonal relationships.

In preparation for recording interactions, students should have been introduced to the procedural measures used to protect the patient's confidential communications, received instruction regarding the fundamental principles of observation, interviewing, and recording, and received specific information regarding what to record to meet the specific purpose. The successful use of the process record as a learning experience is dependent on the cooperative teacher-student analysis of the data. The best results are obtained by those teachers who make themselves available for consultation as needs arise in addition to the regularly scheduled individual conferences. By raising questions the teacher furnishes leads for students to explore in determining the cause-and-effect relationships of given responses with a view toward changing their course of action. Through these individual discussions students grow in self-awareness by recognizing misunderstandings of behavior, glaring omissions of responses to patients and vice versa, and certain emerging patterns of behavior that significantly affect the interaction.

When students learn to recognize these recurrent patterns of behavior, the teacher assists them in validating their clues; this leads to sound conclusions regarding self-understanding and ways of improving interactions with others. The self-evaluation process inherent in the use of this technique can be a valuable adjunct to the student's continued growth. The very act of recording and analyzing the data related to interactions can furnish clues to help the students look more objectively at themselves and difficult situations. Whether or not this feature is used by the teacher as an additional tool depends on the situation and the ability of those involved to view it objectively. The self-knowledge gained by the experience is sacred to the student, cannot be taken away, and need not be shared with anyone unless the student so desires; but it serves as a primary motivating factor in the future effectiveness of that student as a human being.

When there is a prevailing climate of permissiveness, group sharing of data analysis can be a rewarding experience. The process recording, properly constructed, exposes the student's feelings in the situation; therefore, the teacher should always seek the student's permission for sharing the process recording analysis with the group. When this is discussed with the group, students frequently overcome some of their anxieties by knowing that others have experienced similar kinds of feelings or difficulties in dealing with nurse-patient interactions.

There has been a tendency for schools of nursing to utilize the process record as an integral and required part of the clinical teaching programs in the areas of psychiatric nursing and public health nursing, but it can be used effectively in any or all of the clinical nursing areas.

The criteria for selection of the use of the process record as a method of teaching lie not in the kind of clinical nursing subject to be taught but in the ability of teachers to use it effectively and in the degree to which it meets the objectives and desired outcomes for the given nursing situation. Like the nursing care study, use of the process record as a method of teaching should be in terms of these criteria rather than in terms of setting rigid requirements for its use within a given clinical nursing situation or within the total curriculum.

Role-playing

The group conference method lends itself for modification in the use of role-playing. Role-playing involves the acting out of roles related to problems involving human relations. The total group is involved in the analysis of behaviors portrayed in the role-playing situation for the purpose of increasing their insights into similar problems and understanding ways of dealing with them. When group members are provided with opportunities to "live through" problem situations, they gain increased understanding of themselves and learn how to establish relationships. Use of this tool in a group-centered classroom environment affords students opportunities to try out new approaches to establishing interpersonal relationships, to make mistakes, and to work with a particular problem until it is satisfactorily resolved without the stress of performing in a patient situation.

Recording role-playing situations on audio or videotape allows the players to review their own actions and reactions, as well as to receive feedback from the audience. Multiple replays of the same role-playing can be used to bring out a broader or deeper understanding of the interaction. The previously described responsibilities of teachers and students in the group discussion technique apply equally to this method.

For best results in meeting the desired objectives of a given role-playing situation, it is desirable to adopt a format using the following steps in logical sequence.

Selection of a problem. The problem should arise from the group and should be clear and specifically related to a human relations situation that serves a useful purpose within the context of the material being studied.

Construction of the role-playing situation. The purpose of the role-playing session serves as the guide for preparing the design by providing enough content to simulate reality and afford players and observers an orientation to the problem. Situations can be planned by the total group in an on-the-spot manner, by a subcommittee who brings the plan to the total group, or by the teacher or leader who may use an actual case to illustrate the problem.

Casting the players. Players should *always* be selected in terms of their willingness to act in order to avoid misinterpretation of the role and to preserve the individual's self-esteem. The most effective casting is obtained by soliciting volunteers, suggestions made from the group, or selections made by the teacher or planning committee. The best rule to follow is to select persons who appear to be able to carry the role effectively without feeling threatened or exposed by it. Spontaneity is the key to success in the use of this technique; therefore, advance preparation of role-players should be avoided.

Briefing. The teacher or group leader should give a brief review of the selected problem, the purposes to be studied, and the general design of the plan for presenting the role-playing. The players are briefed regarding the role each is to play relative to the purposes of the presentation, but under no circumstances should there be an attempt to instruct the players in what to say or how to act or any form of a script provided. The pattern for briefing the players, whether singly or together, depends on the purpose of the problem situation and the resultant kind of data needed for analysis. Sometimes the objectives are accomplished better if each player is unaware of the role each will play; at other times all players may need to work together to present the data needed for analysis by the group. To preserve spontaneity, a period of 5 minutes is all that should be allowed to help the players warm up to the action. This can be provided while the teacher is briefing the audience.

Briefing the audience consists of advising them regarding the kinds of things to be observed to evaluate the outcomes. Observations may take on many forms: reactions and actions taken by each player, description of the role played by each player, evaluation of the effectiveness of each player's contribution to the total purposes of the demonstration, or reversal of roles that occur, either intentional or nonintentional. Audience participants may be asked to observe for a specific kind of data or for an analysis of the critical issues. Certain individuals may be asked to observe behavior exhibited by a particular player, allowing them to identify with that person. There are unlimited opportunities for flexibility in both the role-playing and the observations, depending on the purposes sought in using this method. Of greatest importance is that the action be spontaneous and that, hopefully, the players can remain in their roles throughout the presentation.

Role-playing action. The scene is played as simply and succinctly as possible. As soon as the purpose is achieved, enough behavior is shown to analyze the problem or to predict what would happen if the action continued, the players have reached an impasse, or a natural closing occurs, the scene may be cut. The timing for most role-playing episodes is not more than 15 minutes, and is often less.

Discussion and analysis of action. Regardless of who is engaged in the discussion, care must be taken to prevent it from centering on the acting abilities of the players; rather, discussion should be focused on the contributions made by the players toward an understanding of the problem they were attempting to solve. Constant effort must be made to relate the discussion to the problem and its purposes. It often is helpful if the role character names are retained during the discussion to help the players focus their thinking about the problem in terms of the role played. Generally the role-players are given the first opportunities to discuss the action in terms of how each felt about the role as he played it at the time and how this ultimately contributes to the understanding of the total problem. In essence the players are analyzing the characters they portray rather than themselves; this sets the stage for audience participants to do likewise. There is additional value in asking the players to discuss their feelings about the situation as they played their roles, in order to gain increased self-understanding regarding the behavior.

From the observer's viewpoint the discussion should be data about their observations in relationship to the purpose of the scene. Particular efforts should be made to avoid discussion of personal opinions concerning what should or should not have been done by the players.

The teacher can channel this discussion in a positive direction through the use of thought-provoking questions and other previously mentioned group discussion techniques appropriate to the situation.

Evaluation. After the group discussion the teacher should conduct an evaluative summary of the group thinking regarding conclusions or generalizations about the behavior observed, leading to greater understanding of human behavior as it affects a given problem and applies to other problems; ways of improving total group practices in the situation; effectiveness of the role-playing scene in meeting the purpose for which it was intended; and suggestions for changes needed to improve the use of the technique. Students also should have an opportunity to evaluate their own feelings regarding their role-playing and its effectiveness in terms of learning value. If the goal is related to the development of certain skills in interpersonal relationships, audiotape or videotape recordings of the role-playing serve as a valuable self-evaluation tool. At the close of the session plans should be made for providing further ways of practicing the basic concepts expressed by the role-playing scene. When indicated, the situation can be replayed using the recommended changes regarding the interaction or a role-reversal approach for further study and evaluation by the group.

The use of role-playing as a tool for promoting understanding of human behavior has a direct application to a wide range of nursing situations. The spontaneity of this technique is most helpful in illustrating behavior problems encountered by students. During clinical nursing care conferences, particularly conferences used to discuss the immediate problems of the day, students frequently express concern regarding ways of effectively handling human behavior problems such as anxiety of newly hospitalized children and adults; reactions of patients fearing procedures, treatments, or surgery; separation anxieties displayed by hospitalized patients and their families; reactions of patients undergoing treatment of conditions carrying a social stigma; reactions of patients to their diagnoses; and preparing patients for self-care activities. The use of role-playing episodes as a means of understanding these kinds of problems allows opportunities for students to identify with the patient and others in the given situation and to analyze the problem, including identifying the interaction precipitating the problem, understanding the basis for the reactions, and determining ways of establishing a more satisfactory relationship. While it may not be possible to improve the presenting problem, active involvement allows for transfer of learning from this particular situation to other similar ones. In other instances role-playing can be used to assist students in developing skill in communicating with patients, either for a specific purpose or for general application to any nursing situation.

For students developing leadership skills, role-playing techniques have uses in helping them develop insights into relationships or ideas for effecting change in human relationships in a wide range of daily activities related to supervisory functions. In this instance nurses have the opportunity to play their own roles, expressing their own feelings and reactions to a given situation; or there may be a reversal of roles so that the nurses play the part of the other person, expressing their own perceptions of that role.

Role-playing has multiple applications to the total field of clinical nursing because it offers dynamic learning experiences designed to minimize misconceptions and maximize individual and group understanding and acceptance of human behavior. Its value lies in its total group involvement, either through observing or through participating in a spontaneous presentation as perceived by the role-players and the observers. Each role-player identifies with a specific person contributing to the situation, while the observers identify with one or more role-players. All group participants have the opportunity to examine their feelings and attitudes while analyzing the total problem as revealed through the actions of the role-players. This technique is negated when the clinical teacher uses it as an entertainment gimmick, provides a script for the players, or fails to follow the episode with a critique.

The seminar

Examination of course descriptions in school of nursing bulletins suggests that there exist divergent and frequently fallacious concepts of the seminar as a teaching method. Strictly, the term *seminar* refers to a small group of graduate students engaged in original research under the guidance of a knowledgeable professor. However, as educational practices change and students become more sophisticated and research becomes more common, the concept of the seminar takes on new meanings and new uses. In general the seminar consists of a scientific approach to the study of a selected problem. It involves a discussion of the problem using a small group of students and a teacher who is an expert in the field of study. The seminar differs from other group discussion methods in that it approaches the investigation of a presenting problem by individual library research, data collection, and analysis to produce tentative findings for the preparation of a written report; oral presentation of the report; discussion of the report by the group participants for further analysis and evaluation of data, lead-

ing to conclusions and recommendations; and directive, evaluative contributions by the teacher. Selection may be a single problem for study by the total group, a problem shared by several group members, or individual subproblems studied by each member and presented as part of the total problem. The nature of the seminar method usually requires a series of sessions for completion of study of the problem.

The effectiveness of the seminar is proportional to the ability of the teacher to direct the total process; the teacher's knowledge as an expert in the field; the students' abilities to employ the problem-solving skills of effective use of the library, data collection, and objective interpretation of the findings as opposed to personal bias; and the students' ability to use group discussion techniques effectively.

The use of the seminar as a teaching method for clinical nursing in the undergraduate curriculum might be best described as *emerging;* that is, its use prior to the 1960s was obscured by the prevalence of pedantic teaching practices. As problem-solving approaches to teaching nursing continue to develop in the direction of increasingly sophisticated patterns of learning, the seminar is emerging as an effective means of providing substance to the "routine" approach to problem-solving. Assuming that there is mutual teacher-student understanding of its use, the seminar has potential as a valuable teaching method, either in its "purest" sense or in modifications of its use within a broader context.

The seminar method could be introduced early in the course of the nursing program by utilizing the students' problems of adjusting to nursing situations as the focus for developing beginning problem-solving skills. In this instance the teacher would play a strong leadership role in moving the problem-solving discussion in the direction of the self-actualization of the students in terms of professional responsibilities, while helping them integrate, synthesize, and apply knowledge from the social, psychological, and physical sciences to the solution of the problem. Each succeeding experience in the seminar discussion could serve to bridge the gap between learned theory and its application to increasingly complex nursing situations.

The senior seminar, albeit a misnomer, has currently become a popular method for teaching in upper division courses. Most commonly it is used in discussions aimed at determining ways of managing problems related to the care, communication, collaboration, and coordination functions of the nurse placed in a leadership position in the clinical areas. The seminar also may be used at this level for the purpose of determining ways of maintaining and improving the health status of patients with complex nursing problems in a variety of clinical settings. An experiment in the effective use of the senior seminar for this purpose is described by Hipps.[18]

Use of the seminar method on a continuum from the beginning clinical nursing course through the upper division courses should allow for the student's progression from the role of a group participant to the role of a student leader. Creativity in the use of this method largely depends on the teacher's ability to assist students in assuming increased responsibility for solving typical nursing problems through the syntheses of accumulated knowledge, skills, and experiences into an integrated whole.

Case analysis method

The seminar and role-playing methods particularly lend themselves to discussions involving case analysis. This method of teaching refers to group analysis of a case history for the purpose of developing skill in reflective thinking by defining problems to be solved, discussing relevant data and various sides of the issues, and verifying facts to make judgments. Learning is focused on decision-making regarding concrete problems related to real-life situations, but the problems can be viewed more objectively because the students are not personally involved.

Use of this method requires a complexity

of thinking and action on the part of the students and the teacher. Students are required to study the case history and do extensive reading as advance preparation for the required analysis and decision-making discussions. They then are faced with the task of analyzing significant factors gleaned from a maze of possible ideas and charged with the responsibility for making their own decisions. All of this involves learning from one another and being able to communicate ideas to others in a way that generates new thought patterns. The teacher has the responsibility for providing appropriate case history material and must be skillful in the use of the seminar technique, keeping the discussion moving without forcing a preconceived outcome on the group, yet ready to summarize the ongoing discussion as necessary to keep it centered on the problem.

The creative teacher in clinical nursing could utilize this method of teaching nurse-patient behavior and leadership skills. But to use it successfully the teacher must meet the following requisites: (1) careful study of the technique involved; (2) extensive exploration of case histories that are realistic, within the realm of knowledge of the group, and contain enough information to permit analysis and decision-making; and (3) careful preparation of the group participants regarding the purpose of the study, the technique used, and needed advance preparation for a given case.

Because of its limited use in the basic nursing curriculum, a detailed description of this technique has not been included. For further assistance in using this teaching method, refer to the References.[19-21]

Case incident method

A variant of the case analysis was originated by the Pigors as the incident process.[22,23] This method is emerging as a promising means of inquiry that can be used effectively in undergraduate curricula to help students develop skill in reflective thinking leading to decision-making. The case analysis method is modified by (1) using a brief statement of a critical incident relative to the current life situation faced by the learner that requires an immediate decision; (2) requiring students to furnish the missing information through a process of inquiry leading to a description of how they would approach the situation along with the reasons for their decisions; (3) group analysis of individual statements to clarify and summarize decisions reached; and (4) application of major findings to the immediate situation along with making generalizations regarding the implications of the findings for the total milieu of the incident.

The Pigors suggest a five-step procedure,[24] which utilizes a number of subtechniques within the structure of the seminar sessions for the purpose of eliciting sound decisions regarding the inquiring into the specific incident:

1. *Studying an incident.* The incident provided by the seminar leader (teacher or student) is studied individually to determine significant factors to be pursued, leading to the decision to be made.

2. *Gathering and organizing information on the case as a whole.* Individuals armed with their own ideas regarding background information meet together to question the leader (who has the facts about the case by virtue of having presented it) about the kind of facts needed and to plan constructive action on underlying issues. The leader summarizes the facts in terms of information needed to build a sound decision for coping with the incident.

3. *Formulating an issue for decision and action.* Group members use the summary of facts to identify key factors of the incident. Visual diagrams of these factors assist the group in interpreting their interrelationships to the incident as a whole. From this information the group formulates a single, objective statement of the issue for decision.

4. *Decision and reasoning.* The process of synthesizing the decision involves four interrelated successive steps: (a) the decision regarding the incident along with the reasoning underlying it is written by individual participants and used as background information for further group study; (b) small groups collaborate in discussing a decision to be made and reasons for the decisions; (c) each small group either reports or role-plays their findings for the total group, followed by a summary discussion of differences and similarities of the decisions and the reasoning in reaching the decisions; and (d) the group leader describes the actual decision, action taken, and immediate results of the incident at the time of its occurrence; the group then appraises the actual situation by comparing it to the suggestions of each small group.

5. *Reflecting on the case as a whole.* The group examines the final decision and reasoning regarding the incident in terms of its broad application to other major issues linked to, yet beyond, the immediate problem.

While the incident process is not designed for use in teaching nursing content, it offers the creative teacher a valuable means of teaching students in the clinical setting to acquire skills in making decisions based on reasoned inquiry. This relatively new approach offers possibilities for the creative teacher who seeks to help students deal more effectively with human relations problems in the nursing setting. Because this method deals with a selected incident, the creative teacher can select the incident and the approaches used to best meet the desired level of skill to be learned. For beginning students the teacher would probably serve as the leader in presenting the incident and in guiding the direction of its application and discussion. As students progress in their ability to supply background information and reach workable decisions, variations in ways of discussing these decisions can be made, and the leadership role can shift from the teacher to the students themselves. Each successive experience in this method of inquiry should serve students to develop increasingly self-directive inquiry leading to skills in making reasoned decisions. As this method of inquiry emerges, it behooves the creative teacher to investigate its possibilities for providing a fresh approach to the teaching of the decision-making aspects of clinical nursing.

In retrospect, all areas of clinical nursing provide a fertile field for various group discussion techniques. But it cannot be overemphasized that their successful use depends on the individual learner's understanding of the process in terms of acceptance of responsibilities inherent in participation and the skill with which the teacher or group leader uses democratic leadership techniques.

EDUCATIONAL COMMUNICATION MEDIA ADAPTABLE FOR CREATIVE TEACHING IN CLINICAL NURSING

Educational communication media refer to the wide range of audiovisual materials used to convey ideas from one person to another through the use of the sensory organs. As part of the total learning environment, they offer avenues for learning, which provide new perceptual understanding and greater conceptual development.

Each educational communication medium must be selected for its use in facilitating the desired changes in a given situation. Collectively educational communication media are chosen for two distinct and quite different purposes:

1. As integrated parts of the total teaching-learning environment they complement the teacher's use of selected teaching methods by clarifying and simplifying the communications, arousing interest and attention leading to motivation for learning, and providing auditory, visual, and other sensory experiences leading to increased concrete understanding and reinforcement of communicated information. They are not meant to be used as substitutes for the teacher or for those methods selected for teaching a given course.

2. They serve as the *means* of providing the selected factual information and directing the routine student activities in the teaching-learning situation. This systematic approach to learning provides optimal opportunities for students to learn through the use of multimedia devices with a minimal amount of personal involvement by the teacher. Detailed discussion of this approach appears later in the chapter.

Limiting the use of educational communication media to teaching clinical nursing necessitates the elimination of detailed information regarding the principles involved in their utilization within the total learning environment. Discussion is confined to basic guidelines for selection and use of educational communication media and descriptions of those media adapted for use in teaching clinical nursing.

With the growth of instructional technologies it is becoming increasingly apparent that every school of nursing needs an organized, service-centered system for coordinating and administering its educational communication media as an integral part of the teaching-learning process. The program should be designed and administered by a specialist in the field whose primary goal is coordinating faculty action to secure maximum utilization of available services. The nucleus of such a program is the production laboratory, which provides facilities, equipment, and supplies for preparing teaching materials. Upon request, the educational communication media specialist consults with the faculty to determine the goals to be accomplished in a given situation and then proceeds to develop the appropriate materials for use. Additional services for the faculty include (1) systematic storage of all types of materials and equipment; (2) a central index registering all holdings; (3) a central index of sources for obtaining additional educational communication media; (4) a checkout system for use of holdings and for keeping a perpetual inventory; (5) continuous maintenance of equipment; (6) opportunities to preview new films, slides, and tapes and test other new devices; (7) guidance in securing proper legal clearance for the production and utilization of educational communication media; (8) technical assistance in producing and using educational communication media and adapting them for use in a particular teaching situation; (9) operation of equipment as needed by faculty; and (10) participation in an organized, continuous evaluation program to determine the extent to which the educational communication media meet the desired objectives and to assess the functional efficiency of the mechanical equipment.

Schools not in a position to invest in this kind of program can seek consultation on technical matters from experts in the local or regional universities, colleges, or secondary schools.

Educational materials produced to meet the total objectives of a course or curriculum area become the property of the respective department or school, to be made available to those responsible for teaching in that particular course or curriculum area. Such an arrangement avoids duplication of time, effort, and materials as well as repetitive use of the same materials. Individual faculty members who contribute to the collection of educational communication media experience the satisfaction that comes from sharing one's resources with others.

Selection and use of educational communication media

As the teaching-learning process shifts from the traditional formal patterns of teaching to the use of informal teaching methods, the following criteria are suggested for use in evaluating, selecting, and utilizing those educational communication media adaptable to the teaching of clinical nursing.

Criteria for evaluation and selection of educational communication media

1. All media should be evaluated carefully to determine the medium most appropriate for meeting the purposes of the nursing program and the specific experiences or problems being considered at a given point in time. The educational communication media must be selected according to the curriculum objectives as opposed to planning the course or clinical experience to conform to the selected medium.

2. The selected medium must be within the range of the student's experience, intelligence, and ability level. This implies evaluation of materials on a continuum from the simple to the complex. For example, does it follow the general pattern of theory and clinical experience to serve as reinforcement? Is it unrelated, advanced material for which students have had no preparation? Is it elementary material offering no new motivation for learning?

3. All educational communication media should be previewed to determine authenticity, recency, validity, reliability, objectivity, clarity, aesthetic discernment, and appropriateness as a model in the use of current, sound educational practices.

4. The educational communication medium must be adaptable for use in a designated situation. For example, one would need to make provision for viewing a closed circuit television program, or because of space limitations one might need to restrict the use of media requiring bulky equipment.

5. Educational communication media selected for use should be readily available. The teacher should plan ahead for reserving necessary equipment and rooms and ordering films, slides, videotapes, and other materials. The effectiveness of the media is negated if they are used when available rather than when needed to meet specific behavioral outcomes.

6. Adequate time periods must be planned in order to receive maximum benefit from a selected medium. For example, a field trip must be planned to allow time for transporting students in addition to the time required to meet the objectives of the tour, whereas a film designed to meet

the same objectives could be shown in much less time.

7. Educational communication media should be thoroughly tested for quality of sound, photography, and working condition before the scheduled use; concomitantly the materials must be used by teachers and technicians who are knowledgeable about the mechanical operational requirements of the media.

8. Decisions regarding the cost of a selected educational communication medium should be relative to the degree of use, availability, and overall ability to meet the essential criteria for selection. The teacher must weigh the relative values of using a costly medium against the use of an inferior but inexpensive medium or no medium at all in meeting the objectives for a given learning situation.

The teacher's decision regarding the selection of educational communication media for use as aids to teaching nursing must be determined first by the specific objectives to be accomplished during the students' experiences. This involves two main tasks: (1) evaluation and selection of educational communication media according to established criteria and (2) planning for use of the selected medium in terms of helping the learners perceive its use in meeting the outcomes sought at a given time—basic knowledge needed to develop concepts of the clinical nursing field, application of principles, recognition of relationships, development of specific skills, ability to solve certain kinds of problems of nursing care or management, or learning to establish more effective interpersonal relationships.

Guidelines for use of educational communication media

1. Selected educational communication media must be integrated into the total teaching program rather than left to chance by "displaying" or "showing" them without further discussion of their application to the nursing situation.

2. Students should be prepared for the use of the selected medium by (a) ad-vance reading assignments when indicated; (b) independent study and observation prior to use if facilities are available; (c) demonstration of the proper use of the medium prior to the time students are expected to use it if this is indicated; (d) provision of written instructions for use of the medium as necessary; (e) discussion of a selected medium relative to its origin, purposes, and potential for improving nursing skill; and (f) requesting students to formulate their objectives for participating in, observing, or using the medium as it applies to the given clinical learning situation.

3. Use of the medium should include student-teacher discussions of the significant features and their relationships to the current learning situation in the clinical nursing experience.

4. Opportunities should be provided for summary and follow-up student evaluations of the learning experience in terms of new concepts formed and effectiveness of the medium in promoting clinical learning.

The proper selection and use of educational communication media *complement* rather than *supplement* the teaching methods use in clinical nursing. The media should be viewed as integral parts of the experiences. As such, they serve as motivating forces for students and provide opportunities for learning concepts. A wide range of media is available for use; selection depends on the need for a desired level of learning experience—direct, vicarious, or symbolic.

Although this book discusses direct teaching of clinical nursing, it is neither possible nor desirable to assume that all learning can take place at this level. Therefore, the use of educational communication media becomes a necessary and integral part of learning in clinical nursing by providing a variety of learning experiences and giving perceptual meaning to abstract learning through the use of symbols. The following descriptions of educational communication media are limited to those appearing to have the greatest potential for use by the creative teacher in clinical nursing.

The field trip

The field trip is an opportunity to observe and study objects, materials, processes, social phenomena, and people within their natural environment. Although this definition could refer to any clinical setting as the site for the field trip, it is generally planned outside the established setting. The community offers excellent opportunities for students to gain firsthand knowledge about prevailing community social, economic, health and welfare conditions and services.

In nursing, a properly conducted field trip offers the following learning opportunities: (1) firsthand information regarding the prevailing housing, industrial, economic, public health, and welfare conditions affecting various ethnic and cultural groups of patients; (2) knowledge about the health and welfare services in the community available for patients; (3) information regarding the nurse's professional responsibilities for providing continuity of patient care; (4) ability in observation skills; (5) interview skills when people are the focus of the field trip; (6) validation of previously learned theoretical information; (7) correlation of subjects within the total curriculum; and (8) source material and background information for developing nursing care studies.

Assuming that the objectives for the selected learning activity lend themselves to the use of a field trip, the creative clinical teacher would do well to consider the following questions before proceeding with the necessary plans. Is the projected time allotment sufficient for providing the total learning activities sought by the use of the selected field trip? Does it offer enough opportunities for learning to justify the time taken from other activities? Can the field trip be accomplished without conflicting with activities being required by other teachers? Can the field trip be planned so that it correlates naturally with the current learning needs of the student? Does it provide educational information and experiences commensurate with the ability and experience level of the students without being repetitious of that which has been taught through the use of another media? Will the size of the facilities permit sufficient opportunities for students to observe, interview, or listen without interfering with one another? Can it provide experiences that cannot be provided in any other way? Can the field trip be carried out economically and safely? Does the selected field trip represent principles from which generalizations can be made in applying the knowledge gained to nursing situations? Is there proper legal protection for the trip?

Satisfied that the selected field trip meets the foregoing criteria, the teacher has a threefold responsibility for its successful completion: (1) careful preliminary planning for the trip, (2) supervision of the field trip experience, and (3) follow-up activities to discuss application of new knowledge to the clinical learning setting and teacher-student evaluation of the total field trip.

1. *Preliminary planning.* The teacher's first task is to make a preliminary survey of existing facilities to determine the educational opportunities of each. A card file of such information can be a valuable resource, but only if all teachers assume responsibility for keeping it up-to-date by sharing data gained either through the preliminary survey of facilities or the evaluations made after the field trips.

With the objectives of the desired field trip well in mind, the teacher must make careful preliminary arrangements with the cooperating agency and with the students. A preliminary visit to the selected agency affords opportunity for a two-way evaluation. The teacher sets the stage for the visit by acquainting the agency with information regarding the purpose of the visit, the objectives to be accomplished through the experiences, the level of ability and understanding of the students, the size of the group, and the nature of the activities they wish to pursue. It affords the teacher the opportunity to know key personnel by name and establish rapport with them; to determine the exact available learning experiences needed to meet the objectives; and to determine the adequacy of facilities regarding freedom of use, size, safety factors, visual and acoustical acuity, provisions for physical needs of students, indirect costs, time and place for meeting with the students, and any special scheduling needed for personnel to talk with the group.

Once these preliminary arrangements have been completed, adequate advance arrangements must be made regarding mode of transportation, finances, legal clearance including parental permission if required, exact time schedules to be followed, and directions for routing. Completed planning details should be communicated to the proper administrative officers of the school. As a courtesy to faculty members, a communication describing the proposed visit may help them in planning their clinical programs to avoid duplication or in seeking inclusion in the tour if arrangements permit. If the timing of the field trip conflicts with class schedules involving other teachers, mutually satisfactory arrangements must be made with them. The students can be involved in many of these activities from the planning stage through to the final evaluation. The teacher holds the responsibility for (a) discussing with the students the objectives of the visit, (b) suggesting specific items to be considered by the students en route to or during the tour, (c) working cooperatively with the students in preparing questions regarding specific items of information and submitting the list to the agency in advance of the visit, (d) providing students with background information regarding the agency or situation through discussion of the objectives of the visit, and (e) helping students determine various ways of documenting the trip.

2. *Supervision of the field trip.* The teacher is responsible for the students from the time they leave the school until they return to it; therefore, the mode of transportation to the field agency should be planned carefully so that students know exactly how to reach the destination, where to park, where to meet, and what time to arrive and depart. Field trips involving longer distances often are more beneficial if group transportation is provided and the travel time to and from the agency is utilized for organized discussion periods.

The public relations value of the field trip cannot be underestimated. One unfavorable incident during a field trip can be responsible for the cancellation of future trips; therefore, the teacher has the right to expect students to observe agreed-upon rules of safety, promptness, and courtesy. The very nature of the field trip removes it from a "sightseeing" activity and places it within the context of a socialized process. Students and faculty alike carry the responsibility for creating a desirable image of the school as a professionally oriented public institution. By the same token the students and faculty, as recipients of hospitality by the various field agencies, can transfer this knowledge and understanding of social adjustment when called on to extend their hospitality to visitors to the school of nursing

Proper planning does much to prepare the students with values whereby the seeking out of learning activities to meet the objectives takes precedence over preoccupation with the physical facilities or the hospitality of the agency. The teacher makes a concerted effort to assist students in meeting their goals by calling attention to pertinent points, asking leading questions, or helping students raise appropriate questions. The teacher can also hold the guide to the agreed-on plan of presentation by occasionally referring to the objectives of the visit; providing students with opportunities to raise questions; checking on students' opportunities to obtain desired pictures, recordings, summarizing information; and offering proper courtesies. In the event that the visit obviously is not accomplishing the desired objectives, the teacher has the right to proceed tactfully toward its termination.

3. *Follow-up activities*. The observations and judgments growing out of the field trip are meaningful only if reported, analyzed, discussed, and evaluated. Soon after the field trip there should be a discussion regarding the application of the information gained to the problems encountered in the nursing setting. Such a discussion conceivably could lead to the development of a whole series of patient-oriented, problem-solving situations based on the analysis of findings of the field trip.

The evaluation of the field trip should reveal such items as (a) degree to which objectives were met, (b) application of knowledge and observations to the immediate situation and total learning in nursing, (c) other values of the field trip beyond its intended purposes, (d) identification of problems arising from the field trip, (e) relative value of the trip in terms of time and expenditure, and (f) recommendations regarding its future uses.

The evaluation process should include both written and oral reports. The creative teacher can use the written evaluation of the field trip to discover a variety of students' views. Left as an open-ended report, it allows for the students' creative expressions regarding those aspects they found significant. A written report, while less creative, reveals valuable data for the teacher in evaluating the effectiveness of the field trip for future use. Regardless of type, the written evaluation report reveals students' abilities to see relationships between actual observable phenomena in other related fields and the daily problems encountered in nursing experiences. Another facet of follow-up analysis is seen in the self-evaluation discussion for the purpose of determining the students' own strengths and weaknesses in the planning and participation in the field trip with a view toward improvement for future similar experiences.

The final decision for using the field trip must be made by the teacher, based on the evaluation of the various factors. For many teachers such items as the necessity for detailed planning, cost, time requirements, and lack of knowledge of community resources have created barriers to the use of the field trip as a worthwhile teaching aid. It is true that there is little need for a field trip that cannot offer any tangible material to be observed or provide outstanding persons to be interviewed. A careful survey of available community resources, an active card index listing available agencies for field trips, and a teacher with imaginative ideas who is unafraid to experiment with this particular tool and is willing to share the experiences with others can plan experiences that enrich the study of patients' total problems.

Three-dimensional materials

While direct experiences in real-life situations provide students with valuable learning opportunities, it is not always practical or possible to make them available. The teacher can provide contrived experiences through the use of three-dimensional materials that offer firsthand opportunities for students to examine, hold, and manipulate real or imitation materials or to design their own materials for study. Such devices as objects, specimens, models, mock-ups, and moulages can be selected and manipulated to eliminate distractors, yet provide the essential information needed to meet specific objectives in a given learning situation.

Three-dimensional materials share the same basic uses of media removed from the natural setting to provide firsthand, multisensory, learning experiences. As teaching aids, they can be distinguished by the following definitions:

Objects are actual articles as they exist (live or otherwise) used in direct study to supply sensory stimuli related to the objectives.

Specimens are sample portions of objects to illustrate the quality and structure of the whole.

Models are the replication of objects to be studied, scaled to a usable size such as miniature, life size, gross enlargement, or sectional views. Some models are constructed to allow students to study them in detail by separating and reassembling the parts.

Mock-ups are models, usually life size, adapted to demonstrate by analogy how a real-life situation functions and may be simplified to emphasize selected aspects.

Moulages are casts or models devised to simulate life objects.

There are many instances in which substitutes for real things offer better learning opportunities than the real things themselves. Like all educational communication media, the selection, preparation, and use of the various three-dimensional materials must be based on the degree to which they meet the desired objectives and must be integrated into the total teaching-learning situation. Once the desired materials have been selected and made available to students, the teaching-learning process extends beyond that of observing and handling the items; provision must also be made for reflective thinking. The teacher has the responsibility for (1) directing students to study the material with a definite purpose in mind, (2) raising pertinent questions designed to help clarify significant relationships, (3) providing supervised practice in the use of those devices designed for such purposes, and (4) helping students develop realistic concepts of size and spatial relationships of the items used.

While the use of three-dimensional materials is more frequently related to formal classroom teaching, there are possibilities for their effective use in enriching the learning experiences in clinical settings. We have a rich source of supply for materials from pharmaceutical companies, chemical industries, surgical supply houses, equipment and supplies manufacturers, electronic eningeering firms, commercial manufacturers of educational materials, materials offered by professional organizations, voluntary health agencies, and local, state, and federal health education and welfare agen-

cies. Creative teachers can combine the use of these resources with their own original materials and those of students to produce materials for use in may learning activities.

The clinical nursing conference can often be enriched by using objects, models, and mock-ups to demonstrate specific nursing care measures required by given patients. Students should be encouraged to make their own models for describing the nursing care measures they used in meeting patients' needs.

The flannel board

With the use of singular representative articles backed with adherents, the flannel-covered board builds an idea by displaying each item in an orderly sequence as it is presented orally. The flannel board serves a lecture much the same as slides. The advantage of using a flannel board is that it assists the speaker in maintaining organization of content by displaying planned, meaningful examples as an inherent part of the presentation. The possibilities for the use of the flannel board in teaching clinical nursing reflect the teacher's inventiveness in the presentation of content and the selection of materials for building the display. Consideration can be given to such items as yarn, pipe cleaners, foam rubber, sponge, embroidery floss, steel wool, velvet, and suede as supplements to the use of pictures or lettered captions. Care must be taken that use is related to desired learning, and not as a gimmick for entertainment purposes. It should be remembered that this can be one of the least expensive aids to use, a boon to many tightened budgets.

To achieve maximum effectiveness in the use of the flannel board, advance planning regarding the following matters is extremely helpful:

1. Be certain that the flannel board is firmly fixed on a solid base in a well-lighted, clearly visible area affording ample ease of access in applying the items.

2. Each item should be arranged in

numbered sequential order of use, ready for instant pickup and application at the time the item is discussed. Delays and interruptions of content to offer apologies for oversights should be avoided.

3. Simplicity is the key to effective presentation. Use of a few simple, meaningful symbols in proper context and sequential order with careful explanations and discussion as they are presented is stimulating without being confusing.

Flannel boards can be manipulated for use in different ways: (1) building concepts by a step-by-step presentation of information and simultaneous use of symbols; (2) presenting the total symbolic picture but manipulating the symbols and pictures during the discussion; (3) using symbols for the study of a technical skill such as learning divided dosage formulas; symbols are used to describe each step in the learning process, then drill exercises are provided to help learners relate the technical information to practical problem situations by manipulating the symbols in new combinations; and (4) presenting symbolic clarification of ideas for learners when using instructional television as the communication media.

In nursing the flannel board affords more room for originality and use of colorful, eye-appealing displays. It also affords unlimited opportunities for students to develop their own flannel board presentations. As an example, a committee of the Indiana League for Nursing developed a set of punch-out visuals, representing food exchanges for use in teaching diabetic patients.* These materials could be adapted for use on a flannel board and serve as a meaningful learning experience, first as a sequence-by-sequence presentation, followed by a drill session in determining food exchanges. Students can teach patients by using this technique. Creative teachers and students are limited only by their inven-

*Available for national distribution through Eli Lilly & Co.[25]

tiveness in adapting materials to various ways of presentation as an inherent part of the content.

USE OF PROJECTED MATERIALS IN TEACHING CLINICAL NURSING

The use of projected materials provides another dimension of sensory stimulation to the teaching of many aspects of clinical nursing, particularly in the areas involving skill learning. The selection and effective use of filmstrips, slides, transparencies, and motion pictures for teaching clinical nursing should be based on the criteria for selection of educational communication media, described earlier in this chapter. However, it must be reiterated that these materials contribute to the teaching-learning situation only when they are planned and used as an integral part of the discussion, they are shown at the appropriate moment to clarify or review a particular concept or skill, the items selected represent the concepts or skills to be learned, they are used as supplementary materials to support and clarify the content to be learned, and the teacher helps the students conceptualize the relationships between the projected materials and the course content.

As teachers are faced with increased class enrollments and increased responsibilities for providing an environment compatible with the complex curriculum goals, the need for seeking technical assistance from experts in the field of educational communication media is increasingly evident. For the teacher to fulfil responsibilities and at the same time use talents to the best advantage, the selection and preparation of projected materials can be left to the specialists. The teacher and the educational communication media consultant work cooperatively by doing what each is best prepared to do: (1) the creative teacher suggests ideas for using various kinds of projected materials for presentation of content; (2) the educational communication media consultant uses creative imagination in selecting and preparing the appropriate materials; (3) the teacher utilizes the prepared materials as an integral part of the teaching plan; and (4) together the teacher and consultant evaluate the effectiveness of the media and recommend needed changes for future use.

The following is a description of projected materials and their adaptation for use in the teaching of clinical nursing.

Transparencies

Transparency is an umbrella term used to describe a variety of materials suitable for projecting a single image, which can be seen by means of a light shining through it. All transparencies share the purpose of providing concrete, learning experiences by visualization of single ideas on a continuum, building understanding to conceptualization of total units.

Transparencies vary in size, composition, and means of projection. The most common kinds of transparencies are 2 by 2 inch slides, 3¼ by 4 inch slides, 7 by 7 inch or 10 by 10 inch transparencies, and filmstrips, as described later.

1. *Slides.* The most commonly used slides are the 2 by 2 inch cardboard framed slides, used with 35 mm. color film. Commercially prepared slides are readily available, although many teachers prefer to prepare their own. The 3¼ by 4 inch slides, usually made of glass, are less popular because of handling and storage problems, but they have the advantage of providing a large image, increased detail and brilliance, and ease of preparation.

Slides allow the teacher to edit or rearrange them as necessary for the planned discussion or modify them as changes in the discussion occur. The teacher can prepare a collection of slides, combining commercially prepared ones with self-made ones. The collection can be edited before use each time it is needed, unsuitable slides discarded, new ones added, or the sequence rearranged to synchronize with the revised narration. Use of slides also provides flexibility by enabling the teacher to stop at any point in the discussion to observe and analyze a particular frame as long as necessary before proceeding to new material. Questions can be easily handled by returning to the specific slide and studying it in more detail.

Slides may be shown by using a slide projector or an overhead projector. They can be stored in a variety of storage trays and loading cartridges. Use of these devices allows sets of slides arranged in proper sequence to be ready for instant use and compact loading into projectors. Another convenience is the push-button control switch or automatically timed control mechanisms for advancing slides, allowing the teacher more freedom during the presentation. The versatility in the use of slide sets has been further improved by such systems as the Sound-on-Slide system* developed by the 3M Company. The system consists of 35 mm. plastic slide frames containing a magnetic disk for recording up to 35 seconds of information on each slide. The message can be instantly erased and rerecorded to provide precise information, and the slides can be changed from one frame to another as the need arises. The "talking slides" are prepared and shown through a Projector-Recorder* unit that combines the magnetic recorder, automatic slide projector, and sound playback system. The device can be used for either classroom instruction or independent study.

2. *Transparencies for use with overhead projector.* Transparencies enlarged to 7 by 7 inches or 10 by 10 inches provide a more refined image and can be easily made from a variety of transparent or translucent materials such as cellophane, acetate sheets or rolls, or translucent colored silhouette paper cutouts. The selection of materials depends on the type of subject matter to be projected and the one best suited to convey the idea. Diagrams and charts can be shown stage by stage through the use of overlays. Each step in the series is reproduced on a separate sheet. The first drawing usually shows the basic information; subsequent drawings are shown in sequence by placing

---

*Trade names of products developed by Visual Products Division, 3M Company, 3M Center, St. Paul, Minn. 55101.

one on top of the other until the entire layout or design is completed. There are many good overlays available, and with additional equipment they can be easily and quickly made to meet the desired objectives. A number of companies have equipment, supplies, and instructions available for those desiring to prepare their own transparencies and overlays; some also offer prepared materials for purchase.

The overhead projector has two distinct advantages over other kinds of projectors: it can be used without darkening the room, and the projector is positioned in the front of the room at desk height, allowing the teacher to use it while facing the students. The projector is positioned to focus the image on the screen above and behind the teacher's head at an angle just over one shoulder and clearly visible to all. Its maximal usage potential is dependent on proper positioning of the projector and the teacher's ability to manipulate projected materials while *facing the group*. The position and construction of the projector provide the teacher with a platform comparable to that of a desk top. The material to be projected is placed on the platform in front of the teacher, allowing underlining, pointing, writing, drawing diagrams, or making illustrations spontaneously while maintaining a face-to-face relationship with the students at all times. The projected images can be reproduced to any desirable size up to 8 feet, so that all can see even the smallest details. Illustrations, diagrams, and charts of more permanent value can be prepared in advance and used numerous times, much the same as other kinds of slides, films, or pictures. A distinguishing feature of the overhead projector is its ability to project almost any item made of clear plastic or glass when it is placed on the platform and the instructor can identify the significant points while discussing it. The possibilities for the use of the overhead projector are limited only by the creativity of the teacher or students who use it.

3. *Filmstrips*. The filmstrip consists of a series of single frame, still pictures arranged in a sequential order on a strip of 35 mm. film, varying in length from 2 to 6 feet. It is used in a slide projector with a special attachment for viewing. The usual size for each frame is ¾ inch high and 1 inch wide. Filmstrips may be either in black and white or color and are available as silent or sound projection. The teacher narrates for each frame of the silent filmstrip; sound filmstrips utilize a disk or tape recording of the narration synchronized with the showing of each frame. The ease with which the filmstrip can be manipulated for showing makes it readily adaptable for use. Its greatest limitation is that one is unable to transpose, delete, or add frames without a complete revision.

The filmstrip is a valuable device because (a) the projector is portable, simple to operate, adaptable for use in half-lighted rooms, and can be projected against a light surface; (b) showing of each frame can be adjusted to the exact desired rate needed by the particular group; (c) frames can be adjusted for close-up views to emphasize the learning of particular skills; (d) each frame remains in view as long as the teacher or students wish to view or discuss it; (e) the filmstrip can be returned to previous frames to clarify or emphasize previous discussion; and (f) it provides for continuity of thought.

While many commercial filmstrips are available, it is a relatively simple and economical matter to prepare original filmstrips that can be used for repeated demonstrations without the necessity of preparing laboratory setups each time the demonstration is needed. The filmstrip should present the sequential steps necessary for the demonstration of a given skill, each frame illustrating one point; the theoretical information should be supplied by the teacher or by the narrative of the sound filmstrip. For filmstrips to be "taught rather than caught," it is necessary for the narrative portion to follow along as running comments for each frame, allowing time for questions, observations, and clarification of questions.

A variation of the filmstrip is that known as the 8 mm. single concept film. Although this device is similar in composition, its distinctive use as an independent study device should not be confused with the use of mass media. The device will be discussed later in the chapter in the section dealing with the multimedia approach to teaching-learning situations.

Motion pictures

Although various kinds of transparencies are more versatile in their application to teaching clinical nursing, the motion picture provides viewers with opportunities to span time and space by depicting continuous action and presenting an illusion of reality in motion. It is the added dimension of motion that provides continuity of action in the simulation of lifelike situations. The use of photography allows learners to view how a particular thing works, how it is done, or how it happened in its proper relationship to how it looks. Film production is an art; those seeking to undertake the task are referred to a description of the basic steps by Frey.[26]

A variation of the motion picture is that of the Technicolor 1000.* The device consists of a portable, lightweight movie projector using a continuous loop cartridge for presentations of up to 30 minutes. It is constructed to be adaptable either for independent study or for projection to a larger group. The completely automatic projector requires just three operations: insert cartridge, press one control button to instantly control sound, light, and film start, press one control button to stop projection. A variety of commercially prepared Technicolor film loop cartridges is available in nursing and other fields, or films can be produced and processed for use in the film loop cartridges.

Because nursing offers opportunities for firsthand, supervised learning experiences involving direct action by students, the use of motion pictures as teaching aids may seem limited. However, there are instances in which selected motion pictures provide added dimensions to the teaching of clinical nursing, such as:

1. To review anatomy and physiology pertinent to the understanding of nursing care measures needed by specific patients. Motion pictures or detailed drawings of selected systems or organs on slides or single transparencies offer excellent opportunities for concentrated study to clarify concepts of the effects of specific disease conditions on the human body in relationship to those observed in specific patients and to the kinds of nursing care they require.

2. When the clinical experience cannot provide the total time period needed to develop certain basic understandings. For example, experiences in relating observable phenomena to the nursing care of patients having chronic diseases, terminal illnesses, seasonal illnesses, or illnesses common to other regions or countries may not be available for all students during the alloted time. Appropriate films or slide collections to supply the needed background information would assist students in developing basic concepts about these patients and the kinds of nursing care required and would avoid relying on "chance" observations.

3. To demonstrate sequential steps of procedures just prior to performance in the clinical situation. Often students need a review of a particular procedure before performing it on the actual patient; or a new procedure emerges in the situation for which students need basic instruction. Motion pictures, filmstrips, slides, and overlay transparencies lend themselves equally well to this purpose because the teacher can supply the necessary commentary and can leave each sequence in view as long as necessary for students to visualize each step. This also eliminates the

---

*Refers to the Technicolor 1000 instant movie projector as developed and described by Technicolor Commerical and Education Division, Costa Mesa, Calif. 94526.

necessity for assembling demonstration equipment each time the procedure is needed and provides consistency in demonstrating the procedure as often as needed to clarify certain points.

4. To show large pieces of mechanical equipment not easily transported to the classroom. The use of motion pictures, slides, or transparencies to acquaint students with mechanical devices such as the heart-lung oxygenator, the respirator, dialysis equipment, and other similar devices can be effective before administering nursing care to patients using such devices. When opportunities for experiencing or seeing these devices as firsthand experiences are limited, all students can have front row seats in viewing them as projected materials.

5. To learn to make nursing assessments and use problem-solving processes in making judgments as the basis for nursing action. For example, when students are either learning the process of problem-solving in nursing care situations or experiencing difficulties in meeting the nursing care needs of specific patients, films and filmstrips can be used to supplement the discussion and offer valuable insights for students in learning to cope with various patients' problems.

6. To develop favorable attitudes toward others, leading to improved social relationships. For example, the use of films describing customs and mores of certain ethnic and cultural groups can promote the students' understanding and acceptance of patient behavior, leading to the establishment of satisfying nurse-patient relationships. Students seeking assistance in working effectively as members of a team may profit by studying some of the excellent films now available concerning team relationships and leadership training.

7. To develop observation skills. For ex-ample, films involving nurse-patient interaction can be used to help students identify problems of interpersonal relationships. One way of developing improved observation skills is to show the film without sound and ask students to observe it for specific behavior patterns or to interpret actions as they perceived them. After the silent showing and discussion the film can be rerun with sound to compare the findings, helping students identify problem areas and develop new insights into their own abilities to observe or interpret behavior of others.

8. To orient students to clinical nursing settings or community agencies prior to assignments or field trips. Projected filmstrips, slides, or transparencies showing physical layouts of agencies or clinical facilities and pictures of personnel concerned with the particular setting as well as services provided can equip students with background information prior to the initial visit.

9. To show health and welfare services and facilities available to patients outside the hospital environment, acquainting students with them without using prolonged time periods in providing a field trip or in instances in which it is neither desirable nor possible to plan a firsthand experience. Students can gain understanding of what it is like for a patient to be referred to a particular agency or of the kinds of services it offers, enabling them to discuss necessary plans with the patient more intelligently than if they had no exposure to the situation.

10. To assist students with patient teaching programs. The same materials used for students can be adapted for use in teaching patients self-care. The patient can look at the visual aid while trying to learn to manipulate the actual device needed in learning self-care, such as learning to give himself insulin.

Creative clinical nursing teachers do not question whether or not they should use these educational communication media; rather they seek a variety of ways to organize and provide meaningful educational materials related directly to the practice of clinical nursing.

With the technological advances in the total educational field the use of these instructional aids is no longer a luxury but an accepted, integral part of the curriculum plan. Teachers have unlimited opportunities for selecting those educational communication media most adaptable for use in the teaching of clinical nursing.

The clinical teacher has the dual responsibility of planning clinical nursing experiences to meet the total course objectives and devising ways of guiding the learning activities that are inherent in and arise from clinical experiences. Spontaneity in meeting students' needs through various projected materials adds new dimensions to the teaching of nursing. The creative teacher who constantly seeks ways of utilizing available materials in new combinations to fit the immediate needs will find it beneficial to develop a stockpile of readily accessible teaching materials for use in the clinical area. Use is obviously dependent on the availability of projection equipment. It would seem that conference rooms should either be equipped with or have ready access to an overhead projector, a slide and filmstrip projector, and a movie projector. Teachers cannot be expected to think of using these projected materials if the projection equipment is so far removed from the clinical situation that the need for the presentation of the material is gone before the equipment can be obtained.

USE OF ELECTRONIC DEVICES FOR TEACHING CLINICAL NURSING
The audiotape recorder

Of the many technological developments in recent years, the magnetic tape recorder is one of the most versatile devices for teaching. It records sound as magnetic fields on monaural or sterophonic audiotapes coated with iron oxide; recordings are made at various speeds, depending on the desired sound.

The audiotape recorder has emerged as an indispensable teaching tool because it can allow one to: (1) preserve live discussions of pertinent information by experts, making the discussions available for use at the psychological or logical moment or for review as often as needed by any one class, by many classes, or by individuals on a local, community, or worldwide basis; (2) record directions, drill materials, or background information for repeated use by students, freeing the teacher to spend more time in other student-teacher activities; (3) permit standardization of instructions or selected content to be repeated at intervals, providing uniformity of presentation of each successive group of students; (4) preserve lectures or speeches heard by a few for sharing with an entire group; (5) capture significant sound effects and preserve them for repeated use; (6) permit recorded material to be edited for rearrangement of content, sound, and exact timing for presentation within a given time sequence or for synchronization with a visual aid; (7) aid in the development of the art of listening; (8) permit students and teachers to record their own actions and interactions, leading to self-evaluation of voice tone, inflections, and content analysis; and (9) reproduce material accurately, easily, and relatively inexpensively.

The effective use of the audiotape recorder is dependent on the same basic steps used with most kinds of educational communication media:

1. *Teacher preparation.* Adequate advance planning is needed, particularly when prerecorded audiotapes are to be used. Recordings should be auditioned to determine the suitability in meeting the desired goals, to gather information for purposes of discussing and evaluating the tape, and to detect areas students might find difficult or might overlook. When students are involved in recording their own audiotapes, the teacher should have in mind clearly defined

objectives and the course of action to be followed.

2. *Student preparation.* Through the use of preliminary comments and questions the student's responsibilities for listening must be clearly defined. The selected taped recording, or use of the audiotape as an evaluation tool, should be properly introduced and accompanied by enough background information to interest the students, posing pertinent questions and suggesting specific items to listen for and to determine their relationship to the current learning situation.

3. *Listening to the audiotape.* The teacher should encourage good listening techniques by expecting students to relate what is said, how it is said, and what it means, whether using a prerecorded audiotape or evaluating their own audiotapes.

4. *Discussing the audiotape presentation.* The teacher should begin with informal questions regarding the students' reactions to the presentation. The teacher should then move to the discussion of points previously mentioned and allow time to clarify points of misunderstanding. It may be necessary or desirable to replay portions of the audiotape to convey its full impact or to clarify multiple understandings by various members of the group.

5. *Follow-up activities.* During the discussion session teachers may furnish students with leads for follow-up study, such as related films or filmstrips, library readings, use of the audiotape recorder at home to experiment with an idea as an outgrowth of the discussion, or radio and television programs to be reported on at a later date. It is possible for many creative ideas to emerge as the students become interested in a particular subject and wish to apply either the method or the concepts learned to other fields for further investigation. When this occurs, it is important for the teacher to ask for progress reports from students from time to time to keep them motivated for further exploration and expression of ideas. Students who have their own audiotape recorders may already have recorded some tapes relating to the topic of discussion or may be stimu-

lated to produce others if the teacher shows sustained interest in them.

There are many potentials for use of the audiotape recorder in the clinical situation. Within nursing the use of the audiotape recorder frequently involves the recording of information from patients, family, or others for use by a wide variety of persons; therefore, it is imperative that the necessary legal clearance be secured before taping lectures, conferences, interviews, or self-evaluations of individual performance. Some examples of possible ways of adapting the audiotape recorder for use in clinical teaching follow:

1. Schools of nursing that have their own collection of or access to audiotape libraries should provide faculty members with a catalogued listing of available materials. Teachers could use these audiotapes as review material for supplementary information or to clarify issues arising out of the clinical experience. Although the audiotapes may have been used during formal class sessions, as students inquire into this information, the audiotapes can be replayed as needed.

2. An audiotaped recording of a clinical nursing conference can be valuable in a number of ways, if used selectively. When large classes must be broken into smaller groups to study essentially the same content, an audiotape recording of one of the conference groups could be used by the other discussion groups to compare their findings with those of the taped conference. It is important that the discussions center around the particular patients being cared for by each group of students, but the use of the audiotapes assists the teacher by preserving continuity in discussing the same basic concepts of nursing care to each group. The opportunity to compare patients' problems and the way they were handled by each group also enriches the learning experience. In using this kind of approach the audiotapes should be limited to 12 to 15 minutes, allowing the remainder of the period to be spent on discussion.

3. The audiotape recorder becomes a valuable tool in providing consistent reporting regarding patients' conditions or team con-

ferences for students and other personnel who report on and off duty at a variety of hours. Repetition of oral reporting by one or more persons is avoided, but of even greater value is the assurance that the message heard by each person will be the original unaltered report. Saving the tapes for several days also allows those who are absent during that period of time to review the audiotapes for pertinent information. Hospital units having changes in the performance of procedures or in the handling of specimens for specialized laboratory tests can use tapes to pass on information. Students find this type of information valuable and appreciate the opportunity to replay the audiotapes to be certain of carrying out the procedures and orders as instructed. The audiotape recorder is available when the teacher is not; hence the possibility of a break in communication is greatly reduced, since the directions can be recorded and available for use. This greatly reduces the time involved by both nursing service personnel and teachers and lessens chances of error or omission.

4. Audiotape recordings of nurse-patient interactions in such situations as home visits, developing interviewing skills, analysis of teaching effectiveness, and process recording assist the nurse in self-evaluation. Students can replay the audiotaped interviews any number of times, evaluating such aspects as the ability to listen or wait for the patient's response, voice tone, inflections, command of language, use of terminology; appropriateness of responses to the patient's remarks, questions, or behavior; ability to assess the patient's needs and deal with the identified problems; and recognition of the effects of their own remarks on the patient.

Clinically the areas of psychiatric nursing and public health nursing have used this technique more than other specialties. However, there are ample opportunities for the use of audiotape recordings in all clinical nursing. An extension of the traditional approach is that involving the use of an audiotape recording to teach students how to teach patients, as reported in a study conducted by Monteiro.[27,28] The teacher pre-

pared and recorded scripts of nurse-patient conversations representative of a number of typical nursing problems involving teaching opportunities. After each recorded incident there was a 30-second pause to be used by the student to record the response to the situation. Immediately following the student's response an appropriate response was given and used by the student for comparison. The completed audiotape could be replayed as often as needed, allowing students to compare their responses, change them, and listen again to the desired response. The student learns by using the audiotape for self-evaluation. The teacher can take a sampling of audiotapes, if used over a period of time, to determine the change taking place in the responses students make and compare the students' taped responses to those given in the clinical situation. Variations in the use of this technique are many. For example, students could be assigned a project to compare recorded incidents and responses to similar types of patients and the actual responses made by nurses to similar questions. The study could be used to analyze the understanding of patients and communicating with them as well as to furnish new material for future scripts. Other kinds of nurse-patient interactions could be prepared for use in a comparable manner for the purpose of helping students assess verbalized needs of patients and deal more effectively with them. An example of such a study was recently conducted by a group of senior students at Skidmore College.[29] Use of the audiotape recorder in these situations has much the same effect on the student as the process recording; therefore, teachers must proceed with caution in using this as a tool for group discussions. The teacher-student relationship must be established when the student feels comfortable enough to use the results to further personal growth, it may be possible to discuss the experience with others if the student wishes to do so.

5. Problem-solving situations encountered in clinical nursing could be introduced in the clinical nursing conference by preparing an audiotape dramatizing the situation and

asking students questions about the presentation to determine how well they listened; or the audiotape could be played without the solution to the problem, asking students to supply the ending, discussing their responses, replaying the audiotape to include the ending, and comparing their ideas with the solution given by the recording.

The increased emphasis on the development of listening skills as an integral part of clinical nursing demands that the creative teacher devise ways of using readily available instructional materials from the world of sound in new and different combinations designed for learning.

The Tele-Lecture*

The technique referred to as the Tele-Lecture is designed to communicate specialized kinds of desired information by renowned or specifically qualified persons to an audience by means of a two-way telephone communication system. The conference or classroom moderator introduces the speaker, coordinates the discussion with appropriate visual aids as directed by the speaker, and moderates a question-and-answer session between the students and the speaker. If portable microphones are available, students direct their questions to the speaker; if one microphone is available, the moderator directs their questions to the speaker.

The use of this system for teaching purposes offers the advantages of availability wherever there are telephones; relatively low installation and maintenance cost plus the cost of the regular long-distance telephone rate from the speaker to the receiver; elimination of travel time for the speaker; and the provision of all technical services by the telephone company.

Schools of nursing can take advantage of the use of this device in three distinct ways:

*Refers to the Tele-Lecture as developed and described by the Bell Telephone Company. Detailed information is available from the local Bell Telephone Company Business Office Communications Consultant.

(1) by sharing a teacher with other schools to offer a complete course or selected lectures; (2) by sharing special lectures offered by resources outside of the schools that would otherwise be unavailable; and (3) by seeking outside resource persons to offer consultation services, lecture, or discussion series to a particular group. The school of nursing could also take advantage of it to reverse the procedure; that is, the school could present a series of educational programs to cooperating field agencies, hospitals, or other interested community agencies. This could be particularly effective as a means of upgrading nursing care practices in the clinical facilities used for student experiences.

While this device is more applicable for use in the formal classroom setting, there are times when clinical nursing conferences could be enriched by consultants from specialized areas. A series of clinical conferences could be planned for each group of students, making experts available through the Tele-Conference, who would serve as consultants in helping students approach nursing care problems presented by patients. Occasionally there arises a problem calling for information or consultation from a source not usually included in the planned series; if adequate time for making arrangements were available, the expert possibly could be brought into the discussion through the use of this device.

Educational television

The science of electronics has produced one of the most intricate, versatile, and universal modes of communicating—*television*. A descriptive, nontechnical definition of television is that of Carpenter:

Television is a multi-dimensional and *general* medium of communication. It is an instrument capable of encoding, transforming, transmitting, or projecting, or re-transforming and then presenting the encoded patterns of meaningful information. These processes are performed so that the information input has correspondence with the information output. Furthermore, the psycho-physical correspondence between the content and the intentions of the communicator and the receptive and responsive behavior of the perceiver can be regulated.[*]

Within this book, discussion is limited to the effective utilization of *educational television*. In nursing, as in other fields, educational television usually flows from two main sources: (1) those programs deliberately planned by a school to meet the necessary educational objectives of a given course or total curriculum and (2) those programs not planned as essential components of the curriculum in terms of meeting the desired educational objectives but used as available to supplement or enrich a particular learning experience.

Educational television programs are transmitted through open circuit or closed circuit systems. Open circuit systems are those commonly used by home viewers; educational or commercial stations transmit programs to be picked up by any receiver within the range offered through the channel held by the station. Closed circuit systems provide private reception of televised programs by transmitting from localized cameras to receivers connected to the transmitter by point-to-point relay, wire, or cable within the closed system. In educational television this usually involves relay of programs from one central source to a number of rooms or buildings within the school complex; or the circuit may be extended to include other places within the same center or within a certain geographic area. For example, it is now common practice for medical centers to originate educational programs, beaming them through closed circuit television systems to numerous centrally located hospitals or other educational institutions in a network reaching across an entire state or region. The federally funded Regional Medical Programs assisted in the development of a number of such systems.

[*]Carpenter, C. R.: Approaches to promising areas of research in the field of instructional television. In New teaching aids for the American classroom, Washington, D. C., 1962, Government Printing Office, p. 74.

Whatever the type of telecast used for teaching, its effectiveness is based on the following characteristics:

1. Images can be multiplied so that information can be shown simultaneously in a number of separate locations and synchronized videotape or kinescope recordings can be made.
2. The camera lens and specialized lens attachments can provide highly magnified, detailed, close-up views of objects and processes ordinarily not visible by the naked eye.
3. Split-screen techniques can allow simultaneous projection of different but related (normal-abnormal) images onto a single viewing monitor.
4. Images can be transported from areas unsuitable or inaccessible for teaching to centrally located viewing accommodations.
5. The simultaneous recording of live programs can provide materials and presentations to be repeated for the same students or for successive groups of students.

The multiplicity of ways in which educational telecasts can be produced increases the possibilities for adapting them to the teaching of clinical nursing. Types of telecasts include (1) live presentations including use of communications satellites for international programming, (2) videotape recordings, (3) motion pictures or film clips, (4) kinescope recordings, and (5) cassette television systems.

1. *Live telecasts.* Programs are seen and heard as they actually occur in the originating studio or location. Worldwide communications satellite systems in operation hold immense potential for international education. Since the advent of Telstar, our total communications system is changing in scope, cost, and immediacy of telecasting.

The extent to which such systems can be used as effective educational tools is dependent on the ways human beings visualize and implement their potential as mass media for education of the world. On a smaller scale, a patient interview, a lecture, or a discussion may be broadcast live to students and colleagues. Although there is often less control of content than in an edited recording, the spontaneity can contribute to the educational value.

2. *Videotape recordings.* Videotape recordings currently are proving to be the most satisfactory means of telecasting because they allow instant replay of the recorded materials *without the intermediate delays of photographic developing and printing.* Individuals or groups can prepare the videotapes at their own convenience and from these master tapes, copies can be easily reproduced for distribution and use by others. The tapes are then available for showing as often as necessary to reach different groups of students at different times. Videotapes provide valuable information for evaluating an individual's performance and for studying ways of improving skills. Because of the relatively reasonable cost of the tape and viewing equipment, together with their versatility, videotape has become the primary mode for telecasts. Videotape recording equipment, including cameras, is available in both studio and portable models, allowing for recording under a wide range of conditions.

3. *Motion pictures or film clips.* A film or portions of a film (a clip) made prior to the telecast may be shown at a convenient time, lending continuity to the content presented.

4. *Cassette television system.* The cassette systems make it possible for prerecorded programs to be shown on a conventional television set in the classroom or home.

The cassette television system has advantages for teachers, including: (1) it may be utilized either as a single television attachment or connected to a master player for simultaneous use in any viewing setting; (2) the system is fully portable; (3) less handling of equipment is required; (4) no room darkening is necessary; (5) it may be used any time; and (6) previews prior to showing are possible.

Although many of us have known a world without television, we should remind ourselves that for most students quite the opposite is true, and television has made its impact on society, ultimately affecting teachers and their teaching activities. As we come to rely increasingly on various kinds of television devices as a means of presenting educational materials, research must keep pace with the teaching efforts to determine more conclusive, evidence that could aid teachers in making the most effective use of time. When used in its proper relationship to the rest of education, television has the advantages of offering the best teaching to large groups of students by preserving presentations done by master teachers on tape; providing observation of real-life situations that would otherwise be unavailable to groups of students; reaching large and widely scattered groups of students simultaneously; providing front row seats for studying small objects, demonstrating use of equipment, or showing interrelationships of items; preserving faculty time by using recordings each time material needs to be repeated to a new group of students; and motivating faculty to improve teaching skills.

For those who claim that television promotes conformity and stifles creativity, it must be reiterated that *creativity resides within the individual, not in the technique or tool used in the teaching process.* The greatest danger in educational television lies in its misuse by those educators who regard it as a panacea for the two-sided problem of faculty shortages and increased enrolment. Quite apart from being educationally unsound, to expect all faculty members responsible for teaching a given subject area to shift from the current teaching pattern into a closed circuit televised lecture or demonstration series creates chaotic teaching-learning conditions. The use of educational television requires extensive planning regarding (1) developing specific objectives to be met through use of televised instruction; (2) devising ways of presenting content within the available time period; (3) preparing, organizing, and utilizing visual aids; (4) determining those resources most adaptable for television presentation and planning for the telecast; (5) working cooperatively with electronics specialists in producing the telecast and providing adequate viewing facilities; (6) advance scheduling of selected resources to assure availability for the telecasting; and (7) implementing a continuous evaluation program.

To rely on educational television's ability to extend the range of expert teachers beyond the limits of the ordinary setting carries with it the responsibility for utilizing competent teachers or, at best, providing teachers with opportunities to develop the skills needed to function effectively in the use of television. Teachers must have an orientation to the total process and all that will be entailed, inservice education programs to acquaint them with needed skills and provide technical advice, and a continuous flow of information regarding the total plan of operation as it is developed. Teachers not directly involved with the studio teaching can learn about the process by becoming involved in other aspects of the program and by observing the teachers' presentations. For the best results television teachers should have opportunities to consult with and to receive assistance from technical advisors and script writers prior to and during the television presentations. The presentation of televised instruction requires teachers who are skilled and knowledgeable regarding subject matter; preparation of material in terms of thought continuity and timing of key points; appropriate use of visual aids to provide a smooth presentation within the prescribed time limitations; and attention to such details as use of vocabulary, speech delivery, use of hands, facial expression, and other body gestures.

Creativity in the use of educational television as an aid to teaching clinical nursing is determined by the teacher's ability to use resources for telecasts hitherto unavailable for teaching purposes, arrange for sufficient time to locate supplies or resources, fessen and prepare original demonstrations and visual aids. While by no means an exhaustive list, the following potential uses of television for the teaching of clinical nursing should be considered:

1. Videotapes can be use for describing facilities and services of selected clinical areas such as the emergency room, operating room, recovery rooms, intensive care units, each clinical area, or hospital departments relating to patient care for orientation purposes prior to the student's assignment to a particular area. The tapes can also be made available for students to replay on an independent study basis to gain more detailed information as needed.

2. Closed circuit television systems provide students with a front row seat in viewing activities in a particular setting that is too small either to accommodate the students or to preserve the safety of the patients or students, for example, telecasts of selected surgical procedures; nursing in an intensive care unit, coronary care unit, or other specialized area; observation of behavior patterns of disturbed children or adults; or selected kinds of nursing care of patients.

3. Demonstrations of procedures can be done either by live or prerecorded presentations or the cassette television system using closed circuit television.

4. A complete series of prerecorded tapes, cassettes, or films can be made to show the long-term processes such as results of group therapy used in psychiatric nursing or changes over the course of a chronic illness. Since students often do not have an experience sufficiently long to observe this total process, the series of recorded films, cassettes, or tapes can give the necessary firsthand information and be used repeatedly for each group of students.

5. Some schools of nursing have limited access to certain kinds of clinical experiences within their school. Through the use of television, available community resources can originate a telecast to the schools so that students can share in learning about these selected areas. For example, one

school may not have access to psychiatric nursing experiences involving short-term patients, but telecasts showing nursing care of patients in such a setting enrich students' background of knowledge by visualizing the actual situation without actual experience.

6. A nurse-patient interview can be used as the basis for a clinical conference discussion involving analysis of the interview technique to recognize patient behavior and the nurse's response; later it can be used to develop a nursing care plan, being replayed as often as needed to clarify information.

7. Reports of a study conducted by the Department of Nursing at Bronx Community College, City University of New York, demonstrated that through the use of closed circuit television and audio equipment one clinical instructor could teach fifteen nursing students just as effectively as his counterpart could teach ten students using the conventional methods of instruction.[30,31] Through the use of a fixed focus television camera and mounted microphone installations in the patients' rooms, the instructor monitored nurse-patient conversations and actions of a group of fifteen students from a special viewing room adjacent to the ward. The student wore a small receiving set in order to pick up necessary directions from the instructor. The students also had access to a signal system, which indicated the need for the instructor's presence. The viewing room allowed the teacher to view each of the fifteen students either by an automatic system of relays or by a manual operation. This experiment revealed many other findings relating to the belief that instructors can adjust their teaching of clinical nursing to the use of closed circuit television systems, that the quality of instruction can be improved, and that supervised instruction can be provided when it is most needed by each student. Another aspect of this study included the use of videotape for recording selected instances of clinical practice for use in the discussion of nursing care conferences and for self-

evaluation of performance. There is great potential for other schools of nursing to experiment with similar projects in various kinds of nursing experiences.

8. Videotaped recordings of patient-teaching sessions can be used for group conference discussions to analyze strengths and weaknesses of the situation. The taping allows for replay to analyze actual points taught or those that may have been missed.

9. Patient-teaching programs can be prepared for use in cassettes for televised instruction of patients in hospital rooms, waiting rooms, and community agencies. This approach could be suggested as a special project to be pursued by students seeking ways of satisfying their own learning needs and creative potential.

10. It is possible to utilize selected open circuit television courses being given on a regularly scheduled basis, either for credit or noncredit. For example, it might be possible to utilize a televised course in physics for students having difficulty with principles of that science.

11. On occasion, commercial television stations offer special educational programs as a service. When such programs relate to the particular nursing experiences, they can be recommended to students. Unless they are arranged as part of the regular class session, they cannot be required; often the mere suggestion made by the teacher or by the students themselves is all that is needed for students to seek out the program. A follow-up discussion should establish relationships between the material presented and the clinical nursing experiences.

Guidelines for use of television in teaching clinical nursing. The use of television as a teaching medium for clinical nursing involves a wide range of activities. Decisions regarding the use of live telecasts, teacher-made prerecorded materials, or readily available prerecorded materials greatly affect the extent to which the clinical teacher becomes involved in the total program. The successful use of television as a teaching medium is dependent on co-operative efforts of each team member—the teacher, the educational communication media specialist, the script writer, the technical crew, the cameraman, and the director.

Effective utilization of television in teaching clinical nursing depends on the same basic guidelines applying to the use of other educational communication media, with the addition of the following specific details of planning:

1. *Teacher preparation.* Detailed advance planning is essential for a smoothly presented telecast that meets the desired objectives within the allotted time period. Teacher-made materials must be carefully prepared and edited; those made commerically or by other schools or professional groups must be previewed to determine their suitability in meeting the objectives and must be reserved in advance for use when needed. When prerecorded materials are selected, the classroom teacher must plan a coordinated presentation to include an introduction and follow-up discussion of the material. Televised presentations of theoretical information must be planned in detail. The use of a script provides the teacher with cues and directs the sequence to be followed. Demonstration equipment should be preassembled, tested, and conveniently arranged. Rehearsals should be done to ensure proper handling and displaying of equipment, positioning, and presentation of a smooth demonstration within the prescribed time limits. While live presentations involving surgical procedures, interviews, nursing care measures, or similar instances in which spontaneity is the prime factor do not lend themselves to rehearsals, the other facets of planning for the presentation should be followed. In many instances it is helpful to prepare study guides for students to follow while viewing the telecast. Advance planning also involves the selection and preparation of appropriate visual aids to be used with projection devices such as the overhead projector; necessary arrange-ments for simultaneous recording of the telecast when desirable and feasible; preparation of physical facilities to provide adequate viewing and hearing; and final testing of all viewing rooms to be certain that all equipment is in operation at the time of the telecast.

2. *Student preparation.* Prior to the telecast the immediate objectives for viewing the program should be discussed with the students. Thought-provoking questions to introduce the telecast provide a frame of reference for the students as they view the program and stimulate them to consider concepts and to see relationships between content presenation and clinical nursing experiences.

3. *Presentation of the program.* To ensure maximum learning opportunities, the physical arrangements for viewing the telecast should provide the degree of light and sound needed to present the program clearly and with minimal distractions. If a live program is being viewed, its effectiveness is enhanced if it is possible to provide a telephone communication system so that students can direct questions to the studio teacher and receive immediate replies. When prerecorded telecasts are used, the teacher must provide the information sought by students; but an added advantage lies in having the material available for replay and further study as needed by the entire group or by individual students. The nature of the program and type of television system will determine whether or not to allow questions during or after the telecast.

4. *Follow-up activities.* The questions posed in introducing the telecast should be discussed to determine the kind of information conveyed by the program, the degree to which objectives were met, new ideas or interests presented, or the need for further information. The discussion should also be directed toward helping students discover best ways to use the information, avenues to pursue in seeking more information, and an evaluation of the program as a whole with significant findings directed

to the responsible persons as feedback for the improvement of future programs. Whenever possible, prerecorded programs should be made available for replay to assist students in clarifying issues raised or in identifying significant aspects previously missed.

Schools of nursing are taking great strides in the direction of televised instruction, although the balance of the programs appear weighted toward the teaching of theory courses. The rapidity with which new technological developments related to television are occurring suggests possible investigation for use in teaching clinical nursing. While television does not purport to take the place of the teacher, the demands placed on the available qualified clinical teachers and clinical facilities by increased enrolments suggest the need for experimentation in the use of educational television for teaching clinical nursing. Through governmental agencies, professional organizations, and private foundations, opportunities are available to creative persons to investigate new ways of presenting materials to students in the clinical nursing setting.

Educational television for schools of nursing will come of age when it can be demonstrated that its use for teaching both theory and clinical nursing can be as good as or better than that provided by traditional means, while meeting the needs of greater numbers of students in providing safe, effective health care for patients.

USE OF PROGRAMMED INSTRUCTION FOR TEACHING CLINICAL NURSING

Although some educators are skeptical of programmed instruction, there is substantive evidence to show that it is effective for producing certain types of learning. Not to be confused with teaching machines, programmed instruction is a method of organizing and presenting individualized instructional material in a systematic fashion to achieve specifically stated behaviors. This systematic application of learning

principles, derived from the theory of learning formulated by Skinner in 1954,[32] incorporates a number of characteristics that distinguish programmed instruction from previously described educational communication media:

1. Learning occurs more easily when there is logical, sequential presentation of subject matter designed to meet specifically defined behaviors. The desired student behaviors must be so specifically described that the subject matter can be broken into small units (frames), arranged in careful sequence, building each successive frame on that knowledge or information gained from the previous frame or frames.

2. For learning to take place there must be action and interaction between the learner and the material to be learned. The process of providing frames of information requiring an answer before proceeding to subsequent frames requires the student to interact with the learning material.

3. Learning is more effective and efficient when the learner receives reinforcement by immediate feedback of results regarding responses. Programs generally include a high percentage of correct responses, providing immediate rewards to motivate the learner. If each response is checked with the correct answer, immediate confirmation reinforces the impression in the student's mind; knowledge of incorrect responses allays attempts to build knowledge on misconceptions and allows the student to correct the misunderstanding before proceeding with new material. Learning can become a pleasure when success or failure is a private affair, not a trial, threat, or competitive arena.

4. The rate of learning varies among individuals and from one subject to another, one situation to another, one day to another. Programmed instruction provides individual students with

opportunities to advance at their own rate of learning. Students have the freedom to proceed rapidly, moving on to more advanced materials, or to spend needed time in mastering particular concepts. By prescribing relative time limits for learning programmed material prior to discussion or application, the teacher can check the answers to determine the degree to which the total group is ready to discuss and apply the information.

5. Revisions in programming and teaching are based on objective analysis of the student responses. Analysis of student responses allows for student-centered evaluation and revision of programs to meet more nearly the ability levels of the particular students. Evaluation can be removed from the realm of "opinions by experts" to that of controlled experimentation.

Types of programs

Although there are no limits to the number of types of programs that conceivably could be developed, there are generally two main types: (1) the *linear* program, which is concerned with the student's ability to recall data; and (2) the *intrinsic* program, which is concerned with the student's ability to *recognize* data. Although these two types of programs share the common purpose of individualizing teaching accompanied by reinforcement, they differ in their approach, intention, and rationale, as pointed out by Crowder[33]:

1. *Linear programs.* Programmed material is arranged in a single sequence, requiring every student to proceed in an orderly fashion from the first to the last frame. Generally this form uses the constructed-response approach associated with Skinner and his colleagues. The constructed-response approach presents easily grasped bits of information, followed by a series of frames requiring short written answers. The student then compares his response with the correct response, is re-warded by knowing the response is correct, and proceeds to the next item. Student errors are considered irrelevant to the learning process; therefore linear programs are designed to maintain a low-level error rate by providing built-in positive responses. Programs rely on the student's ability to recall information with step-by-step repetition of words or ideas emitting automatic responses. This built-in feature has advantages and disadvantages, governed primarily by the type of material to be learned and the level of ability of the group to be reached. The greatest problem is that of maintaining sustained interest in the program when it is oversimplified by repetition.

2. *Intrinsic programs.* Programmed material is arranged to provide alternate routes determined by the student's responses. Program branching simulates a diagnostic approach by using the feedback for each particular student to determine the route to be taken. That is, when a response indicates mastery of certain points, a number of subsequent questions may be skipped; when a response indicates a need for review, the student is directed back to an earlier portion of the program for further study before proceeding with new content. This method consists of the use of a short narrative presentation of each new idea, followed by multiple-choice questions. After making the response the student is directed to the source providing the correct response, which often includes an explanation of the answer and a suggestion regarding remedial information if the answer is incorrect. Thus, the student is asked to pursue the remedial work before proceeding with the program. This approach provides a means of helping students to recognize errors made and determines reasons for making them.

Devices for presenting programmed material

The foregoing description refers to the ways in which teaching materials are arranged to form a *program,* but a vehicle for presenting the program is needed. The wide range of available devices for presenting programmed materials generally can be classified under two main categories: (1) programmed textbooks and (2) teaching machines.

The programmed textbook enjoys popularity because it is less expensive than machines, is readily available, and has the possibility of being constructed by the teacher who needs a program to meet objectives of a particular course for which no program is available. Textbooks are available in vertical or horizontal linear programs or branching programs.

Some believe that the programmed textbook is less effective because it provides opportunities for students to look ahead at the correct answers. Others reply to this charge by pointing out that the goal is to promote learning; if this approach on the part of the student does in fact produce the desired learning outcomes, it does not matter how the student accomplished the task. Of more importance in the use of programmed textbooks is the matter of providing the stimuli necessary for sustained student motivation to reach the desired goals. This is a matter of using the teacher's creative abilities as a human being to supplement the programmed material so that the student is stimulated to use it to its fullest potential.

Programmed textbooks are appearing for all types of learning in all kinds of how-to-do-it subjects related to self-improvement, homemaking tasks, hobbies, and tasks requiring higher levels of thought processes. Virtually all branches of education, including nursing, now have some programmed textbooks. Many schools of nursing have produced programs tailored to meet their particular needs; other schools of nursing have "borrowed" published programs from the medical sciences and other related fields, using them with varying degrees of success. Nursing journals occasionally include a programmed instruction unit covering one or more topics of current interest. These can be utilized in conjunction with other teaching devices and reference sources.

The term *teaching machine* is used arbitrarily to distinguish the mechanical programming devices from the textbook programs. Clearly the teaching machine is useless without suitable programmed materials; the machine merely represents the hardware needed to convey the program to the learner. When a teaching machine and a valid program are in harmony with one another in terms of format, the end result should provide individualized instruction much the same as the previously described characteristics of programmed instruction.

During the past decade computer-aided instruction (CAI) for virtually all grade levels in a wide range of subject matter has been used to provide individualized instruction with a thoroughness difficult to match by a teacher. Computerized teaching systems have the capabilities of presenting material in a variety of forms ranging from simple typewritten programs of information and multiple choice questions to the projection of text, pictures, or films on a television screen along with controlled tape-recorded information on signal, and the use of oscilloscopes and programmed printouts of electronic recordings of the body's reaction to various kinds of stress situations for study and analysis. Students have the opportunity to respond to the programmed information by using an electric typewriter or by touching a "light pen" to a cathode ray tube, or more simply by an oral or handwritten response. The totally computerized systems can be highly individualized because they enter into a conversation with the student, responding patiently to each response, either by correcting him or praising him for correct responses and referring him to more difficult materials utilizing the branching technique. The computer can electronically record data about each action of each student relative to the time needed to answer each question and the path followed in arriving at a response; teachers can then use this information to study the individual student's learning problems and reprogram the course of study accordingly. Although the costs of computer-aided instruction are prohibitive for many in nursing education, computerized systems are being installed in many universities across the country. Nursing education administrators may investigate these possibilities for their faculty.

The selection of prepared programs suitable for use in a situation exerts an effect on the desired outcomes. Therefore, the teacher should give careful consideration to the following questions when previewing such programs: Are the objectives of the program compatible with the objectives of the learning experience? Is the content up-to-date? Can the program be adapted for use in clinical teaching? Are the examples and applications comparable to those in the given situation? Is the program constructed in accord with the principles of programming? Is the form—linear or intrinsic—suitable for accomplishing the desired goals? How can the program be presented—textbook, requiring a particular machine, requiring a computer attachment, or adaptable for use with a variety of devices? Is it reusable? What is the cost per student? How has the program been validated? What results were obtained from using it experimentally? What are the qualifications of the author in terms of subject matter and skill in programming?

By the same token the teacher must give careful consideration to the selection of the device to be used to present a given program. Although it is difficult to evaluate these devices at face value, the teacher can look for cost per student, number of kinds of programs it will accommodate, types of programs it will accommodate, size and portability, auxiliary equipment needed to operate it, adaptability for use in the clinical situation, ease of operation, and availability of service and parts for nonfunctioning equipment. The rapidity with which the use of programs and programming devices has grown makes it highly unlikely that teachers can have enough background in-

formation to evaluate these devices effectively; therefore, it is recommended that the teacher conduct a preliminary investigation to determine the answers to the foregoing questions, then consult a specialist to assist in the ultimate evaluation and selection of the program or equipment.

The values derived from developing programs to meet the needs of a given situation cannot be underestimated. In nursing education there are multiple opportunities for the development of individual programmed learning materials. Teachers who are entertaining ideas about producing their own materials should give careful consideration to the requirements of effective programming. It is safe to say that the best programs have been those produced by teachers highly competent in the given subject matter and who have had training in program writing and have received advisory assistance from psychologists trained in programming. The highly diversified art and science of programming is emerging as a specialized area of education worthy of detailed study; thus, any attempt to provide teachers with detailed principles and techniques of program construction would be incompatible with the basic purposes of this book. Teachers who seek to write their own programs should refer to the References for needed background information.[34-39]

While programmed instruction has been more readily adapted for the classroom portions of nursing education, it is time for teachers to determine creative ways of adapting programmed instruction to the teaching of clinical nursing. The following examples are by no means conclusive; they are meant as a springboard for determining other applications of programmed instruction to the teaching of clinical nursing:

1. Programmed materials used for many of the theory courses such as pharmacology, chemistry, anatomy, mathematics, or theory related to the various clinical areas can be made available to students for review as an integrated part of the clinical experience. For example, those portions of pharmacology

that relate to each clinical area could be reviewed as necessary for students just prior to and during the time they are in a given clinical situation.

2. As new developments occur that require the teaching of new kinds of equipment, even during the life of the current program, they can be programmed and made available both to students and to graduates to be studied in more detail following the initial demonstration.

3. Prior to the clinical nursing experience a laboratory demonstration model of procedures, along with programmed materials giving detailed instructions regarding the step-by-step performance, can be set up for continuous viewing and independent study and practice by the student.

4. Programmed booklets containing step-by-step instructions for various treatments and procedures can help to bridge the gap between the time the material was presented in the laboratory and the time of acutal performance. Because of the increased number of students and the rapid turnover of patients, there is often an unexpected lag in the time interval between theory and practice; or the opportunity for administering the procedure may arise at a time when the teacher is not available for assisting the student. Quick reference to the programmed material may enable the student to proceed, followed by an evaluation conference with the teacher, using the program as a self-evaluation guide.

5. Geis and Anderson have built a strong case for the use of programmed instruction in teaching the deveolpment of motor skills, so that all students reach essentially the same point of readiness for applying them in the clinical situation.[40] Although students have been exposed to the classroom demonstrations of various procedures, this in no way guarantees that the procedure has been learned. Programmed instruction to supplement the classroom demonstration can be used effectively by requiring students to work through the programmed workbook for the particular procedure within a given time period before they will be expected to apply this knowledge or skill in the clinical situation.

6. Programming various kinds of motor skills can be accomplished by using a teaching machine designed to accommodate synchronized slides with a tape-recorded narrative, while simultaneously providing the opportunity for the student to practice the skill. This approach frees the student for active physical participation in learning the skill when provisions are made for (a) built-in automatic controls or foot-pedal controls for moving the sequence of steps forward without interruption of manual activity and (b) projection of the pictures of each step of the procedure so that the pictures appear as an extension of the student's own hands. Although this type of programming is still in its infancy, there are published reports describing its use in the teaching of nursing procedures.[41,42]

7. Bitzer reported a study on the use of the Plato system for teaching clinical nursing in a simulated clinical laboratory situation.[43] The Plato system (Programmed Logic for Automatic Teaching Operations) is a computer-controlled automatic teaching device designed to present problems automatically, weigh answers, provide help when needed, and give electronic analytic feedback to the student. Nursing care situations related to myocardial infarction programmed by the computer offered students opportunities to determine needed data, then proceed at their own rate of speed in selecting problem-solving approaches from a variety of programmed alternatives, ultimately leading to a plausible solution. Aside from utilizing the learning by self-discovery concept, the simulated laboratory approach provided students with opportunities to make mistakes that might endanger patient safety in the real-life situation.

This experiment suggests that schools of nursing could adapt this teaching machine or other similar devices to teach problem-solving approaches to nursing care as an intermediary step between classroom theory and direct nursing experience. Progression from use of the programmed approach to the direct experience would be in accord with the individual student's ability to master the programmed material. This approach to learning has added benefits in that the anxiety factors involved in trying to relate positively to patients while learning new nursing care measures are absent when the student is allowed to approach the problem in the simulated laboratory setting.

8. Currently there are available a variety of programmed teaching devices such as those designed specifically for developing skill in recognizing various patterns of arrhythmias and in treatment measures such as defibrillation, countershock, and pacing. The devices range from programmed texts to various kinds of tape cartridges for showing on ocilloscope reading. There are also a number of simulated devices that can be used in a variety of ways in the development of skills related to heart and lung disorders. One of the most versatile and valuable is the Arrhythmia Trainer and Torso.* This device has capabilities for programming various kinds of arrhythmias through the use of manually controlled continuous loop, eight-track cartridges and simulated EKG readings programmed through the Trainer and Torso to be read simultaneously on an oscilloscope and an EKG printout, allowing students to study the results until they become firmly fixed in their minds as recognizable normal and abnormal heart rates and rhythms. The Trainer and Torso also can be programmed to produce a variety of arrhythmias through a manually controlled panel, followed by practice in providing the necessary treatment without the need for providing laboratory setups or selected patients. The Trainer and Torso can be used either on an independent study basis or in a group discussion–drill session by simple manipulation of the control panels to provide any number of kinds of arrhythmia patterns in accord with the immediate learning needs of the students and the creativity of

the teacher. The teacher also can arrange program testing situations as needed by the students and can determine students' competencies in defibrillation, countershock, and pacing procedures.

9. Use of the computer in the development of programs that call for more complex problem-solving as opposed to the step-by-step approach to programmed instruction is under development. Teachers of nursing would do well to consider how they could be adapted for use in programming the development of skills related to nursing assessment and intervention. As nurses become more certain of their own judgments and actions, it will become easier to plan for programmed instruction of material beyond the level of psychomotor skills, which now predominate.

Guidelines for effective use of programmed instruction in clinical nursing

However programmed instruction is used in clinical nursing, it is so designed that it adds new dimensions of precision and efficiency to the process of instruction. The following guidelines for the use of programmed instruction in clinical nursing may be helpful in clarifying the role of the teacher:

1. The clinical teacher must have a thorough knowledge of the entire content of each programmed unit, inasmuch as self-paced programmed instruction produces a wide range of variations in progress of students and a resultant need to assist students with learning difficulties in various sections of the program. Thus the teacher must have knowledge of the subject and readily available instructional materials to meet individual needs of students in terms of enrichment or remedial follow-up programs.

2. The use of programmed instruction as an independent study device at some point should provide additional time. Teachers should avoid the temptation of using the free time to provide further programmed materials and use it in group discussion sessions, in additional patient care time, or other student-teacher interaction.

---

*Trade name for the device manufactured by Hewlett-Packard Medical Electronics, 175 Wyman St., Waltham, Mass. 02154.

3. Programmed materials should be supplemented by experiences beyond the verbal response level. Students must be taken beyond the point of reading, writing, and reciting answers; the teacher must supplement the material through the use of perceptual experiences that relate directly to the verbal experiences. In clinical nursing this is so simple a task that it may become overlooked. That is, the obvious pattern is to follow the programmed instruction with clinical experiences; but the teacher must help students relate the verbal knowledge to the perceptual knowledge as experienced in the clinical nursing setting in order for the total concept to be formed.

4. The rigidly controlled process of stimulus-response-reinforcement sequence followed in programmed instruction tends to standardize the teaching-learning process without utilizing the unique background of experience each student brings to the situation. Therefore, the teacher should become particularly sensitive to the unique abilities, talents, interests, or other background information each student possesses. These characteristics must be nurtured by providing opportunities that lead to creative learning and furnish leads into other clinical experiences to help the student to grow to his true individual capacity, whether or not these abilities are indicated by the results of the programmed instruction materials.

5. Teachers using programmed instruction in any form must understand and appreciate the principles of programming, accept the process as a serious educational business, and increase students' confidence in its use by keeping them fully informed regarding the nature, purpose, and expected results of the particular program being used. Students also should be encouraged to participate in the evaluation of the items or frames making up the program, and their suggestions should be carefully considered as a part of the final evaluation of the effectiveness of the program.

6. Programmed instruction materials are designed for use in teaching, *not as testing devices*. Although students are required to submit written responses to given questions on the program, these responses provide the student with knowledge through self-discovery. They are used primarily to determine when the total group has reached approximately the same level of learning, which students need more assistance, and which students would profit by additional inquiries into other more advanced materials or other kinds of clinical experiences.

Programmed instruction is not meant to be viewed as the answer to all educational problems or become the core of the total educational system. It must be remembered that the very basis for a successful programmed unit is the definition of specific behaviors desired of the student; where this cannot be determined, programmed instruction cannot be used. When programmed instruction is appropriately used, it provides the students with personalized and private interaction with the learning material, permits them to proceed at their own rate of learning, and gives immediate reinforcement. The use of programmed instruction in the teaching of clinical nursing is only as effective as the teacher using it. Its use in some form or another presupposes that it provides teachers with released time to work directly with students. Indeed, the demands placed on the teacher in terms of preparing programs, knowing the content thoroughly enough to diagnose learning difficulties and give help to a variety of students in various stages of the particular programmed unit, planning remedial work, and guiding students into further avenues of interest can be met only by the most creative of teachers! This should leave little doubt that a teaching machine by any name can ever replace a teacher.

CREATIVE TEACHING IN CLINICAL NURSING THROUGH USE OF THE MULTIMEDIA APPROACH

The previous discussion of the adaptation of educational communication media to the teaching of clinical nursing suggests that each medium has a unique contribution to make, depending on the teacher's ability to use it creatively. Left to be used without some systematic arrangement, educational communication media often suffer from disuse or misuse leading to piecemeal learning. Increasing enrolments without concomitantly increasing faculty members invoke the need to identify and organize optimal combinations of teaching methods and educational communication media to provide integrated, independent learning experiences producing the desired student performance. This requires teachers who can use a creative approach to the selection and integration of the appropriate combined media and teaching methods for independent study and who have the ability to interact with students. This approach to learning involves the combination of two broad concepts aimed at providing learning opportunities to satisfy requirements of each individual: (1) tutorial study and (2) multimedia approach to learning.

Tutorial study refers to the means through which teachers provide opportunities for individual students to progress at their own rate, with freedom to think and study a defined task at various depths and breadths, providing tutorial assistance as needed. Tutorial study takes place within a structural framework providing for scheduled sessions of individual study and group discussion. It is based on the concept that responsibility for learning resides with the student, implying that all students possess potentialities for self-initiative, self-discipline, creative productivity, and self-evaluation.

Multimedia approach refers to the concept of instructional technology that uses a multisensory stimulus-response approach to the integration of subject matter and educational communication media in a systematic unit of study to meet specific objectives. The combination of these two concepts provides course content that is structured for individual students to pursue at their own rate of learning with a minimum of teacher involvement in the routine classroom functions. Such an arrangement frees the teacher to function on a tutorial basis with some students who indicate a need for additional help in meeting the desired behaviors, while other students progress more rapidly into new avenues of learning.

All the previously described teaching methods and educational communication media become multimedia devices when they are used in combinations designed to elicit multisensory responses from the student. Organized in meaningful combinations, they are no longer supplements or aids to learning but become the very core of the teaching program by providing motivation for learning through the use of independent study. Learning involving the multimedia approach seeks to define the goals and to select those educational communication media and teaching methods that *together* can best accomplish the goals. It might involve words and writing by the teacher, audiovisual stimuli of various devices, stimuli from programmed materials and textbooks, laboratory experiences, and other forms appropriate to the given situation. To complete the learning sequence the teacher must coordinate the available learning resources and use them to produce maximum learning. The organization and utilization of various media into a meaningful frame of reference for study depends on the teacher's understanding of the learning resources and ability to use them creatively.

Learning centers that provide facilities and the necessary hardware for equipping individual study carrels, laboratory facilities, library facilities, lecture rooms, and seminar rooms are beginning to emerge in higher education. For the most part the approach to the use of the independent laboratory concept has been on a limited basis. One pioneer program in higher education was initiated in 1961 by Postlethwait of Purdue University, who experimented with the use of audiotape materials to supplement a freshman botany course. From this experiment the concept of the integrated experience approach has been developed for use in all science laboratory courses at Purdue University.[44] Another example of this approach has already been demonstrated by Oklahoma Christian College, which has completely revamped its education system to provide an electronically equipped dial-access independent study carrel for every student as the heart of its learning center, which also houses the library, seminar and lecture rooms, and lounges for students to carry on their own discussions.[45]

The rapidity with which education is moving toward a multimedia, tutorial study approach to learning is forcing schools of nursing to consider this approach. The adoption of the multimedia concept of teaching requires rethinking on the part of the schools' administrative officers, faculty, and students regarding curriculum revision, effective utilization of faculty, integration of the total range of media into the teaching plan, flexible scheduling of classes and clinical experiences, and the provision of physical facilities and equipment needed for adequate independent study opportunities for students, based on reasonable research studies within the situation. The Nurse Training Act of 1964, Project Grants Section (Nursing Education and Training Branch, Division of Nursing, National Institutes of Health, Department of Health, Education, and Welfare) has been an impetus to the development of audiotutorial approaches to learning by many schools of nursing. Descriptions of those programs developed for the use of the multimedia concept of learning reflect many commonalities, but each has its own unique features adapted to the individual school, its students, and its faculty. An example of one such project is that developed by the Indiana University School of Nursing in 1968.* The project, *Development and Evaluation of a Systems Approach for Improving the Teaching-Learning Process in Nursing,* was originally developed for use in the sophomore year. Plans call for extending the program into the junior and senior years, based on the assessed outcomes of the current program. The setting contains study carrels providing for a variety of media such as synchronized slide sets and audiotapes to be used on an independent study basis, a separate study area for viewing televised

*Supported by PHS NU 0024-01, Project Grants Section, Nursing Education and Training Branch, Division of Nursing, National Institutes of Health, Department of Health, Education and Welfare.

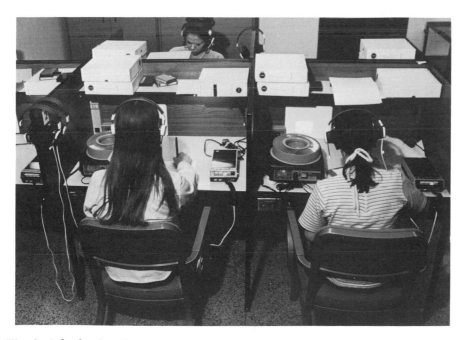

Fig. 2. A bank of study carrels at Indiana University School of Nursing, illustrating the use of synchronized slide sets and audiotaped units of study. (Courtesy Mr. Gilbert Edo, Indianapolis, Ind.)

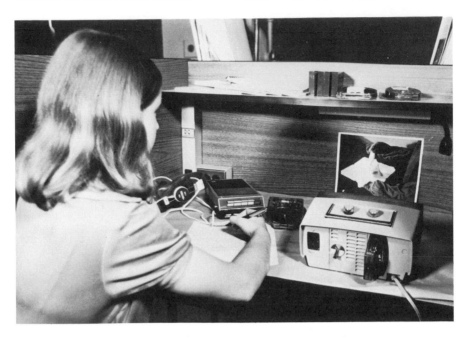

Fig. 3. A close-up of the use of the single-concept film for demonstrating the steps of a procedure. (Courtesy Mr. Gilbert Edo, Indianapolis, Ind.)

materials, a five-bed unit equipped with all of the materials needed to practice the development of nursing skills. The total learning approach follows that designed by Postlethwait[44] with adaptations made to meet the objectives of the program and to utilize the available physical facilities and the type of educational media that would best meet the objectives. There has been evidence to indicate that the use of this systems approach is effective and is well received by the students.

The federal funding cuts of the middle 1970s have severely limited resources for developing totally new multimedia centers. Rather than instituting but poorly using such resources merely because they are fundable, schools are now forced to consider carefully where and how the new concepts are most appropriate and financially feasible.

Guidelines for adapting multimedia approach to teaching of clinical nursing

The teacher who elects to use the multimedia approach to the teaching of nursing can help students explore a variety of sources for answers to problems arising from the clinical setting. For too long nursing educators have viewed the clinical setting as a place to "practice" nursing procedures. While it is true that the multimedia approach lends itself particularly well to the teaching of fundamentals of nursing, there is need to apply this approach to a broader context. The many kinds of problems arising out of each daily clinical nursing assignment could benefit from the use of this concept as an integrated approach to the teaching of clinical nursing in any area of content.

To adapt the multimedia approach to the teaching of clinical nursing, the following suggestions may be helpful:

1. The clinical teacher should develop a statement of specific behaviors to be achieved by the student in order to successfully complete the course or unit requirements. The more definitive the behaviors, the easier it is to select the appropriate approaches or media in their proper relationships and sequence in meeting the desired outcomes.

2. The clinical teacher should determine

the total time allotment for each course or unit. That is, the time allotted for class, laboratory, or clinical experiences plus the allotted amount of study time should be used as the formula for planning the kinds of learning activities that can be used to meet the objectives. Time patterns may be established by a given school, but the traditional pattern of allotting two hours of outside study for each hour of class time seems to be fairly standard though it suffers from lack of validation. It then becomes the individual student's responsibility to spend either more or less time in the prescribed program as needed to meet the desired behaviors.

Determining various patterns of student contact hours per week involves time allotments for clinical nursing and theory classes. Background theoretical knowledge necessary for functioning in the clinical situation may need to be examined to determine those portions best suited to large lecture sessions, those that could be taught by independent study, and perhaps those that require supervision in terms of using films, recordings, or writing examinations but could be handled by teaching assistants, freeing the faculty member for other tasks. Time allotments for the use of the laboratory for learning certain procedures should be reexamined. Combining independent study with the use of a laboratory that is fully equipped and under the supervision of a qualified nursing assistant over an extended period of time must be considered along with laboratory experiences requiring the presence of the teacher for a short period of time. Time allotments for clinical experience should be determined according to that needed for actual experience and that which can be learned just as effectively through independent study. Time could be compressed to a minimum in the teaching of more complex skills, if opportunities were available for students to study them independently. Time also must be allotted for clinical nursing conferences, which provide vital teacher-student contact. This aspect is an integral part of the multimedia approach because it provides students with opportunities to express themselves in a "live" and "knowing" environment. The teacher, a knowledgeable clinical nursing expert, can guide them in their problem-solving activities, diagnose their learning difficulties, refer them to needed review materials, or lead them into new avenues of learning.

3. The clinical teacher should explore the variations of teaching methods and educational communication media along with the different possibilities for arranging classes, clinical experience, and independent study within the allotted time schedule.

The dial-access, electronically controlled listening equipment used in some study carrels provides for greater flexibility of use of tape recordings. The prerecorded tapes are located in a central electronically controlled system for broadcasting. A directory of available listening hours for each tape is given to the student; the student selects the time, reports to the study carrel, dials a number as listed in the directory, and at a specified starting time the tape begins. Should the student be late, the program must be picked up "in progress." A less complicated approach, which may be used for smaller numbers of students, allows them to listen to a selected program by dialing it at any time.

The simultaneous use of teacher-prepared workbooks to accompany the taped directions, lecture, procedure, or problem-solving situation provides both audio and visual stimuli. The workbook becomes the student's notes; the teacher determines student progress by periodically reviewing the workbooks with the student.

Possibilities for learning skills by drill, practice, and repetition should be investigated relative to combining the use of prerecorded exercises, teaching machines, and clinical experiences to accomplish the desired results. The availability of prerecorded materials such as these affords students opportunities to sharpen their skills without relying on the presence of the clinical instructor or postponing the practice until the opportunity presents itself in the clinical setting.

The various combinations of teaching techniques and educational communications media to provide a multimedia approach to the teaching of clinical nursing could proceed ad infinitum. Clearly the multimedia approach to the teaching of clinical nursing represents a *blending* of previously discussed teaching methods and educational communication media. Teachers should refer to the discussions on applications of each teaching method and each educational communication medium to the teaching of clinical nursing. Rearranging and combining these methods and devices to provide multisensory stimuli for the learner have endless possibilities, depending on the specific behavioral objectives being sought and the teacher's own creative ideas.

4. The clinical teacher should plan a detailed program to be followed by the students in reaching the desired outcomes. Such a program should give a step-by-step sequential breakdown of the specific teaching methods and educational communication media to be used by the student within specified time periods. Results of this kind of total planning can be outlined to show specific operationally defined behaviors expected of the students, time schedules listing kinds of experiences to be utilized, and evaluation measures for determining the extent to which the behaviors are accomplished.

While the multimedia approach admittedly was devised as a means of providing improved learning conditions for greater numbers of students by allowing them to progress at their own rate on an independent study basis, it by no means eliminates the teacher! This approach to learning changes the *roles* of the teacher. As the multimedia approach to learning becomes implemented, the teacher will be expected to (1) prepare or select available material to meet the desired behavioral outcomes adequately; (2) coordinate the teaching materials into meaningful learning units; (3) diagnose individual learning problems; and (4) remedy problem areas through individualized instruction, group discussions, and furnishing a variety of sources for students to explore in finding the answers they seek. As more sophisticated educational practices are adopted by schools of nursing, the teacher will be aided in the diagnostic and remedial aspects of the tutorial functions by computerized information regarding any particular student's progress at a given point in time.

The teacher remains the central figure in planning and implementing the instructional program. Only experience and continued experimentation will determine how educational technology can sustain creative teaching and how the various technological devices can best be used to generate increased student achievement while maintaining personalized instruction.

There is no one best way of presenting instructional materials that will guarantee the creative teaching of clinical nursing. The "mix" of educational approaches, devices, and methods must be studied in terms of how well they meet the desired objectives, their accessibility, and the teacher's ability to use them creatively. In the final analysis it is the individual teacher's understanding of the total teaching-learning process and the degree to which each teacher is willing to invest the self in the teaching process that are responsible for the teacher creativity that begets student creativity.

REFERENCES

1. Mereness, Dorothy: Freedom and responsibility for nursing students, American Journal of Nursing **67**:69-71, Jan., 1967.
2. Schulman, Jerome L., and others: Observation of a hospitalized child as a teaching technique in student nurse education, Journal of Nursing Education **5**:7-13, Nov., 1966.
3. Marschak, Marianne, and Call, Justin: Observing the disturbed child and his parent, Journal American Academy of Child Psychiatry **5**:686-692, Oct. 1966.
4. Learning about death and dying, American Journal of Nursing **71**:56-57, Jan., 1971.
5. Brown, Amy F.: Curriculum development, Philadelphia, 1960, W. B. Saunders Co.
6. Bergevin, Paul, Morris, Dwight, and Smith, Robert M.: Adult education procedures, New York, 1963, The Seabury Press, Inc.
7. Cartwright, Dorwin, and Zander, Alvin: Group dynamics, Evanston, Ill., 1968, Row, Peterson Co.

8. Kemp, Paul C.: Perspectives on the group processes, Boston, 1964, Houghton Mifflin Co.
9. Knowles, Malcolm, and Knowles, Hulda: Introduction to group dynamics, New York, 1959, Assocation Press.
10. Phillips, Gerald M.: Communication and the small group, Indianapolis, Ind., 1966, The Bobbs-Merrill Co., Inc.
11. Racy, John: How a group grows, American Journal of Nursing 69:2396-2402, Nov., 1969.
12. Richardson, Stephen, Dahrenwend, Barbara, and Klein, David: Interviewing, its forms and its functions, New York, 1965, Basic Books, Inc., Publishers.
13. Zaleznik, Abraham, and Moment, David: Dynamics of interpersonal behavior, New York, 1964, John Wiley & Sons, Inc.
14. Heller, Vera: Handicapped patients talk together, American Journal of Nursing 70:332-335, Feb., 1970.
15. Melody, Mary, and Clark, Genevieve: Walking-planning rounds, American Journal of Nursing 67:771-773, April, 1967.
16. Hall, Benita F., and Little, Delores E.: Group project and learning outcomes, Nursing Outlook 17:82-83, June, 1969.
17. Hepler, Ruth: An experience in creativity, Nursing Forum 9(2):146-150, 1970.
18. Hipps, Opal S.: An approach to senior seminar, Journal of Nursing Education 6:19-21, Jan., 1967.
19. Andrews, Kenneth, editor: The case method of teaching, Cambridge, Mass., 1956, Harvard University Press.
20. Heidgerken, Loretta E.: Teaching and learning in schools of nursing, Philadelphia, 1965, J. B. Lippincott Co.
21. Dautz, Lois: Interpersonal processes in nursing: case histories, New York, 1970, Springer Publishing Co., Inc.
22. Pigors, Paul, and Pigors, Faith: Case method in human relations; the incident process, New York, 1961, McGraw-Hill Book Co.
23. Pigors, Paul, Pigors, Faith, and Tribou, Marita: Professional nursing practice; cases and issues, New York, 1967, McGraw-Hill Book Co.
24. Pigors, Paul, and Pigors, Faith: The incident process—a method of inquiry, Nursing Outlook 14:48-50, Oct., 1966.
25. Dymelor Diet Demonstrator, Indianapolis, Ind., 1967, MI-92-70, Eli Lilly & Co.
26. Frey, Myra: Basic steps in film making, Nursing Outlook 17:50-60, May, 1969.
27. Monteiro, Lois A.: Tape recorded conversations: a method to increase patient teaching, Nursing Research 14:335-340, Fall, 1965.
28. Monteiro, Lois A.: The tape recorder as a teaching machine, Nursing Outlook 12:52-53, Oct., 1964.
29. Boguslowski, Marie, and others: Tape recording patient recordings: a minimester project, Nursing Outlook 17:41-45, May, 1969.
30. Griffin, Gerald, Kinsinger, Robert, and Pitman, Avis: Clinical nursing instruction by television, New York, 1965, Teachers College, Columbia University.
31. Griffin, Gerald, Kinsinger, Robert, Pitman, Avis, and Kessler, Eunice: New dimensions for the improvement of clinical nursing, Nursing Research 15:292-302, Fall, 1966.
32. Skinner, B. F.: The science of learning and the art of teaching, Harvard Educational Review 24:86-97, Spring, 1954.
33. Crowder, Norman A.: On the differences between linear and intrinsic programming, Phi Delta Kappan 44:250-254, March, 1963.
34. Mager, Robert F.: Preparing objectives for programmed instruction, Belmont, Calif., 1962, Fearon Publishers.
35. Mager, Robert F.: The instructional technologist, Educational Technology 7:1-4, May 15, 1967.
36. Craik, M.: Basic considerations for writing objectives, Educational Technology 6:5-13, Feb. 28, 1966.
37. Lysaught, Jerome P., and Williams, Charles M.: A guide to programmed instruction, New York, 1963, John Wiley & Sons, Inc.
38. Brethower, Dale M., and others: Programmed learning: a practicum, Ann Arbor, Mich., 1965, Ann Arbor Science Publishers, Inc.
39. Perry, Lucy C., and others: An experience in preparing programmed instructional material in nursing, Journal of Nursing Education 8:27-32, Jan., 1969.
40. Geis, George L., and Anderson, Maja C.: Programmed instruction in nursing education: applying principles of the technique in producing materials, Nursing Outlook 11:662-665, Sept., 1963.
41. Anderson, Maja C.: A new aid to teaching and learning, Nursing Outlook 9:677, Nov., 1961.
42. Becker, Mary, and Mihelcic, Marilyn: Programming a motor skill, Journal of Nursing Education 5:25-30, Aug., 1966.
43. Bitzer, Maryann: Clinical nursing instruction via the Plato stimulated laboratory, Nursing Research 15:144-150, Spring, 1966.
44. Postlethwait, Samuel N., Novak, Joseph, and Murray, Hal: An integrated experience approach to learning, Minneapolis, 1964, Burgess Publishing Co.
45. North, Stafford: Learning center gives each student a study carrel, College and University Business 40:46-49, May, 1966.

SUGGESTED READINGS

Beauchamp, E. A.: Breathing manikin facilitates teaching of respiratory care, Heart and Lung 1:621-625, Sept./Oct., 1972.

Brown, James W., Lewis, Richard B., and Harcleroad, Fred F.: A-V instruction: media and methods, New York, 1969, McGraw-Hill Book Co.

Budd, Ruth: A picture is *still* worth more than a thousand words, Nursing Outlook 17:48-49, May, 1969.

Collart, M. E.: Computer-assisted instruction and the teaching-learning process, Nursing Outlook 21:527-532, Aug., 1973.

David, Janis, and others: Listen: the student, Nursing Outlook 15:48-49, June, 1967.

de Tornay, Rheba, and Searight, Mary W.: Microteaching in preparing faculty, Nursing Outlook 16:34-35, March, 1968.

Drage, Elaine, and Lange, Blanche: Ethical considerations in the use of patients for demonstration, American Journal of Nursing 69:2161-2165, Oct., 1969.

Faris, K. Gene, and Moldstad, John: Organizing a program for creating instructional materials, Bloomington, Ind., 1966, Indiana University School of Education.

Frerichs, Marian L., and Frerichs, Allen H.: Don't overlook class discussion, Journal of Nursing Education 5:3-6, Nov., 1966.

Geitgey, Doris: Some thoughts on team teaching in nursing education, Nursing Outlook 15:66-68, Oct., 1967.

Hornback, May, and others: Party line for nurses, Nursing Outlook 16:30-31, May, 1968.

Jacobs, Paul I., Maier, Milton H., and Stolurow, Lawrence M.: A guide to evaluating self-instructional programs, New York, 1966, Holt, Rinehart and Winston, Inc.

Landurath, L. J., and others: Computer nursing education, Hospitals 47:99-100, March, 1973.

Lange, Crystal M.: Autotutorial techniques in nursing education, Englewood Cliffs, N. J., 1972, Prentice-Hall, Inc.

Martz, K. V., and others: Computer-based monitoring in an ICU: implication for nursing education, Heart and Lung 1:90-98, Jan./Feb., 1972.

McGinty, D., and others: The homeostatic nursing care plan, Journal of Nursing Education 12:14-19, April, 1973.

McKnew, Donald, and Easterly, Judith: Psychosocial seminars for nursing students, Nursing Outlook 17:44-46, July, 1969.

McPhetridge, L. Mae: Nursing history: one means to personalize care, American Journal of Nursing 68:68-75, Jan., 1968.

The national survey of audiovisual materials for nursing, New York, 1970, American Journal of Nursing Company, Educational Services Division.

Pearman, Eleanor, and Suleiman, Louise: Test of a programmed instruction unit, Nursing Research 15:258-262, Summer, 1966.

Poshek, N.: Multimedia approaches to teaching and learning in a baccalaureate nursing program, Journal of Nursing Education 11:36-43, Aug., 1972.

Robinson, Geraldine, and Kataoka, Winifred: How to develop an audio-visual aids bank, Nursing Outlook 14:49-50, July, 1966.

Robinson, Vera: Humor in nursing, American Journal of Nursing 70:1065-1069, May, 1970.

Roth, D. H., and Price, D. W.: Instructional television: a method for teaching nursing, St. Louis, 1971, The C. V. Mosby Co.

Silva, M. C.: Nursing education in the computer age, Nursing Outlook 21:94-98, Feb., 1973.

Smith, Dorothy: Perspectives in clinical teaching, New York, 1968, Springer Publishing Co., Inc.

Stein, R. F., and others: A multimedia independent approach for improving the teaching learning process in nursing, Nursing Research 21:436-447, Sept./Oct., 1972.

Stoten, S.: Film-making: experiencing the patients' point of view, Imprint 19:12-13, Dec., 1972.

Sumida, S. W.: A computerized test for clinical decision making, Nursing Outlook 20:458-461, July, 1972.

Taylor, Calvin W., and Williams, Frank E., editors: Instructional media and creativity, New York, 1966, John Wiley & Sons, Inc.

Wiedenback, Ernestine: Meeting the realities in clinical teaching, New York, 1969, Springer Publishing Co., Inc.

Wittkopf, B. W.: Self-instruction for student learning, American Journal of Nursing 72:2032-2034, Nov., 1972.

9 Evaluation of teaching-learning experiences in clinical nursing

The preceding discussion of teaching technologies and their application to the teaching of clinical nursing should stimulate new ideas and questions and may lead to new problems, particularly within the realm of evaluation processes related to clinical nursing. We should not be satisfied with testing that reveals only students' abilities to recall factual knowledge and perform rote skills. There is need for organized research regarding the process of evaluation so that we can have valid and reliable information regarding student progress. It is necessary to measure individual growth and the worth and workability of newer technologies to the teaching of nursing. The process of evaluation in clinical nursing continues to pose a dilemma for nurse educators. Recognition of the impossibility of equating competence in theory with competence in clinical practice compounds the problem. Evaluation is determined by the degree to which students achieve the desired behaviors for a given nursing area. Those who have a knowledge of the behaviors to be learned during a particular experience must develop the tools. It must be remembered that although this is a discussion of clinical teaching, it is fallacious to assume that professional nursing can be clearly divided into theory and practice. Any evaluation of the student in the clinical setting must be logically consistent with and related to evaluation of the student's performance in related theory courses or nonpatient care experiences.

The discussion in this chapter does not provide answers to all of the questions that can be posed by teachers regarding the planning and implementing of clinical evaluation programs. Rather, it is designed to stimulate the thinking and actions of teachers as they strive to grow beyond the point of using subjective evaluation of clinical performance.

CLARIFICATION OF TERMS

The focus of this chapter is on the evaluation of individual student achievement in clinical nursing; but this area of evaluation becomes a part of the total evaluation to determine the effectiveness of the course in meeting the desired objectives, the success of various teaching methods, and teacher effectiveness. To avoid confusion it is well to distinguish between *evaluation* and *measurement*.

Evaluation is a continuous process of collecting data to be used as a basis for making a judgment. It involves not only consideration of that which occurs but also the worth of the behavior through the exercise of judgment.

Measurement is appraisal to determine a quantitative factor (extent, degree, or capacity) without value judgments. In its strictest sense measurement implies the assignment of a value on a scale of equal units for each characteristic to be measured.

These processes are significant as methods teachers devise to evaluate clinical nursing competencies. Perhaps the tendency to rely on the concept of measurement has perpetuated the use of checklists now in use but perhaps inadequate for evaluating student performance in clinical settings. A flexible concept of evaluation can encourage a more sophisticated approach to the appraisal of student performance.

PURPOSES OF EVALUATION IN CLINICAL NURSING

While educational evaluation performs many functions, its chief goal is to promote continuous improvement in the learner, the teacher, and the curriculum based on evidence discovered through a systematic appraisal.

The evaluation in clinical nursing varies in relation to the objectives set by any program. The trend is toward an ongoing evaluation program aimed at determining student growth in becoming a skillful practitioner. However, each teacher must avoid the tendency to view evaluation in broad terms such as "total nursing performance," or "teaching the whole student." Such an approach results in repetitious, global evaluations from one assignment to another with little evidence regarding the degree to which students met the objectives for the given assignment. Within this context evaluation processes should serve the following purposes: (1) to determine the background ability each student brings to the situation; (2) to determine the progress by each student at frequent intervals during the assignment; (3) to determine the ability of students to use nursing theory as a whole while progressing in the development of clinical skills; (4) to discover learning difficulties of individual students and the group in order to adjust the teaching, including remedial or advanced assignments as needed; (5) to provide reinforcement of learning for students; (6) to foster development of self-evaluation; (7) to determine the readiness of students to become self-directive; (8) to determine the effectiveness of teaching techniques; and (9) to obtain data for conducting research studies relating to student achievement.

EVALUATION PROCESS ADAPTED FOR TEACHING CLINICAL NURSING

Educational evaluation theory provides us with steps to be followed in effective planning, implementing, and interpreting the evaluation of clinical nursing. However, before embarking on a full-scale plan of evaluation it is important to consider the following questions: What do you wish to evaluate? Why do you wish to evaluate certain kinds of performance? Who should be involved in evaluation? When is evaluation most effective? How do you propose to accomplish the evaluation? How do you intend to use the evaluation? With answers to these questions in mind the teacher is better equipped to proceed with an evaluation program suited to appraise nursing performance.

The evaluation program for a given area of nursing should follow the same basic format as that planned for the total curriculum; that is, it should include the following processes:

1. *Stating the objectives for the given clinical course.* As has been stated, the teacher must determine the specific objectives (behaviorally defined) for experience in the nursing area. The statement of objectives should (a) include the cognitive, conative, and affective aspects of the desired changes; (b) be realistic regarding clinical situations, allowing for flexibility in accord with patients' needs; (c) be consistent with the objectives for related subject matter, the total curriculum, the conditions of learning, and the educational philosophy adopted by the school of nursing and the university; (d) be attainable within the time prescribed for the given program; and (e) be flexible enough to allow for progression of individuals according to their abilities.

2. *Stating the specific changes to be expected as outcomes of reaching each objective.* For each objective of the clinical nursing course there must be defined behavioral changes for each level of attainment (such as sophomore, junior, or senior level). The key to the success of the entire evaluation system lies in the statement of these behavioral outcomes in a manner that can be measured, that provides for levels of attainment, and that provides evidence of behaviors sought by each objective. It

is well to spend considerable time and study in the development of behavioral outcomes. Since this book does not permit a lengthy discussion of this process, further information will be found in the References.[1-5]

✶ 3. *Describing learning experiences that include desired behaviors.* The defined outcomes should be accompanied by examples of the behaviors that students are expected to attain in a given experience. Situations germane to the particular experience should be used to define how the teacher expects the students to act, but there should be flexibility in the use of these situations to provide for individual variation.

✶ 4. *Providing adequate sampling of experiences including desired behaviors.* To provide a reliable measure of behaviors in the clinical experiences, there must be an adequate sampling of experiences representative of all desired behaviors. Students faced with the variables inherent in nursing need a range of opportunities to accomplish an objective.

✶ 5. *Selecting methods of evaluation appropriate to the desired behaviors.* Appraisal of the identified behaviors should utilize a variety of tools and techniques. Just as diagnosis is established on the basis of data from a variety of sources, so the teacher needs a variety of ways to determine students' ability. Individual differences necessitate a variety of appraisal methods to determine a student's progress. However, standardization is needed to determine criteria for quality of performance, as reflected by the terms in each evaluation tool. Creative teachers of clinical nursing should be sufficiently familiar with the various kinds of evaluative tools and techniques to use them in accord with the learning needs of individual students. It is not enough to plan an evaluation system calling for the routine use of these various techniques. They must be used in terms of their ability to yield the desired information as individual students reveal varying patterns of learning. The end results should be a total picture derived from organized use of a variety of tools and techniques, regardless of the sequence and frequency of their use.

✶ 6. *Selecting evaluation devices in accord with established criteria.* In using the variety of devices for the evaluation and measurement of achievement in nursing, teachers can choose between those that use purely subjective decisions and those that give some degree of reliable, valid information regarding student progress. It is imperative that teachers involve student representation along with total faculty participation in the development of evaluative tools that meet the major criteria of reliability, validity, adequate sampling, and minimal personal bias. Nursing faculty should combine their expertise with that of education and evaluation specialists in devising or selecting a complete program of evaluation.

✶ 7. *Assigning criteria for measurement.* The use of rating scales and similar devices for evaluating student progress poses the problem of defining terms indicating levels of achievement. The terms should have enough variance for students to achieve without denying their individual differences. The development of a scale to describe the expected achievement at various levels should be based on the principle of defining the number of distinctly discernible differences using clear terminology. For example, words such as "excellent," "average," "satisfactory," or "poor" have ambiguous meanings for both evaluators and students. The establishment of terms such as "satisfactory" or "unsatisfactory" must be based on mutual faculty agreement regarding descriptive behaviors exemplifying typical performance that is either satisfactory or unsatisfactory for each grade level of students—sophomore, junior, or senior. One example of providing better observer objectivity and reliability in rating clinical performance is that described by Anderson and Saxon.[6] They devised a performance evaluation scale for a selected procedure consisting of two parts: (1) an observation sheet for recording observable behaviors during performance of the selected procedure, and (2) a criteria sheet defining the activity and describing criteria for successful performance and for failing performance. The teachers referred to the criteria sheet *after* having observed, comparing the criteria with the previously recorded observations. The teachers then assigned a performance value of "successful," "unsatisfactory but acceptable," or "failing." This approach eliminates some of the bias and wide variations of observations made from one clinical teacher to another; it bears consideration by other faculty groups seeking to develop more equitable evaluation tools for use in clinical nursing. In attempting to do so, however, groups should carefully consider the new biases introduced. It is not clear from the labels, for example, how one can be both "unsatisfactory" yet "acceptable."

Another means of determining measures of satisfactory or unsatisfactory behavior has been developed by Fivars and Gosnell,[1,7] using Flanagan's Critical Incident Technique to determine the work habits and characteristics of a large group of nursing students. These were then classified into effective and ineffective incidents in twelve major categories. This approach serves to help define descriptive terms for use in constructing a reliable and valid rating scale.

A problem of great concern to clinical teachers is the practice of assigning a letter or numeric grade for clinical nursing experience. We may not have arrived at a point of evaluating clinical performance with sufficient objectivity to justify a grade. Heslin strongly suggests that no rating scale that implies varying degrees of attainment can justify the assignment of a grade, and that for those faculties who are committed to providing a grade for clinical performance, there should be an accompanying statement indicating that the grade represents the *opinion* of the evaluator.[8] This is a crucial area for faculty members to consider in developing criteria for differentiating between good and poor clinical performance sufficient for assigning a grade. Some programs have separated clinical and theoretical portions of course evaluation. Pass/fail ratings are only given for clinical performance; the final grade depends on achieving a pass.

8. *Providing a learning environment conducive to evaluation.* Cooperative student-teacher planning of learning experiences includes providing an atmosphere in which students are encouraged to continuously evaluate themselves and feel free to seek help and accept guidance accordingly. The clinical teacher's concept of evaluating student progress must be built on sensitivity to student needs and understanding of student behavior as it relates to each nursing experience. Students who learn from their first experiences that the teacher serves to guide them in improving or developing their skills in a nonauthoritarian relationship accept the various phases of evaluation as integral parts of the total learning situation. Many barriers to effective performance are reduced, and assessment of growth becomes more reliable.

9. *Appraising data to determine total progress of students.* Data regarding students' progress in clinical nursing should be assembled and reviewed in terms of relative values each item contributes to the total profile. If done well, the appraisal reveals a composite picture of the student's progress in achieving the desired competencies while simultaneously providing information regarding the effectiveness of the teaching program, the methods used to implement the program, and the teacher.

10. *Interpreting student progress as revealed by data.* Student-teacher evaluation conferences for interpreting student progress must be based on mutual trust and respect, leading the student into greater knowledge of self and motivation for continued efforts. While there is a need for scheduled, formal conferences for purposes of discussing progress, there is an equal need for teachers to carry on continuing evaluation conferences during every contact with students. If information revealed by evaluation devices is to be of value as

a learning tool, it must be discussed with individual students as it occurs, serving as a guide in directing subsequent activities.

For those who hold the theory that the teacher needs more than one observation of specific behavior before making a judgment, it must be pointed out that the teacher, in reality, does not see the student at all times and that the incident may, in fact, be a typical performance. Therefore, day-to-day conferences to discuss all data gathered by both teacher and student during that time allow the student to clarify the actions taken and to continue to grow in areas needing alteration before a pattern of "undesirable" performance can develop. There should be a joint discussion of how each perceived what happened, reasons and progress made since the previous experiences, with opportunity for joint formulation of goals for subsequent experiences. To provide the needed reinforcement of learning, these discussions must include positive aspects as well as needed areas of improvement. Periodically scheduled formal evaluation conferences with students may serve the purposes for which they are designed. However, in the face of increasing enrollments a realistic appraisal of time involved reveals that it is often difficult for the teacher to conduct these conferences and be available in the clinical situation in order to collect the desired data. Frequent, on-the-spot conferences with students allow the faculty to continue to be present in the clinical situation, keeping students up to date on their progress. If teachers allow students to take advantage of the information when it is noted, students are provided with ample time for improvement of performance, and those who have mastered a given task can progress to other more challenging learning opportunities.

A uniform record system should also be established. This should provide a profile of the progress made by students in terms of desired outcomes and a record of actual data. Data recorded for permanent use reflects growth as the student progresses, reactions of students to specific incidents, and changes in attitudes or approach. Concern for the individual rights of students has forced all educational institutions to exercise considerable care in the quantity and quality of information recorded. This awareness has come about because of instances in which highly subjective, prejudicial comments added to a record have prevented progress by the student either in school or after graduation.

Criteria for selection and use of devices for appraising clinical nursing performance

The first step in the development of evaluation programs in clinical nursing is faculty recognition and acceptance that the process of group decision making *is* time-consuming but is necessary for establishing more reliable and valid criteria for measuring nursing performance.

Assuming that course objectives and behavioral outcomes have been established, it is reasonable to assume that each teacher will provide the group an adequate sampling of objectives to be evaluated in order to measure the degree to which they are attained. However, the lack of clear, accepted standards for judging nursing care gives rise to an overwhelming need for experts in nursing to identify some criteria. These can be used in judging the quality of student performance.

Validity refers to the degree to which a particular device measures that which it is intended to measure. Validity is tested in terms of the degree of relevance between the items on the evaluation device and the purposes for the specific group of students. Although the desired objectives and specific behaviors for a given group of students may be defined, the process of validation in nursing practice becomes difficult because we lack criteria on which to base measuring devices. Nursing research studies describing performance by nurses can be used as the basis for determining such criteria; however, the degree to which a given faculty can use valid instruments to evaluate clinical nursing performance is variable. Nurse faculty members can make a concerted effort to arrive at a consensus regarding content validity by determining the relationship between the objectives of the course and the items used to evaluate the student's performance.

A rating device can be considered a valid measure of performance when a large percentage of those using it are in agreement regarding each component of the device. Therefore, faculty within a given school of nursing should correlate results from measuring devices used with many groups of students and results revealed by using more than one form of the same type of device. Another approach is to correlate the results with those obtained by another school of nursing considered to have developed a device with some degree of validity.

Reliability refers to the consistency with which results can be obtained each time the device is used under comparable circumstances. If a measuring device used repeatedly in comparable situations produces similar results, it is deemed reliable. To ensure reliability the measuring device must contain adequate sampling and must produce comparable results when evaluated or scored by equally competent persons. The teacher of nursing can test for reliability by using the same device several times with the same group of students under the same conditions or by submitting results to several competent persons for scoring. In either case if results remain relatively fixed, the device is said to be reliable. For the more discerning, measurement devices can also be tested statistically for reliability. However, it must be pointed out that high reliability by itself is meaningless if the measuring device is invalid. A measuring device can be so designed that it produces accurate results, but it may not pass the validity test because it does not measure the behaviors specified.

Nurse-educators give lip service to the term *objective evaluation,* but little evidence is available to explain how this, in fact, is accomplished. The very nature of evaluating clinical nursing performance means that the evaluators, the students, and the setting in which the evaluation occurs deal with human beings. As such, one can hardly eliminate subjectivity in evaluation One part of a more realistic approach is for evaluators to examine ways of eliminating personal bias by gaining insight into how their own needs, feelings, prejudices, abilities, and misconceptions tend to influence their value judgments in evaluating students. Some teachers rely too heavily on ratings recorded by previous teachers, so that preconceived notions regarding students form the basis for judgments. Other teachers tend to set themselves up to evaluate student performance on what they *think* students can do rather than confining the evaluations to what students *demonstrate* they can do.

Subjectivity resides more with the evaluator than with the evaluation device, because it is generally the evaluator who has prepared the device or who will interpret it. Therefore, it is well to consider how subjectivity affects which evaluation devices are selected, used, and interpreted. Teachers must rely on observations in judging effective or ineffective nursing performance. Each observing teacher, however, has a set of beliefs and standards that prohibit a completely objective view. Only sound mastery of the subject taught, widely accepted standards for performance, and constant sharing of work with others can offset this bias.

One factor responsible for bias in evaluation is that referred to as the "halo effect." It has many aspects, including (1) teachers who overrate students in the desire to gain their approval; (2) teachers who rate students high in order to let the ratings reflect their success as teachers; (3) teachers who have expert ability to perform a skill or apply knowledge, and who give high ratings to students with comparable abilities or qualities; and (4) teachers who allow their judgments to be influenced by the students' nationality, family heritage, social status, attitudes toward the learning environment, temperament, or habits relating to the management of their personal lives.

Other teachers develop biases resulting from misconceptions regarding the process of evaluation. For example, (1) teachers who confuse effort with achievement by overlooking the causes of failure in students who constantly "try hard" but make minimal gains toward the desired outcomes; (2) teachers who believe that students should receive ratings according to length of time in school, beginning with seniors and decreasing to lower levels; (3) teachers who hold to the normal curve for rating all students, regardless of size or abilities of the group; and (4) teachers who excessively allow students to operate outside the prescribed standards of performance in deference in their rights as individuals. Closely allied to this area of bias are the great differences between the way in which teachers interpret the meaning of traits to be evaluated and the observed behaviors. While subjective analysis of performance may not be wrong, it is hazardous unless a number of persons express their judgments of the observations, contributing to a decision regarding that which was observed.

From the student's point of view the very act of being observed or evaluated often produces variations in performance, deviating from that practiced under different conditions. Some students succeed at being their most gracious, efficient selves, whereas others are so emotionally insecure that they cannot coordinate their movements or thoughts into their normal pattern of operation. Closely allied with this problem is that of being judged in a setting in which the patients continually offer new variables with which students must cope. Unless the teacher considers these various factors in their proper perspective, the resultant value judgment will tend more toward subjectivity than objectivity. It can be seen that eliminating bias in the use of methods and tools for evaluating students in clinical nursing is a complex and rarely completed process.

TOOLS AND TECHNIQUES USED IN EVALUATING CLINICAL NURSING PERFORMANCE

Evaluation of clinical performance involves a variety of ways of securing evidence related to the behaviors described by the objectives of the course. Providing an appraisal of nursing performance involves the selection of tools and techniques that best measure the desired behavior in a situation. The range of choices includes direct observation using critical incident reports, anecdotal records, sociograms, or rating scales; pretests, post-tests, or other tests; and appraisal of products such as models, mock-ups, nursing care studies, term papers, projects, or demonstrations. Regardless of the devices selected for use, teachers are responsible for building in reliability and validity in the process of clinical nursing evaluation through *the way they use them,* as well as by *selecting reliable, valid devices for use.*

Observation techniques and tools

The principal means of evaluating clinical nursing performance is by direct observation with devices for recording and interpreting the observed behaviors. The problem lies in reducing the previously discussed bias affecting the observation for appraising student performance.

The strongest influences of the teacher's observations are those related to the teacher's background, experiences, abilities, and attitudes. The degree to which each objective at each level of the clinical nursing experience is defined provides the particular patterns to be observed. Observations can be more readily made when a definite purpose is fixed. It should not become a question of how often to make observations; they should become an integral part of the daily teaching-learning process in clinical nursing. Constructive use of observations should result in (1) seeing relationships among various kinds of data, leading to conceptualization of the situation as a whole; (2) recognizing the significance of observed behaviors requiring suspended judgments until the situation is carefully analyzed; (3) beginning to interpret the "why" behind the observed behaviors, and (4) basing recordings and interpretations *only* on that which is observable in a given situation. In essence, to effectively use observations for purposes of evaluating clinical nursing performance, the teacher must observe each incident in terms of "where," "when," "what," "how," "why," and "with whom." Observations provide the clinical teacher with valuable information in assessing students' nursing of patients and group interaction in a variety of settings.

Observation continues to be regarded as an effective means of evaluating nursing performance, but teachers responsible for these activities must have a thorough knowledge of the exact behaviors to be accomplished during a given experience, along with an analysis of the level of each performance to be rated according to a standardized scale. The faculty in each area is responsible for establishing behaviors to be observed and the criteria for successful completion of assignments. A feature of the process should be providing students with information sufficient to explain the behavior and the degree of attainment needed to complete the given program successfully.

Observation should be an integral component of the experiences of students in the clinical setting under normal conditions. The creative teacher can use various ways of recording observations in an effort to establish and preserve data for appraisal of clinical performance, including verbatim descriptions, symbolic descriptions, graphs, flow charts, videotape recordings, audiotape recordings, remote control television cameras, anecdotal notes, critical incident records, rating scales, sociograms, or other comparable devices. A definitive but by no means exhaustive description of these devices follows.

Anecdotal notes. Anecdotal notes, properly used, indicate behavior development for individual students in demonstrating application of knowledge in the performance of skills, the ability to give nursing care and to interact with others, attitudes or habits revealed during the performance, and ability to plan and organize work. The essential elements of an anecdotal note consist of the identification of the student, the date and time of the observation, the narrative report, and the signature and role of the observer. While there is a tendency for anecdotal notes to be stated in subjective terminology, which decreases their validity and reliability, it is a relatively simple matter to reverse this defect for use as valuable and simple tools of assessment. If observers record anecdotal notes in accord with the basic concept of photography, by which the camera records *the actual occurrence as it happens,* the anecdotal record would be a *word snapshot of the incident.* That is, the incident is recorded as it occurs, without the use of modifying expressions reflecting the observer's interpretation of the incident.

In the event that there is need for interpretation of a given incident, a separate notation indicating this to be the opinion of the evaluator should accompany the anecdotal note. Anecdotal notes should include recordings of a wide range of incidents, representing the most typical behavior of the student. Recording should include incidents describing both favorable and unfavorable departures from typical behavior as well as progression made toward improvement. Because of variables the teacher is wise to follow up on atypical incidents to determine whether they are, indeed, atypical or are the usual pattern of behavior previously unobserved. Used properly, anecdotal notes can be submitted by head nurses, supervisors, and others in a position to evaluate student performance, lending greater validity to the final interpretation of data.

The flexibility with which anecdotal notes can be used is both an advantage and a disadvantage. Accurately and objectively written, anecdotal notes allow observers to describe behavior without making a forced choice (as on a checklist) and supply evidence for helping students improve their clinical performance. But the flexibility with which the notes can be written may reflect personal conflicts between the student and the teacher without providing objective data regarding actual behavior; or there may be gaps in the recordings that make it difficult either to determine a pattern of behavior or to explain reasons for some behaviors but not others.

Organizing, interpreting, and summarizing the data revealed by the anecdotal notes, along with individual student conferences to determine the meaning of some of the observations, suggest areas that could be strengthened, and indicate direction of growth become a time-consuming task. The effectiveness of the anecdotal notes lies with the individual teacher's ability to prepare and interpret them while reducing personal bias.

Critical incident technique. Another means of collecting information based on direct observation is that of recording what is known as a critical incident. This consists of a sample of observable human behavior in a given situation that clearly demonstrates either positive or negative factors contributing to the effective or ineffective completion of the activity. Such a definition raises the question of who determines those behaviors deemed critical to student development.

Before this particular technique can be applied successfully to the evaluation of nursing performance, all teachers in the school must reach agreement regarding a list of critical behaviors developed from the observations of many students by many qualified observers. The resultant observations must then be categorized and classified into a workable number of agreed-on behavioral areas dealing with work habits, performance abilities, and personal characteristics considered advantageous for the successful accomplishment of the clinical nursing program.

Each behavioral category must then be described in terms of the most commonly observed effective and ineffective behaviors. This process involves detailed analysis comparable to a research study, which, if undertaken by a faculty, yields valid, reliable criteria for evaluating observable clinical nursing performance with a greater objectivity. However, Fivars, Gosnell, and Flanagan have developed a form known as the Clinical Experience Record for Nursing Students, which provides a listing of twelve behavior categories, with subcategories of effective and ineffective behaviors for each behavior, derived from a survey of over 2,000 incidents of student performance.[9] The nature of the record makes it adaptable for use by any nurse-faculty group desiring to use the Critical Incident Technique as the means of recording observations of student performance. The record serves only as a guide by providing space for recording observed critical incidents, which can then be compared with the twelve major categories described in terms of effective and ineffective behaviors to determine a classification for each recorded critical incident.

As critical incidents for each student are recorded and classified, a pattern of behavior in all categories of performance begins to emerge. It must be reiterated that this device is not intended for use as a rating instrument for any one course; it is a guide for use in classifying behavioral trends as observed by the teacher. In the event that this particular record does not provide an adequate framework for defining behaviors needed to appraise students' abilities in a specific clinical experience, the faculty can revise, delete, and add the needed information. This readily available record offers teachers multiple opportunities to record and interpret observations of performance in more objective terms, leading to more reliable and valid clinical nursing evaluations. The crux of the effectiveness of this technique lies in the clinical teacher's ability to observe and record critical incidents. Observers must develop lists of behaviors that are important to the successful performance of nursing care in the given area, along with a set of criteria for successful completion of assignments.

The same technique used in recording anecdotal notes is used to record critical incidents. The recorded incident must then be examined to determine whether or not it is critical, classified according to behavior, and judged as effective or ineffective behavior according to each student's expected level of performance and the established criteria. Incidents should be recorded during every experience as soon after occurrence as possible and transferred to the performance record at regular intervals to provide a profile of the student's progress during the total experience. The records should then be studied to ascertain behavior patterns for given areas of performance. Findings should be used to determine subsequent progression of experiences comparable with individual student's abilities. To complete the cycle of student-teacher planning and selection of experiences, this record is used as the basis for individual student-teacher discussions in helping students visualize their own behavioral patterns relative to their progress and their plans for future action. Frequent individual conferences of this nature offer opportunities for the teacher to provide reinforcement by indicating strengths and to provide encouragement for development in areas of weakness, especially if not clearly recognized by the student.

This record is an integral part of the total evaluation program used to assess the student's performance during the clinical experience. The device does not lend itself to a definite grade assignment, but it does provide students with specific facts regarding their strengths and weaknesses in clinical performance.

Rating scales. Rating scales represent a standardized method of recording qualitative and quantitative judgments of observed performance. The scale generally lists traits, skills, and attitudes to be evaluated according to a value scale ranging from low to high, expressed either through the use of numerical scores or descriptive phrases. Rating scales are frequently used for describing observed performance of skills, but they also may be used for evaluating a single process or procedure, a written assignment, or an oral presentation such as a nursing care study. Unless great care is taken to construct rating scales that accurately describe the desired behaviors, skills, or performance required for meeting the course objectives, the devices will be unreliable and invalid in the estimation of the actual level of student performance. There must be faculty agreement regarding the standards to be used for each rating to correspond with each objective. Unfortunately there is always the chance that the observer's personal feelings, such as disinterest or dislike for the rating device, lack of time, personal bias regarding students, or individual variables producing halo effects, will influence his ability to make objective judgments about student performance. Accuracy of ratings is increased in proportion to faculty understanding of the behaviors and common agreement regarding the descriptive phrases used for the ratings of each behavior.

In the use of rating scales students can be the recipients of unjust evaluations unless a research approach is used in the development and implementation of a scale that does, indeed, represent a sufficient degree of reliability and validity. Simultaneously teachers responsible for using the device should be given expert guidance in how to eliminate bias when rating student performance.

As research continues to provide more valid and reliable measures of assessing clinical nursing performance, creative teachers will use this knowledge to devise their own evaluation tools for measuring clinical performance in accord with the new technologies. For example, it is possible to collect critical incidents as the basis for defining a set of descriptive behaviors for use on a rating scale. To complete the rating scale the faculty must establish a mutual agreement and understanding of the descriptions of typical ratings for each merit rating category. After the scale has been developed and tested, it should be used by a number of qualified raters who are competent to make appropriate judgments, revised in accord with their findings, and used experimentally with several groups of students. Perhaps this time-consuming process has contributed toward perpetuation of the use of unreliable, invalid rating scales by clinical nursing teachers. Dwyer and Schmitt[10] have described how one faculty worked for two years to construct a rating scale for evaluating students in maternal and infant nursing, classifying behaviors into five categories and assigning numerical weights to each. All faculty then used the agreed-on scale to evaluate the students. At the end of the semester the results were recorded on a standardized optical scanning sheet for computer processing, calculating the student's total performance in T scores. Although the system is not without drawbacks, it does offer a more reliable and objective form of clinical evaluation for students who are being evaluated by a number of clinical teachers in the same clinical area.

The sociogram. While the sociogram may not be classified as an orthodox evaluation tool, it can be an effective means of recording and analyzing student attitudes and social interaction. The sociogram consists of a diagram recording the existing interaction and interpersonal relationships of individuals within a group during a given session.

The clinical teacher can use the sociogram for evaluating clinical nursing performance in two distinct ways: (1) to evaluate an individual student's ability to function effectively as a member of a group, such as a nursing or multidisciplinary team, in the planning, organizing, and implementing of care; and (2) to evaluate an individual student's ability to participate with others in group discussions such as clinical nursing conferences, nursing clinics, role-playing situations, seminars, and case analysis discussions. In either case the sociogram provides the clinical teacher with information regarding an individual student's leadership abilities and ability to use processes of group interaction; it pinpoints problem areas by indicating the pattern of interaction established by each student in the group and indicates an individual student's attitudes toward others in the group and toward the discussion itself. The dynamics of group interaction are affected by many variables in the nursing environment as well as the individual variables of behavior; therefore, the best results are obtained when the clinical teacher uses the sociogram at frequent intervals, sampling various types of group activities.

The preparation of a sociogram involves making a schematic drawing to represent the position of each group participating, indicating the frequency of contributions made by each member along with the direction of flow for each interaction. The completed sociogram provides raw data for analyzing the interactions responsible for the resultant group action in terms of individual and total group behavior. The teacher can then provide assistance to students in establishing effective human relationships. The creative teacher can use many variations of this tool, such as (1) observing a particular group for one particular trait; (2) using frequent observations to diagnose problem areas affecting the group functioning; and (3) assessing individual contributions made by students over a period of time in order to determine each student's patterns of behavior in establishing interpersonal relationships and the composition of the relationships; this can include nursing teams with various levels of nursing personnel or interdisciplinary team relationships, in which students may exhibit an entirely different pattern of interaction. A collection of sociograms from observations made in these situations provides a composite picture of students' attitudes, values, and social sensitivity affecting their behavior in the group setting. Individual conferences help students recognize their strengths and weaknesses; often the evidence provided by the sociogram assists them in verbalizing their feelings regarding their ability to interact with others, their feelings of rejection or withdrawal, their desire to function in leadership roles, or problems of great concern to them regarding barriers to interaction with particular group members.

Together the teacher and the student can discuss means and select clinical experiences best suited to overcome the problems or lead the student into areas related to particular aptitudes such as leadership roles in various group situations. The clinical teacher can use the data analysis for understanding the cause of certain behaviors exhibited by students, making the best use of those having leadership abilities, providing additional experiences for those needing assistance with particular problems related to interpersonal relationships, and removing barriers to interaction whenever possible. The sociogram can also be used as a tool in evaluating the effectiveness or ineffectiveness of a group conference by presenting the raw data to the group and asking them to analyze and discuss possible reasons for the interactions as indicated by the diagram. From this discussion students and teachers can examine the problems underlying interactions with others and can plan ways of improving their behaviors during subsequent group meetings.

While the sociogram does not lend itself to a grading system, it provides concrete evidence that can be used to discuss problems related to learning to interact effectively in group situations, and it helps the teacher determine areas of strength and weakness in order to provide clinical learning experiences directed toward the development of effective human relationships.

Testing devices

Most schools of nursing rely heavily on either teacher-prepared tests or standard-ized tests in measuring progress and in assigning grades. However, these tests do not represent valid measurements of performance in clinical nursing *unless they clearly are constructed for that purpose.* Creative teachers have sought ways of broadening clinical evaluation to include testing devices designed to accomplish that purpose. The discussion of the following testing devices is based on the assumption that each device would be constructed to meet validity and reliability requirements and would be prepared, used, and interpreted in accord with established processes.

In the evaluation of clinical nursing, performance testing devices include pretests to determine the background knowledge and skills students have as they enter a new area, tests to determine students' progress and readiness to assume responsibilities, and achievement tests to indicate degree of progress during stated intervals and at the conclusion of the experience. Preoccupation with evaluating clinical performance in terms of mastery of skills has tended to overshadow the devising of tests to measure the student's ability to organize information, think creatively, and make value judgments relative to nursing care. Evaluation of creative abilities evidenced by divergent patterns of thought in clinical problem-solving situations should include essay tests, completion tests built around nursing care problems, and other similar devices for measuring creative clinical nursing performance.

Essay tests. Bagley[11] views the evaluation of clinical performance as closely related to the use of the essay test. He maintains that both seek to determine the student's ability to integrate, organize, and apply knowledge in demonstrating understanding of a high order, except that nursing situations present more variables in solving problems of real-life situations. Essay questions can be used to advantage in determining how students organize the basic information provided by a test item describing a clinical nursing problem and the degree to which they utilize critical thinking abilities in providing a workable solution to the problem or discover that there is more than one way to solve the problem. Inherent in the use of essay examinations for aspects of clinical nursing is the student's conscious or unconscious expression of attitudes, values, and appreciations regarding specific clinical nursing experiences. For example, the use of an essay test to determine the student's ability to solve nursing problems related to the geriatric patient may reveal the student's basic attitudes, values, or appreciations regarding geriatric patients because of the image they represent to the student. The answers also reflect the student's ability to understand or appreciate the cultural, social, economic, or age factors as they affect the student's approach to the presenting problem.

The difficulty with essay examinations lies in two areas: (1) the construction of questions designed to elicit free expression of ideas regarding a solution to a problem without seeking *exact right or wrong* answers to specific questions, and (2) the scoring of the questions by distinguishing between data revealing the student's ability to solve problems and the student's personal attitudes and ideas about the problems. In both instances the teacher of clinical nursing must determine those broad areas to be tested regarding the student's ability to organize information, make generalizations, and use creative thinking in making value judgments to solve the problem rather than give specific answers to the question. To score the test items it is necessary to develop a systematic approach to the analysis of data, leading to certain conclusions, as opposed to seeking definitive, factual answers. While the attitudes, ideals, values, or appreciations revealed by students serve as a means of helping teachers understand student behaviors, they cannot, in fairness to the student, be considered as a part of the grading criteria for the test unless changes in them have been clearly stated as objectives for the experience. Brown's description of an experiment to determine the extent to which tests and grades motivate learning underscores these aspects of measurement leading to the adoption of a pass-fail, or a satisfactory-unsatisfactory grading system.[12]

Written situation tests. The use of periodic written situation tests drawn from nursing situations is another means of evaluation of clinical performance.[13] A description of a "case," or nursing care problem, is used as the basis for testing students' abilities to apply theoretical knowledge to lifelike situations. Following the written description of the situation to be tested, several approaches may be used to secure the desired information: (1) the student is requested to solve the problem by supplying answers to a series of simple completion test items; (2) the student is requested to list the steps to be taken, using an essay approach to the question; (3) the student is given the opportunity to determine solutions to the problem by using appropriate books and journals, which could be considered a simulation approach because it is one frequently used in the actual working situation when problems arise; or (4) the student makes a selection from a number of possible solutions listed in multiple-choice form. The creative teacher of clinical nursing can use this method to great advantage because the clinical situations provide the needed information for creating descriptions of nursing situations to be solved by the students. This method of evaluation provides a means of discovering the creative potential of individual students and of determining their readiness to progress in accomplishing the desired outcomes. Such tests could well be used as self-evaluative devices by allowing students the opportunity to discuss areas of strength and weakness with the teacher and to retain the tests for self-study purposes.

Situation tests using educational communication media. Situation tests, as just described, have been developed by others, whereby the situation itself is presented to students through the use of simulated teaching devices such as the previously described Arrhythmia Trainer and Torso, or slides, films, audiotapes, or videotapes, followed by a series of related questions. This same concept of learning is utilized by many of the programmed instruction devices developed for specific purposes in nursing education. The use of such media can convey the situation to the students in more meaningful ways, providing for greater standardization in the presentation of the situation and leaving less chance for variations in students' interpretations. The judgments regarding what they have seen or heard provide the basis for the students' decisions as they answer the test items. As we move increasingly into the area of independent study and use of multimedia approaches to learning, this type of testing on an individual as well as a group basis will, of necessity, become an integral part of the clinical nursing evaluation program.

Observational situation tests. Another situation-type test lending itself particularly well to the evaluation of nursing performance is that described by Fivars and Gosnell[1] as the Observational Situation Test. This test substitutes the use of simulated situations with that of controlled observations of student performance in the actual nursing setting. The technique requires either that the teacher of nursing become adept as an observer or that trained observers be utilized in gathering the needed data for evaluating the desired behaviors. The purpose of the Observational Situation Test is to determine the extent to which students can demonstrate ability to solve patients' problems in the live situation. Given a set of conditions determined by the teacher, the teacher-observer records the student's actual behaviors while functioning in the clinical setting, introducing additional variables to be overcome as the student demonstrates his particular way of coping with the problem.

Although it may be argued that patients' problems vary widely, it is possible to select problems having comparable outcomes. These can be used for observing students' abilities to follow through with appropriate actions, regardless of the range of individual conditions likely to occur when dealing directly with patients. There are various way for observers to record the student performance, but the use of the Critical Incident Technique appears to be quite satisfactory, since it does not require subjective judgments regarding degrees of quality of performance. The observer merely records the incidents as effective or ineffective according to the outcome of the total action, using the predetermined behavioral categories for recording each incident. Available valid and reliable rating scales, checklists, and similar devices may also be used for scoring this type of test.

Another variation of this method employs a more sophisticated approach by using data processing for determining specific items to be tested. Each task to be tested is placed in a sealed envelope; during the testing period students are given the envelope, which provides the procedural instructions for accomplishing the given task. Trained observers are available to record actual performance by using one of the aforementioned devices, providing the needed data in arriving at a final score. This approach has been used by the American Institute of Research[14] and has implications for use in schools of nursing. Some teachers of nursing might inquire into the processes involved in this evaluation approach and devise their own research for adapting it in evaluation of clinical nursing.

Evaluation of assigned materials and products

Throughout the clinical course students are usually requested to give demonstrations, prepare oral or written nursing care studies, and prepare workbooks, diaries, exhibits, posters, models, mock-ups, and other similar devices. When these items bear a direct relationship to the clinical program, they can provide a new dimension to the total experience. But unless the teacher of clinical nursing makes a provision for evaluating these materials as a part of the total program, they tend to lose their educational significance and value. These projects and products reflect many of the same desired outcomes as the direct nursing experiences; therefore, comparable approaches to their evaluation should be considered by the clinical teacher.

The teacher should determine criteria for judging major components of each project or product, determine the weight to be assigned to each criterion, and define descriptions of merits to be assigned for each category of rating, such as satisfactory or unsatisfactory. When there is an agreed-on plan for evaluating these materials, the faculty should assume responsibility for keeping students informed regarding the criteria to be used for judging their completed projects or products. The dangers of placing too much value on such tangible assignments, along with using a disproportionate grading system, can be controlled by the clinical teacher's continuous evaluation of these course requirements in relation to the desired outcomes for the total course.

Interpretation of evaluation system to students

Whatever the grading system used by a faculty of a school of nursing, the teacher of clinical nursing holds responsibility for communicating the meaning of the grades in terms of individual student progress. Students have the right to be kept informed regarding the quality of their performance as indicated by any test or other measure of evaluation. If grades are presented, students should be given the complete range of scores made by the total group as an indication of how they stand in relation to others in the class. Grades in themselves are useless unless students are advised of their level of performance as indicated by specific items on the evaluating device. Rankings, percentile scores, or letter grades alone do not provide students with information they need in terms of areas requiring remedial assistance or areas in which they excel and may wish to pursue further. Interpretation of results of the total evaluation system used in the clinical nursing situation should be a cooperative venture between student and teacher who continually seek opportunities for professional growth and development based on mutual respect and understanding.

STUDENT SELF-EVALUATION

Evaluation is an integral component of the teaching-learning cycle. Therefore, if the teaching program in clinical nursing has been built on the democratic philosophy of providing students with opportunities to assume responsibility for their own learning, it follows that they also need opportunities to appraise their own progress through self-evaluation. As in the case of the previously described methods of clinical nursing evaluation, student self-evaluation begins with the identification and clarification of the desired objectives for the given experience and the formulation of a plan for attaining them.

One of the prevailing themes of this book has been that of promoting teacher-student cooperative planning in the setting of goals for learning and in determining needed learning activities. It follows, then, that there must be an opportunity for students to explore the attainment of their goals with a teacher who is a good listener. When students can express and analyze their reactions to nursing situations and their learnings needs and can appraise their progress toward their goals, they are able to proceed at their own rate, using their own approach until they are willing to accept assistance from the teacher. Learning is a highly individualized process in which much information on the degree of progress made toward goals is known only by the student. Therefore, it is highly important that the students learn to carefully evaluate themselves through various self-evaluation tools. The subjective element of self evaluation is present to the degree that students respond to the ratings in terms of self-defense or self-enhancement. If teachers of clinical nursing attend to the students' responses, they will establish a learning environment that offers help at the time students are ready for it. An open-door policy will allow students to seek help any time they need it and to express themselves regarding their daily needs, plans, and progress. The way in which this is accomplished will be determined by the individual teacher's self-awareness and use of self.

To be effective, self-evaluation practices should be introduced with the first course in clinical nursing, becoming progressively more refined as students advance to independent action in the achievement of personal and professional goals. Whatever format is adopted, there should be a plan of consistent self-evaluation providing for periodic reports of progress toward meeting goals, along with opportunities for cooperative teacher-student discussion of problems encountered and means of resolving them, with the aim of furnishing students with greater insights into their own problems.

A number of devices may be used in the total process of student self-evaluation. The following, which were described in Chapter 8, are mentioned because they can serve a vital role in self-evaluative processes, and some have been widely used by nurses. They include process recordings, audiotape recordings, videotape recordings (indicating action as well as verbal skills), and programmed instruction materials. Other devices more commonly used are self-rating scales, narrative reports, and anecdotal records. Self-rating scales may be used as a final summary of progress made toward meeting the desired objectives and specific behaviors. An example of such a rating scale can be found in a publication of Guinee.[15] This type of rating scale can be used by comparing the students' ratings of themselves with the teacher's ratings of the students. Widely variable results indicate a need for the teacher and the student to reexamine the total learning situation. The student may have misunderstood the assignment or have resorted to the use of ratings as self-defense or self-

enhancement mechanisms. The anaysis may provide an opportunity for the student's becoming more accurate in self-evaluation; this in itself should be considered an indication of the student's psychological growth. From the teacher's viewpoint the results may reveal that the teacher misinterpreted the student's actions, introduced certain elements of the halo effect, failed to convey the expected outcomes in a manner understood by the students, or relied entirely on this device at the close of the clinical nursing experience without having had an ongoing program. Students do not respond favorably to self-evaluation processes at the time that a grade is near at hand or if they have had no previous information from the teacher regarding their progress during the experience.

Narrative reports and anecdotal records are closely related, but they differ in format and degree of use. The narrative report lends itself to use with beginning students in recording running comments and notes regarding their goals and the way they believe they should perform in order to accomplish them. Each successive narrative builds on the previous ones as students become more involved in nursing experiences; reflective thinking is required as the students describe feelings about their performance and determine ways of directing their activities toward improvement. Students may tend to write the narrative report for the sake of fulfilling a requirement rather than using it as a guide to reflective thinking, or they may tend to respond according to what they think will satisfy or please the teacher without really representing the student's feelings. If, indeed, we expect students to be self-directive, creative individuals in their approach to the learning situation, we must provide them with enough flexibility to adapt a given requirement to meet their individual learning needs best. While it is true that some students need a "crutch" in order to produce a narrative report, these students must learn to exert their powers of critical thinking and develop the habit of analyzing a situation without the help of others.

The very process of self-evaluation means the risk of exposing one's true self to the teacher; therefore, the teacher must maintain a position of acceptance of whatever the student chooses to reveal. The teacher uses this information to move the student in the direction of growth by accepting it for what it means to the student. The teacher must pose questions that will allow the student to determine his own strengths and weaknesses as revealed by the information and must develop a plan of action to move in a positive direction. Regardless of the degree of growth during initial phases of the process or the teacher's personal feelings regarding the issue, the ideas expressed represent the best that the student is capable of at that particular time. Given encouragement, acceptance, and clues to needed changes, the student can grow through the experience and become increasingly self-directive in determining a pattern of action best suited to meet his goals.

Narrative reports assist teachers in gaining insight into individual student needs as they function in the clinical nursing setting, provide valuable information regarding the direction in planning or revising needed learning experiences, and indicate the need for inclusion of new areas of learning or for remedial learning experiences. The process of self-evaluation assists students to grow in their experiences and abilities to think about their performance, resulting in the development of self-awareness regarding their ability to understand, interpret, and accept their own behavior in their continued growth.

Anecdotal notes, whether written by students for purposes of self-evaluation or by teachers, utilize the same basic principles described earlier in the chapter. Their use as a self-evaluation tool over an extended time period can encourage students to draw their own conclusions regarding their ability to perceive their behavior as a whole during the clinical experience and to analyze specific incidents as they occur.

The use of these data assists the teacher in helping students analyze and accept their behaviors by their own recognition rather than convincing students to view themselves as the teacher views them. There are various ways of utilizing anecdotal notes as a self-evaluation device, depending largely on the objectives desired. Palmer's extensive study in the use of anecdotal notes as a self-evaluative device describes several ways of seeking the desired information.[16] Studies of this type are needed in other schools of nursing if we intend to develop reliable and valid methods of evaluation and self-evaluation related to clinical nursing performance.

Through the use of process recordings, audiotape recordings, videotape recordings of performance, or programmed instruction materials, students can review their performance on an independent study basis before analyzing their strengths and weaknesses. The narrative reports, anecdotal notes, and self-rating scales, along with comments or suggestions made by the clinical teacher, should offer students ungraded comments or suggestions for consideration in terms of assessing their strengths and weaknesses and determining means of improving their performance. Opportunities to explore these, with ample time for study and analysis, aid students in coming to terms with themselves and in formulating their plan of action to improve their performance.

Throughout the total process of self-evaluation, regardless of the techniques or combinations of devices used in the self-analysis, the teacher of nursing should be available for individual or group conferences as students seek them. Teachers must create an atmosphere of learning that encourages students to seek assistance in analyzing their strengths and weaknesses, discussing professional goals and ways to attain them, discussing problems that they encounter in the clinical situation and offering encouragement in maintaining ideals and high standards in the practice of the profession. In addition, students need individual guidance relative to proceeding in accord with their assessed level of performance. Those who sense that they have accomplished the desired competencies seek opportunities to broaden their scope of learning; the teacher is responsible for helping those students to assess further their abilities and needs to that end. Students having great difficulties, who become aware of their own capabilities and limitations, sometimes find it easier to accept the fact that either they must seek additional help or they cannot satisfactorily complete the program. These frequent conferences, along with cooperative teacher-student evaluation processes, strengthen relationships between student and faculty as they share their observations and work together in an effort to contribute positively to the total teaching-learning process.

EVALUATION OF TEACHER EFFECTIVENESS IN THE CLINICAL NURSING SETTING

A school of nursing evaluation program would be incomplete without some consideration of teacher effectiveness. Such an appraisal has not proceeded smoothly nor advanced rapidly because of many of the same variables inherent in other kinds of evaluation. But if we cannot distinguish between good and poor teaching in the clinical nursing setting, how can we expect teachers to know the way to help students achieve desired goals? Furthermore, if teachers of clinical nursing wish to give serious consideration to changing their teaching approaches in terms of the various innovations suggested throughout this book, there must be more than juggling clinical experiences and student schedules. Clinical teachers must rethink ways of integrating classroom subject matter into the nursing experiences, act differently while teaching in the clinical nursing setting, and relate differently to the students. The responsibility for the improvement of teaching rests with the faculty of a school; the faculty must agree on identifiable criteria

for determining good teaching as distinguished from poor teaching before improvement can be made and before the administrative officers of the school can reward good teaching. The following are some unanswered questions regarding the role of the faculty in appraisal of teaching effectiveness: (1) How does a faculty identify good teaching? (2) Do teachers really want to teach? (3) Should the faculty give equal attention to identifying poor teaching practices? (4) How can teaching and learning aids be used to improve teaching practices? (5) How should teaching excellence be recognized and rewarded? (6) How does identification of clinical teaching quality affect a faculty member's rating, which usually includes evaluation of research and service skills as well? Although we lack the immediate solution to many of these questions, we cannot fulfil the purposes of the school unless we can evaluate the performance of teachers who are delegated the responsibilities for students.

While many approaches are being taken to measure teaching effectiveness within programs, this discussion is confined to an exploration of possible ways of evaluating teacher effectiveness in the clinical nursing setting. The approach is discussed within the confines of three broad categories: (1) student evaluations of teaching effectiveness, (2) teacher self-evaluations, and (3) colleague evaluations.

Student evaluation of teaching effecti/eness

The impact of contemporary culture discussed (in Chapter 1) keenly affects the evaluation of teachers by students. It is coming to be an accepted feature of the American academic scene; however, teacher evaluations conducted by student groups with varied motives lead to inaccurate appraisal and do little to change teacher performance. On the other hand, properly obtained evaluations of teacher effectiveness result in: (1) a means of teacher self-improvement leading to changes in teaching approaches and course objectives, (2) strengthening student-teacher relationships, (3) renewed recognition of the student as an individual and as the basic reason for the existence of the educational institution, and (4) greater commitment to teaching.

The limitations of student rating devices such as developmental level of students involved in the rating, cultural biases, student fears involving grades, and rating scales heavily loaded with items calling for reactions to personality factors, mannerisms, and teaching styles affect the degree to which one can establish positive correlations between student approval and teaching effectiveness. Teachers fear that official requests for ratings from administrative officers invite students to become hypercritical and even rebellious regarding their teachers and courses. However, it would appear that there is a need for these teachers to supplant fear with courage by inviting student evaluation of their teaching. It is the very act of not acting that causes administrative officers of a university to gain control by seeking this information if it is not available by any other means. In spite of the limitations of student ratings of teacher effectiveness, individual teachers can use student ratings profitably by analyzing their own teaching patterns, styles, mannerisms, and greatest strengths and weaknesses and by examining broad samplings of such student responses over an extended period of time.

There are many ways of devising tools for student evaluation of various aspects of clinical nursing such as (1) appraisal of the objectives of the particular clinical nursing experience and the extent to which the teacher provides for their accomplishments; (2) organization and management used in planning clinical nursing experiences; (3) quality of the teacher's supervision of students in the clinical setting; (4) teacher-student relationships in cooperative planning, implementing, and evaluating of clinical nursing experiences; and (5) the teacher's ability to function as a knowl-edgeable, expert clinical nursing practitioner. Rating devices calling for justification of stated opinions are of greater value to the teacher than those indicating a scaled reaction ranging from excellent to poor and should follow the same basic rules used by teachers in evaluating students.

In addition to rating scales other devices are available such as (1) forms asking students to complete sentences best describing their feelings or complete drawings to illustrate their thoughts regarding a particular incident, (2) use of Q-sort questionnaires, (3) narrative descriptive forms following the use of a few lead questions, or (4) attitude inventories designed to measure students' attitudes toward a course rather than toward a teacher. Even when teachers believe that they have made a rating scale or similar device that excludes some of the previously stated limiting factors, the teachers themselves must be able to view the results with detachment regarding their personal feelings. Students who are honest in their evaluations can provide teachers with valuable information, but if teachers themselves are emotionally insecure, the results can be disturbing to their self-confidence. On the other hand, a word of caution is needed for those teachers of clinical nursing who tend to rely too heavily on students as their source of gratification and ego strength. What is needed is a middle-of-the-road approach to the analysis of such evaluations. The results should be weighed in terms of the known limits offered by such evaluations, yet teachers should be motivated to continue their effectiveness in teaching because of the support evidenced by the data as well as the suggested areas of improvement noted by the students.

Teacher self-evaluations

While teachers may glibly state that they evaluate their success according to the degree to which students effectively achieve the outcomes established for a given course, teachers should know about their own performance of teaching functions in order to maintain or improve their effectiveness. To arrive at a destination without knowing how one got there is comparable to saying that the students accomplished the objectives of the course but the teacher is not quite certain *how* they did it.

Teachers of clinical nursing who are genuinely concerned about continuing to develop professionally seek the answers to such questions as: How do teachers plan learning experiences to meet the desired objectives? How do teachers allow for individual differences while supervising students in the clinical settings? How do teachers provide for student progression to independent action? How do teachers promote student self-understanding? How do teachers provide a democratic learning environment conducive to the release of the student's creative potentials? How do teachers use their own creative potential in providing ways of helping students meet the desired objectives? What kind of student relationships seem to be most conductive to learning in the teacher's particular clinical experience? There are many other questions that need answering if teachers are to continue to function creatively in clinical nursing.

Clinical teachers can use televised recordings, videotapes, audiotape recordings, films, and other devices for examining their own performance. In addition, each teacher of clinical nursing needs periodic opportunities for reflective thinking and self-evaluation of teaching practices. Sometimes this analysis can be augmented by using a rating scale or checklist as the criterion for the self-evaluation. Heidgerken suggests a criterion for self evaluation that is general in nature and could be adapted for use in the teaching of clinical nursing.[17]

Evaluation by colleagues

While the primary purpose of appraising teaching effectiveness is that of improving teaching in terms of the total profession, this overall purpose frequently suffers from the individual teacher's concern for self-improvement. In fact in schools of nursing there is an apparent unwillingness of teachers to concern themselves with the improvement of a colleague's effectiveness in teaching clinical nursing. But if teaching effectiveness appraisals are to contribute to the improvement of teaching in clinical nursing, individual teachers must initiate the necessary action for appraising the teaching practices of their colleagues, a practice commonly used in colleges and universities. A more equitable evaluation can be made by a colleague who is studying similar teaching techniques and patterns and is interested in teaching improvement as opposed to evaluation by administrative personnel, who can evaluate faculty members for purposes of promotions without real regard for the improvement of instructional programs. Once the purpose and criteria for peer visitations and evaluations are made clear to all faculty members, there can be increased feelings of cooperation in looking for ways of improving the nursing program. Just as we allow students the freedom to select certain experiences, so should teachers of clinical nursing be permitted to request colleagues to visit each other's class in order to clarify ideas and seek suggestions regarding ways of improving certain areas of teaching.

This kind of evaluation can be helpful but will flourish only in an environment in which teachers want to improve their teaching and have participated in setting up the criteria and methods of evaluation to be used. The teacher should always be consulted prior to any visit regarding its feasibility and purposes to avoid undue emotional conflict in the teacher while being observed. The observer should be familiar with the teacher's background and purpose of the visit in order to make best use of the observation time. The observer should be unobtrusive; however, the teacher should extend to the observer the same courtesies extended to any visitor. After the visit the observer should (1) make a permanent record of the visit in accord with its purpose and (2) arrange to have a conference with the teacher. In conference, the two can clarify observations, identify specific strengths, outline suggestions for improvement, and arrange continued reciprocal help regarding handling of problems that are of concern. If teachers of clinical nursing or other faculty members of a given school of nursing object to evaluative observation visits by colleagues, the responsibility for substituting constructive suggestions and actions lies squarely with them. By tradition the faculty contributes to policy-making by the university; by the same token the faculty must assume responsibility for identifying good and poor teaching practices in an effort to improve teaching effectiveness.

Ability to accept information about oneself is a complex phenomenon; but it helps if one believes the information to be objective, valid, and given in an effort to help rather than harm. Teachers who are able to translate understanding into action as a part of the teaching process, to experiment with their own behavior, to obtain objective information about their own behavior, and to evaluate this information in terms of teachers' roles are attaining self-insight.

REFERENCES

1. Fivars, Grace, and Gosnell, Doris: Nursing evaluation: the problems and the process, New York, 1966, Macmillan, Inc.
2. Barc, Carole: Behavioral changes through effective evaluation, Journal of Nursing Education 6:7-11, Nov., 1967.
3. Tyler, Ralph W.: Basic principles of curriculum and instruction, Chicago, 1950, University of Chicago Press.
4. Let's examine, an annotated bibliography on measurement and evaluation, Part I, Nursing Outlook 16:70-72, May, 1968.
5. Let's examine, an annotated bibliography on measurement and evaluation, Part II, Nursing Outlook 16:52-53, June, 1968.
6. Anderson, Diann, and Saxon, Jean: Performance evaluation of nursing students, Nursing Outlook 16:56-58, May, 1968.
7. Flanagan, John C., Gosnell, Doris, and Fivars, Grace: Evaluating student performance, American Journal of Nursing 63:96-99, Nov., 1963.
8. Heslin, Phyllis: Evaluating clinical performance, Nursing Outlook 11:345, May, 1963.
9. Flanagan, John C., and others: The clinical experience record for nursing students, Pittsburgh, 1960, Psychometric Techniques Associates.
10. Dwyer, Joyce, and Schmitt, John: Using the computer to evaluate clinical performance, Nursing Forum 8(3):266-274, 1969.
11. Bagley, Norton R.: Merits of the essay test in the evaluation process, Nursing Outlook 14:67-68, Sept., 1966.
12. Brown, Margaret: How much do tests and grades motivate learning? Nursing Outlook 16:60-62, Oct., 1968.
13. de Tornay, Rheba: Measuring problem-solving skills by means of the simulated clinical nursing problem test, Journal of Nursing Education 7:3-8, Aug., 1968.
14. Gorham, William A., Lichtenstein, Stanley, and Marchese, Angeline C.: Specific nursing behaviors related to patient care and improvement: measuring nursing performance, Washington, D. C., 1959, American Institute for Research (AIR-B-24-59-FR-204).
15. Guinee, Kathleen: The aims and methods of nursing education, New York, 1966, Macmillan, Inc.
16. Palmer, Mary E.: Our students write their own behavioral anecdotes, Nursing Outlook 11:185-187, March, 1963.
17. Heidgerken, Loretta: Teaching and learning in schools of nursing, Philadelphia, 1965, J. B. Lippincott Co.

SUGGESTED READINGS

Armington, C. L., and others: Student evaluation—threat or incentive, Nursing Outlook 21:789-792, Dec., 1972.

de Tornay, Rheba: Measuring problem solving skills by means of the simulated clinical nursing problem test, Journal of Nursing Education 7:3-8, Aug., 1968.

McIntyre, H. M., and others: A simulated clinical nursing test, Nursing Research 21:429-435, Sept./Oct., 1972.

Moore, Marjorie: A point of view of evaluation, Nursing Outlook 16:54-57, July, 1968.

Morton, B. F.: Nursing service and education in a comprehensive health care center, Journal of Nursing Administration 3:23-26, May/June, 1973.

Murphy, Juanita: The nub of the learning process, American Journal of Nursing 71:306-310, Feb., 1971.

Simpson, M. June: The walk-around laboratory practical examination in evaluating clinical nursing skills, Journal of Nursing Education 6:23-26, Nov., 1967.

Stevens, Delphi: A tool for evaluating clinical performance, American Journal of Nursing 70:1308-1310, Jan., 1970.

Stewart, Ruth F., and Graham, Josephine L.: Evaluation tools in public health nursing education, Nursing Outlook 16:50-51, March, 1968.

Strom, Robert, and Galloway, Charles: Becoming

a better teacher, Journal of Teacher Education 18:285-291, Fall, 1967.

Topf, Margaret: A behavioral checklist for estimating the development of communication skills, Journal of Nursing Education 8:29-34, Nov., 1969.

Wientge, King M.: Adult teacher self-improvement through evaluation by students, Adult Education Journal 18:94-100, Winter, 1968.

Wood, V.: Evaluation of student nurse clinical performance, International Nursing Review 19(4):336-343, 1972.

Unit IV   Professional responsibilities for fostering creative teaching in clinical nursing

Professions, like nations, can only flourish through an individual sense of corporate responsibility.

FLORENCE NIGHTINGALE

10 The creative teacher of clinical nursing: responsibilities to the profession

RESPONSIBILITIES AS A PROFESSIONAL NURSE

Popular usage of the term *professional* has reduced its meaning from that described by experts in the professional fields to apply to almost any occupational endeavor reflecting performance beyond that of the amateur. Nursing continues to grapple with the knotty problem of defining the meaning of professional nursing. It is not the intent of this chapter either to compare various proposed concepts of the term or to offer another definition. Rather, the discussion is confined to the nature of the responsibilities expected of *professional nurses who are teachers of clinical nursing.* Darley reminds us that the use of one's intellectual capacity, educational background, and sense of moral values in making highly responsible judgments is the hallmark of the professional person. He further suggests that the professional person, dealing as he does with unpredictable human situations, must make judgments based on standards set by the person himself, which transcend the rules, regulations, and codes of ethics set by one's professional group.[1]

Responsibilities for development and maintenance of professional nursing standards

The term *professional* implies the provision of a highly individualized and personalized service to others administered in accord with standards without being limited by criteria and qualifications. The profession of nursing holds the responsibility for providing an effective service to the society it serves by developing and enforcing professional standards in the selection, preparation, and practice of nurses. The Standards of Nursing Practice developed by the Congress on Nursing Practice of the American Nurses Association[2] have provided a more definitive statement of the parameters of our practice than was available previously.

Clearly, however, it is not enough for the teacher of clinical nursing to rely on a set of standards as guidelines for recommending students for graduation and licensure. The individual teacher, regardless of position in the organizational pattern, must acknowledge accountability to society for setting and maintaining professional standards by (1) recommending admission standards commensurate with qualities and knowledge found necessary to practice nursing effectively; (2) continuously appraising student performance; (3) continually evaluating the curriculum, using experimental studies in deriving valid information for recommended changes in standards; (4) setting personal standards of practice and ethical behavior that exemplify the goals of the school and the profession, and (5) working actively with other professional nurses to meet the societal expectations.

The nursing profession is directly responsible for the administration of its standards; it has primary responsibility for developing and enforcing standards of selection, preparation, and performance of students and faculty and in the administrative organization of the educational institution. States have shared this responsibility by mandating licensing boards to monitor both the education and practice of nursing. Nursing organizations, particularly the National League for

189

Nursing, participate by accrediting schools of nursing and certain practice agencies. Good teachers of nursing are willing to divorce themselves from the "they" concept regarding standards to be met to attain school accreditation and professional licensure for students. They recognize that part of their nursing responsibility is to contribute ideas and findings to the appropriate controlling bodies. The end results then reflect the "we" concept in the coordinated actions of professional nurses striving to maintain professional standards. Teachers cannot be responsible for graduates of their programs. They can, however, provide effective role models of conscientious practitioners and encourage their students to strive toward the same. The failure of health professionals in effective self-critique has led to increased external, often governmental, study and control. If we see control as a means of ensuring social well-being, we can work toward effective implementation of multiple review techniques.

Responsibilities to professional nursing organizations

The comment made by the late President Kennedy applies equally in this situation—ask not what your professional organization can do for you, but what you can do for your professional organization. Teachers of clinical nursing share with all professional nurses the same rights and responsibilities as members of their professional nursing organizations. But by virtue of their position, clinical teachers are in much more accessible circumstances for supporting and contributing to professional nursing organizations as role models for students in helping them to develop their sense of responsibility regarding the profession and its supportive organizations.

While a professional organization is chiefly concerned with the improvement of professional services to society and the provision of improved educational and working conditions for its members, its basic intent is *not* that of thinking and acting *for* the individual professional nurse. We have now reached a point at which the pressures of social, economical, educational, and health changes are leading to shifts in power distribution among vested interests of political groups. There has been a growing tendency for individual professional nurses to allow those in control of their professional organizations to do their thinking and acting for them, yielding to conformity with the group, or to ignore professional groups altogether and act individually. As professional nurses function within the framework of their organizations, individual members and, in particular, teachers of clinical nursing have an obligation to inform themselves of various facets of the issues at hand and to think and act in a way that represents rational participation and individual integrity in the resolution of multiple problems. The teachers of clinical nursing should consider themselves valuable to the profession and should make a sustained effort to support and contribute to professional organizations in ways other than monetary. There are endless ways of contributing actively to nursing organizations, whether on local, state, national, or international levels.

Our rapidly growing profession can scarcely afford the luxury of having many wait on the sidelines to be asked to serve. The necessity to move with expediency often dictates the choice of those who can be relied on to contribute, but those who volunteer in various activities are welcomed with open arms. The danger here lies in allowing oneself to become involved with too many projects, resulting in time pressures that interfere with competent work based on sound judgments. Used in its proper perspective, the ability to say "no" is as important as the ability to say "yes." The professional nurse must seek balance in activities and personal and professional responsibilities in a manner that allows for individual satisfaction in each undertaking.

When the ability to play an active role in professional organizations becomes limited, the teacher can keep informed about the organizations' activities, basic beliefs, stands taken regarding current issues, legislative matters affecting nurses and nursing, and standards affecting educational and patient care practices. Subscribing to and reading the professional publications, attending professional meetings in which ideas and issues are raised, and discussing these ideas with others within the immediate environment have an enlightening and unifying effect, producing informed, cooperative actions of an organization that more truly represents its constituents. Once adequate information and discussion have been afforded members and action is taken, it is incumbent on every member to give support to changes that are made. This means the recognition that the view an organization has chosen may continue to arouse emotional responses. These must be handled by those who recognize the need for changes and are willing to involve themselves to ensure implementation of such changes.

When one considers the numbers who make up our professional organizations and the percentage of occupational groups within nursing that is representative of this membership, it becomes apparent that teachers in clinical nursing are a minority group. In active involvement they may appear the majority because of employment that allows or encourages flexibility of time to attend meetings, support committee work, and other activities. If the teachers are not in close touch with a wide range of practitioners, their work could lead toward further separation, rather than unification, of action.

While our pattern of professional organization may be no more complex than that of some other groups, there is a tendency to use our complexities as deterrents to the interpretation of the functions, qualifications, and standards of varying levels of nursing contributing to the profession. To the public there are few crucial differences between the licensed practical nurse, the nursing aide or graded assistant, and the registered nurse graduated from an associate of arts program, a diploma pro-

gram, or a collegiate program of nursing; between the various levels of educational preparation and experience of teachers of clinical nursing; or between economic security programs for nurses and nurses' unions, the ANA, and the National League for Nursing (NLN). There are such questions as the following: Why is there a shortage of nurses? Why must hospital costs reflect the nurses' demands for increased salaries? Why do we contribute to hospital building fund drives when there are insufficient nurses to take care of us now? Why should students spend four years in a school of nursing when they can become a registered nurse in less time in other kinds of programs? What is going to happen to all of the nurses who are graduates of diploma schools of nursing? What will become of the licensed practical nurse if we move toward two levels of nursing personnel—professional and technical? What is meant by the extended or expanded role of the nurse and how do we plan to provide educational experiences to this end? Why does the nursing profession support two professional organizations? What is the difference between the two professional organizations? How do these two organizations work cooperatively without encroaching on each other's objectives? What does the ANA or the NLN do for me? What services do these organizations offer society?

Questions similar to these could be asked ad infinitum by those concerned with nursing as a profession and as it affects society. The teachers of clinical nursing is responsible for setting the example in working toward answers that will lead to a better nursed and better informed public. Perhaps the slogan should be *speak out again and again!* Maybe the time has come for us to seek the assistance of public relations experts with mass interpretation regarding these issues, which are not to be ignored if we, as a profession, wish to be recognized as individuals of worth to the society we seek to serve.

The best opportunities for promoting membership and participation in our professional organizations lie in our ability to present a role model that motivates students, new graduates, and other graduate nurses to emulate us. It is indeed a paradox when one witnesses the excellent, business-like means used in making sound judgments regarding major issues faced by the profession that are displayed by the students who are involved in their own local, state, and national nursing organizations; yet when these students become graduate registered nurses, so little of this talent is seen represented in the memberships of the professional organizations. There is little doubt that the success of the National Student Nurses' Association (NSNA) can be attributed largely to the need for peer groups such as this to meet together to discuss issues in nursing and nursing education as they see them. Perhaps teachers of clinical nursing, along with countless other nurses, have failed to convey the true meaning of our responsibilities and contributions to our professional organizations.

As early as 1967 the NSNA took action at their national convention indicating their deep commitment to nursing and to its future as a profession. The report of this meeting reveals a request by the group that they have the opportunity to assist the ANA-NLN Committee on Careers in informing prospective students about trends in nursing and nursing education and that ANA professional credentials and personnel service forms and ANA membership applications provide space for listing NSNA activities. In addition the organization pledged its members to seek opportunities to cooperate with state nurses' associations in efforts to interpret the professions' standards for nursing education and practice to state agencies and legislative bodies, and the entire group pledged itself to prepare its members for joining the ANA as soon as eligible on graduation.[3]

While teachers in clinical nursing may say, "This is nothing new—we have done these things in our school and our local organization for quite some time," the crux of the matter lies in the realization that this convention represented some 4,300 students from fifty states and Puerto Rico, who evidently believed enough in the necessity for assuming their responsibilities to their professional organizations to establish their own mechanisms for achieving these goals. This leads us to believe that as practicing professional nurses, we have failed to help students fulfil these needs. These students are to be commended for their foresight and courage in proposing such an action approach to some of the time-worn problems. It now becomes imperative that we, as nurse-educators—administrators, teachers, nursing service personnel, and others concerned about the nursing profession—accept these suggestions in the spirit in which they were meant. We, because of our closeness to students, can provide some of the necessary machinery and individual support that is needed to help these men and women as they inherit a lifetime of work in implementing the decisions we have been so busily making for them! Teachers of clinical nursing would do well to use with students the same principles that they use in establishing satisfying interpersonal relationships with patients. Students are telling us that they do indeed want a voice in shaping the profession, but they also see things in new combinations, which means that we must be willing to accept change and listen to some of their approaches and ideas before we reject them or, even worse, fail to seek their participation. Students who have participated in their own organizations and have served on faculty committees are better prepared to make the transition as contributing members of the ANA and NLN.

It is important to recognize the need for seeking new members for the organization as a constant building process; we cannot wait until we have drained the life blood from an organization and then expect to recruit new members to replace the "regulars." This means that we must provide an environment that motivates students to participate as they become graduates. Another dimension of promoting membership and participation is that of constantly being aware of professional associates who either are not members or are not actively contributing to their professional organizations and those who are new in the community, particularly international nurses, who, for want of an invitation, are most eager to attend and contribute to organizational meetings. While it is understandable that some nurses believe they are unsuccessful "salesmen" when it involves soliciting memberships for organizations, the most valuable tool these nurses have is their use of themselves in showing by example of words and actions how to assume the responsibilities and rights associated with the professional nursing organizations.

Liaison responsibilities

It is an assumption that the school of nursing is organized on a philosophy that encourages informing personnel at all levels regarding the objectives, plans, current operation, and progress toward long-term goals, along with open discussions of issues as they arise. Given this assumption, the teacher of nursing should be active with the administrative officers in these matters. Students in the school of nursing should be the first to know the status of their school regarding current and long-term goals, curriculum patterns, accreditation status, underlying principles of the accreditation process, and information regarding any major change affecting them as students and the reasons for the change. By the same token students should be given the opportunity to question actions, suggest alternatives, share ideas with the faculty by participating on appropriate committees, and seek faculty members who will be willing to help them individually and in groups. The clinical teacher can function as a liaison between the school of nursing as an organization and the student body and by example promote assumption of responsibilities for furthering the profession.

Today nursing literature, as well as that of other professional fields, abounds with discussions regarding the fragmentation of services provided patients and the need for determining exactly how each person in contact with a patient contributes to care. While many of the health professions believe that they understand the expectations and limitations of their own responsibilities for patient care, they are reluctant to recognize or accept that which other groups suggest as their roles. Nursing has had a particularly difficult time with this process, in part because of changes in nursing practice, and in part because nursing has been predominantly a woman's field. Nurses have often done more talking than actual fact finding regarding the definition of their roles in the care of patients. The absence of positive statements by us has led those in other disciplines to decide for us those things we should accept as our responsibilities and those that remain taboo.

Presently we are attempting to fit our ideas about nursing into the milieu of each clinical setting that involves a multiplicity of health team members. Nurse practice acts, medical practice acts, and common practice are not consistent from one hospital setting to another in the same geographic area, much less nationwide. Many physicians have begun to state (officially or unofficially) that they have responsibilities with nurses and other professionals; other physicians are seeing that a partnership for providing comprehensive, intensive care for patients should involve nursing. Some of the paramedical groups—for example, inhalation therapists—now assume responsibility for pulmonary resuscitative measures or therapies for chronic lung disorders. Some hospital chaplains believe that the patient who seeks emotional and spiritual help should be directed exclusively to the chaplain because the nurse is not equipped to offer supportive assistance.

Clearly the problem lies in interpreting the contribution each group can make and using this information to establish understanding and effective interpersonal relationships among all health personnel. This task is a responsibility for each profession;

evidence of such action is emerging as in the American Medical Association–American Nurses' Association Joint Practice Commission. Insofar as the teacher of clinical nursing is concerned, it would seem that the following responsibility is involved:

1. Creating a positive image of the actions a professional nurse can take in meeting health needs in our complicated social system. The teacher of nursing must show by *example* that the nurse can be relied on to observe patients, make an assessment of health status, diagnose nursing concerns, refer problems elsewhere appropriately, and use sound judgment in proceeding with needed care. It follows, then, that the teacher also assumes responsibility for teaching students to function in a like manner in accord with the level of their abilities. Until we, as nurses, are willing to accept responsibility for what we *can do,* we will remain in the dilemma in which we now find ourselves. From active teaching can come the new knowledge we seek for determining our roles and responsibilities as professional nurses.

2. Gathering data regarding the contributions made by other health workers. The teacher of nursing who makes a concentrated effort to determine how each group sees itself as functioning in meeting the health needs of society can help students function within nursing while working with other groups to obtain for patients those components of care they seem best equipped to handle. But beyond this the teacher of clinical nursing is charged with providing educational environments for students. By understanding the roles of these various groups, the teacher can serve as a liaison between groups or can demonstrate the constructive use of conflict to arrive at improved definitions of caregivers' roles.

3. Participating actively in intergroup communications. It is all too easy to teach nursing students in a vacuum, protecting them from contacts with others and limiting one's own interaction. Unless beginning practitioners learn that productive exchange with other groups is an expected part of the profession, they will have difficulty learning to practice it during their careers.

However each teacher of nursing goes about establishing relationships among nursing personnel and others, the success of such a program rests on the nurse's willingness to speak and act in a way that positively identifies the role of the nurse in providing for the health needs of society.

Responsibilities for seeking new knowledge about the practice of nursing

Progress in scientific and technological knowledge has influenced health care and teaching throughout the world. The foregoing chapters have merely scratched the surface of how these changes affect the teaching of nursing. Careful study of these suggestions for the creative teaching of clinical nursing will indicate the need for the teacher to be a constant student of the profession. Teachers of clinical nursing must assume responsibility by seeking various ways to continually increase their knowledge and competence. Wisdom develops as clinical teachers engage in thoughtful review of ideas and adjustments needed to meet the changing educational practices and needs of society. Self-confidence is generated in realizing that one's present knowledge has grown from that learned during a formal educational program. Continuing education is as necessary a part of the nurse's professional life as the basic educational program; there are so many educational opportunities available today that no nurse has a valid excuse for not seeking ways of continued self-development. To enter into any pursuit of continued learning, the teacher must *feel* a deep commitment toward self-growth in clinical competence, problem-solving, reasoning, experimentation, and application of principles to a variety of situations. The direction can be to help students to master these same competencies or to add to the body of nursing knowledge.

Two important factors stand out in considering continuing educational opportunities for teachers: (1) the use of "not having time" as a crutch for failure to continue learning must be eradicated; every individual has the same number of hours in a day, but the way in which the time is used makes the differences; and (2) the pursuit of knowledge for the sake of knowledge is meaningless; it is the way in which one uses the new knowledge in future practices that counts.

The concept of continuing education should be viewed in its broadest sense, including many avenues of learning available for those who seek them. The following are some examples of kinds of experiences that can contribute to continued learning:

1. Reading books, professional literature, research reports, and the newspapers contributes toward continued education. While it seems unnecessary to mention reading literature related to one's particular specialized area, it is important to recognize that one must pursue these readings with an open mind, and, even more importantly, one must limit the amount of reading done *only* in nursing, *only* in a selected area of teaching, or *only* in a selected area of clinical nursing. Growth also comes from reading materials in related sciences and other professional fields and contemplating these ideas as they are or could be related to a particular area of nursing.

Readings selected from different areas of the human experience are another essential of such a reading program, providing teachers with greater perspectives about total life experiences. The social expectations of a profession involve the capacity to view human beings broadly and to place discrete events appropriately into an understanding of the environment. Those seeking wisdom pursue these readings purposefully for understanding of life situations of their own and other, as well as for

enjoyment. The backgrounds that students bring including travel, home environment, elementary and secondary education, and life experience require teachers who can provide intelligent information to help students or other professional nurses within the immediate environment. Some of this information is available through other means, including visual and performing arts. Health workers more identified with mental, as opposed to physical, health have used this wealth of material more directly than others.

2. Attending and participating in professional meetings—either business meetings or those designed to add new information in a particular area—increase a teacher's learning. The rapid growth in scientific and technological knowledge has encouraged professional organizations and agencies to offer frequent institutes, workshops, and discussion groups on a broad spectrum of topics. Unfortunately, may of these programs offer information but do not result in learning that produces measurable effects on the practice of nursing. It is important that the clinical teacher select programs that have the potential for facilitating application of the new knowledge and stimulating further independent study.

For the teacher of clinical nursing, there are several responsibilities for participation in such programs. Not only is it necessary to further one's own learning but also to generate ideas for such meetings. The teacher of nursing must assume responsibility for *contributing* to these programs. It is a different kind of teaching and learning that occurs when teaching colleagues who study the material, weigh its uses and applications, appraise its value, and contemplate ideas suggested by the material. Interaction with a wide range of practicing nurses broadens the faculty member's horizons beyond the specific courses usually taught, or beyond the beginning level at which some must function so often.

3. Visiting other schools of nursing or nursing situations to investigate ways of accomplishing a particular learning task. The potential for learning constructively

from one another by visiting with faculty peers is facilitated because it is possible to enter into a discussion in which differences are recognized, there is rational understanding of ideas, and creative insights and growth are developed.

4. Experimenting in the clinical setting by challenging one's own practices and judgments can lead to new inferences and concepts on which to base practice. The creative teacher of clinical nursing finds the time to engage in this kind of activity. This is not to prove to others that one's own ways are "right" or "the best" but to examine one's own actions in order to discover errors and to devise better ways to proceed.

Not all such study and experimentation can be classified as research. However, there is a professional obligation to utilize scientific inquiry, and clinical practice can provide multiple opportunities for data collection and analysis. Close collaboration with practitioners in a setting used for teaching can facilitate jointly conducted studies, both small and large.

5. Enroling in formal courses of study will assist teachers in updating their practices and broadening their scope of knowledge. There are so many courses open that it is primarily a matter of personal goals that determines which one to pursue. These include noncredit courses in specialized areas, credit courses leading to advanced study, graduate education programs, correspondence courses, tele-courses, and research-oriented courses. The liberal arts courses also offer the kind of background information in the humanities and sciences often needed by clinical teachers seeking to enrich their knowledge of a particular area of nursing.

Responsibilities for contributing to new knowledge about the practice of nursing

Professional writing involves two facets: writing for the profession and writing for the public. Writing for the profession involves writing about nursing for nurses,

employers, and colleagues of nursing. Writing for the public involves the presentation of nurses to the general public. Given a professional obligation to develop and share information, most nursing faculty are at a level of their profession that entails the use of written communications. Some of the writing will be informal: reports, proposals, materials for students. Other writing should be more formal: papers, articles, books that can be shared with many. Teachers of nursing must start writing; as competency is attained, writing becomes easier.

In writing for nurses, possible topics include (1) new theories regarding the practice of nursing, (2) scientifically tested advances in providing nursing care, (3) setting and maintaining professional standards, (4) approaches to learning that creative teachers are using, (5) ways of using various methods of independent study approaches to learning, (6) new developments in nursing education and their implications for the future, (7) legislative measures and their effects on nurses and patients, and (8) ways of improving the economics of health care.

In writing about nurses and nursing for the public, the writer should consider the specific audience to whom the material is directed because that will determine not only the kind of material but also the level of understanding to be reached and will suggest which medium of publication is the best vehicle. There are two prominent needs for writing about the profession to the public: (1) to interpret nursing in its proper perspective in order to counterbalance the often inaccurate accounts written by non-nurse writers and (2) to secure public understanding and support regarding our relationships to the total health programs of the nation and our recruitment and financial needs.

Editors usually actively seek and encourage new contributors to the nursing journals. However, the writer must be willing to risk enough to seek an avenue for publication; be exposed by expressing thoughts, feelings, or findings regarding a particular subject area; be willing to cooperate with the publishers in preparing the article; and be capable of withstanding disappointment when rejected by a particular publisher. While it is true that publishers seek out specific individuals they believe capable of producing the material they wish to publish, nurses should approach editors to determine possibilities for publishing a given article. It is wise to make inquiry of a publisher by describing a proposed article and the group it is intended to reach prior to submitting the entire manuscript. (Most publishers of periodicals and textbooks have directions for preparing manuscripts, along with policies for selection or rejection.)

Probably the two greatest barriers to writing and publishing are hesitancy to submit unsolicited articles to publishers and a reluctance to *begin* to write, which is often a matter of procrastination rather than lack of initiative. If nursing is to continue to grow in the direction of a true profession, nurses must become involved as contributing writers! The more extensive undertakings and supported research projects have a built-in feature of reporting results that almost assure publication. But it is the practical suggestions or new approaches to old ideas that perhaps only you have discovered or thought about and that, if shared, may be of inestimable value to the practice and teaching of nursing in particular and to the profession as a whole.

Faculty job descriptions and contracts usually specify some contribution to research or the advancement of knowledge as an expected activity. Because of the limited numbers of nurses with doctoral preparation, committees on faculty appointment and advancement have often eased this requirement. However, such leniency is disappearing, and nurse-faculty are increasingly being scrutinized for levels of research activity and competency comparable to that of colleagues in other professions.

Apart from those research activities considered the responsibility of a college faculty, the creative teacher usually engages in research of a less formal nature. Most nursing faculty would not argue the fact that by virtue of their position they are charged with some professional responsibility for patient care. In providing an environment for students' experiences, the teacher becomes actively concerned with the presenting problems of patients. It is within this realm that clinical teachers should study nursing care practices. There is no place for the still too prevalent practice of complaining about nursing care practices but doing nothing to improve them.

There appears to be a threefold responsibility for teachers in the clinical nursing setting: (1) investigating nursing care problems occurring in the clinical situation, either independently or with the help of the students and nursing personnel; (2) studying one's own nursing care practices to see if the problem lies in the situation itself or in the approach one is attempting to follow; and (3) participating in clinical research activities being conducted by the agency. This later contribution is particularly important in hospitals or other agencies that have a nursing research department engaged in clinical research. Students need a thorough orientation to any ongoing project, avoiding the introduction of unwanted variables into the controlled situation.

Providing a teaching-learning environment in which research is considered an integral part of the total nursing services involves interpreting the purposes of research to the students and providing them with reports as the study progresses and results become available, followed by discussions regarding implications of findings for the improvement of nursing care practices. The teacher of nursing, by virtue of preparation, background, and close association with specific problems, shares responsibility with other nursing colleagues for encouraging professional research activity and contributing to ongoing projects. The contribution should, of course, be relative to the teacher's specific preparation. It is incumbent on each teacher to exercise sound judgment in determining the area in which to make a contribution.

Clinical studies often reveal information worthy of validation by others in various clinical settings. Teachers of clinical nursing must assume responsibility for communicating the results of these studies so that their potential can be realized. For every research study reported in *Nursing Research,* there are numbers of unpublished reports of small studies gathering dust in departmental libraries or on someone's desk after having served their initial purpose. This gap between studies that have been done and those that have been reported is already of such import that we stand to lose a high proportion of findings that might be significant and that could be utilized in validation instead of duplication.[4]

The far larger gap is that between what is known from published and unpublished studies and what is applied routinely in care settings. It is the responsibility of educators to remain abreast of findings and incorporate them as regular practices that students are expected to master.

RESPONSIBILITIES AS A UNIVERSITY FACULTY MEMBER

As collegiate schools of nursing achieve autonomy and equal status with other schools in the university, they are faced with the problem of maintaining a faculty qualified to meet the accepted standards of the university professor. The increasing number of NLN-accredited schools of nursing offering programs leading to baccalaureate degrees in nursing and beyond raises the question of who are the faculty members in these schools. Approximately 80% of the full-time faculty in these schools possess a master's degree and less than 10% possess a doctorate degree. These figures, along with the knowledge that large numbers of university nursing faculty have been "transplanted" from teaching programs in diploma schools of nursing or are

entering teaching for the first time in a collegiate program, lead to concern regarding the academic respectability of some collegiate schools of nursing.

Historically, nursing has been criticized from without for reliance on "good bedside nurses" to teach the nursing components of the curriculum; these teachers passed on their knowledge and experience by teaching both good and bad practices that they have learned from their teachers in the basic nursing program. From within, criticism has focused on use of new "textbook" teachers who do not understand the complexities of day-to-day nursing practice. Neither of these practices exists full-blown in today's schools of nursing. However, there still do exist a number of faculty who tend to be skill-oriented even though the professional nursing curriculum must be built on other knowledge of nursing practice. On the one hand, school administrators desire a faculty who recognize their responsibilities as well as their rights in discharging their functions as college or university faculty members. On the other hand, limited formal educational opportunities have been available to teachers who are seeking to learn how to function in a community of scholars as well as in a school of nursing. The following discussion is aimed at providing a minimal frame of reference for helping teachers of clinical nursing carry out their responsibilities as nurse faculty members within the organization of a college or university.

Functioning in accord with the philosophy and purposes of the university

The teacher of clinical nursing, like any faculty member, is obligated to teach in accord with the established philosophy and purposes of the school of nursing and those of the university. It means that all faculty carefully examine the philosophy and purposes of the educational institution to determine whether or not they can personally function within it. Too often, teachers eagerly seek teaching positions in collegiate schools of nursing but look only briefly at the framework used by the school. While the school of nursing should have established its philosophy and purposes in accord with those of the university, the teacher who chooses an academic environment is accountable to both the school of nursing and the university.

Functioning in a collegiate setting affords teachers certain privileges that encourage creativity. However, the university holds the right to expect its teachers to fulfil their responsibilities implied by its basic philosophy and purposes. The most commonly stated purposes of colleges and universities are teaching, research, and community service. The degree to which each of these purposes is to be met is dependent on the individual institution, but to satisfy needs of society the teacher must be able to function in a manner that embraces to some extent all three. It is interesting to note that there are differences in the basic purposes of junior or community colleges and those offering a basic college degree. For example, research is not considered a purpose in some junior colleges; therefore, a teacher vitally interested in research would find it difficult to function in such a collegiate setting.

Observers of universities occasionally note a change in orientation of faculty members from the institution as a community of scholars to their department and the related profession that it serves. New faculty members should not only be aware of and able to work within the university's philosophy but should be prepared to join campus-wide committees and activities to further its goals.

Responsibilities for maintenance of academic excellence as a member of a community of scholars

To become a member of a community of scholars means that nursing faculty members must actively contribute to the scholarship characterized by all those within the educational institution. The skilled, creative teacher possesses the scholarly tools needed to function as an inquirer, analyzer, reporter of new phenomena, and synthesizer; but the true scholar also relates his discoveries to the age in which he lives and to the society he serves. It is this last attribute that is so essential to the process of teaching. It is one thing to be a learned professor, but one must also be skilled in communicating ideas to others and in directing others in a manner conducive to creative learning. While the scholarly teacher of nursing is expected to know a great deal about a particular area, he also is expected to know how this area relates to other aspects of nursing and to other disciplines. The climate for scholarly learning is enriched by cross-disciplinary interaction among faculty members, fostering an environment in which students feel free to cross departmental barriers in seeking the knowledge needed to pursue a problem.

The rights afforded faculty members in freedom to manage time according to responsibilities and the opportunity for obtaining nine- or ten-month appointments carry with them the responsibility for pursuit of continued learning, recognizing that being a scholar is not an end in itself but a dynamic approach to life. The mark of a true scholar is the way he approaches self-growth activities. When individual faculty members recognize and accept both the teacher's rights and the university's responsibilities for promoting self-growth, there exists a community of scholars. The scholar who believes in self-growth and considers it a part of his existence has the self-respect and respect for others needed to pursue additional avenues of learning. Furthermore, he does not consider the educational endeavor as a task to be done because the university stands to gain from it; rather he considers that which he stands to gain in becoming a better teacher and person. This is not to say that a university *should not* underwrite the teacher's expenses while pursuing educational experiences. An institution that provides academic freedom and has respect for its teachers as scholars will provide as much financial support as possible for its scholars.

There are any number of opportunities for faculty members to pursue in continuing their own growth. Many universities offer sabbatical leave programs for their faculty members. There usually are available a variety of programs sponsored by learned societies, workshops, institutes, short courses dealing with specialized subject matter, and departmental programs within the university. Faculty appointments in an academic year generally are arranged by a university to provide its faculty with time to enrich themselves by keeping abreast with changing concepts and new knowledge or with opportunities for personal growth. Some of the activities to be considered are (1) obtaining a summer appointment to teach in another university or educational institution; (2) obtaining a nursing position involving patient care, either in a generalized area or an area suited to the teacher's background or practice specialty; (3) enroling in postgraduate study; (4) attending short courses or workshops; (5) volunteering services to some health, welfare, or community center agency; and (6) traveling to visit another program, culture, or country. Regardless of the chosen means, the rewards are of value and contribute to the scholarly image when the teacher integrates these experiences into subsequent teaching and practice.

Responsibilities for participation in academic affairs

Participation in academic affairs implies the teacher's responsibility to teaching and scholarly activities contributing to the education of the student. Professors should also be involved in the determination of philosophy, purposes, and programs for the education of the student. If faculty members are encouraged to pursue and teach the truth, they must also be offered the opportunity and assume responsibility for the academic affairs of the total university. Such faculty rights and responsibilities must be viewed in their proper perspective. It is easy for professors to become so involved with administrative responsibilities that they have little time for teaching, let alone for continuing other scholarly activities. Teachers should not be involved with such detailed administrative duties that they neglect their first responsibility—the teaching of students. On the other hand there are those who have become so involved in their teaching areas that they avoid all responsibility for academic affairs. It becomes the responsibility of the individual faculty members to develop sensitivity and responsiveness to the institution by participating in academic affairs affecting the daily lives of students and faculty.

Inherent in this responsibility is that of interpreting the philosophy, goals, and programs of nursing education to others within the university. It seems exceedingly difficult to break the barriers between general and professional education. Every contact a nurse faculty member has with a non-nurse faculty member should be utilized to improve understanding of the goals and problems of each. This is an added responsibility of nurse faculty members that seems to be crucial to the way in which we, as a professional group, learn to work within the framework of the university; if we concentrate our efforts in this direction, we may not have to consider it a responsibility in the years ahead.

When faculty members work together to provide an academic program, the unified efforts provide the strength that cannot be achieved when faculties work as independent units. While most nursing teachers are well oriented toward working cooperatively in the school of nursing program, these same teachers have the responsibility of working with the university faculty to implement the educational program of the university. Academic affairs involve not only curriculum planning and teaching but also planning ways of providing for the economical, social, and professional needs of its faculty members.

It is important, then, that school of nursing faculty recognize that they have a responsibility for participating with other faculty on campus-wide committees, comparable to that which they have already assumed in relation to the school of nursing. In assembling faculty members representative of the various schools within the university for the purpose of studying a particular aspect of academic affairs, nurse faculty members' contributions are welcomed along with those from other areas. If it occasionally appears that nursing interests are underrepresented, it may be because of ourselves. The lower incidence of nurses with doctorates and the high rate of turnover in a nursing department often mean a lower proportion of faculty with the necessary rank and length of service to qualify for committees and councils.

Responsibilities for participation in student affairs

In addition to the responsibilities of teaching and research, the teacher of clinical nursing is further responsible for participating in student affairs. Here again, the traditional realm of the school of nursing teachers have been accustomed to assisting students in planning recreational and social events, assisting them with class projects, and counseling them individually and collectively regarding personal and professional problems. The degree to which teachers are responsible for providing these services depends on the university's adminstrative pattern. However, there is always some responsibility for providing recognition and support for students as they pursue their curricular and extracurricular activities in an environment that fosters growth and understanding.

At the policy-making level it would seem particularly important for nurse teachers to participate in planning for admission, progression and graduation standards, orientation and testing programs, health services, financial aid, records and grades, and placement and follow-up programs. Other student activities programs are complex, with the teacher playing a supportive role. The teacher who contributes for purposes of personal status disrupts the organizational plan and hinders the end results; it is the interests of students that take priority in the way in which the program is organized. The teacher

can derive personal satisfaction by contributing to the total learning environment as a part of the campus, which works as a community to provide the students with programs in both the classroom activities and out-of-class activities, leading to the goal of developing a contributing member of society.

Responsibilities for interpreting and promoting university programs and activities

The university is at once responsible for providing leadership in the preservation of our heritage and for taking the initiative in making needed changes to modify human institutions, economics, and politics while operating within the framework of legal and social controls of the existing society.

It is incumbent on each teacher as a faculty member to assume responsibility for the interpretation of university-wide programs to its public, giving evidence of the contributions of the existing educational programs. Such things as achievement of graduates and the services made available to the public as a result of the experimentation, research, and progress made in various fields become the foundation for building a strong bond between the public and the university. A faculty recognizing that each is responsible for the end results also assumes that the university is greater than the sum of its parts. Each faculty member is responsible for being sufficiently conversant with the purposes and accomplishments of the university and school of nursing to be able to interpret actions, programs, and policies to the public.

The image of the university is affected by the conduct of its faculty and students, as evidenced by their research, learning, and public service. Educational programs, athletics, recreational activities, and social programs all contribute to education. The university has as many public relations promoters as it has students and faculty members; the model they represent can facilitate the interpretation of the school's services and needs to the general public and to those concerned with finance and educational policy.

To participate in or promote the university and its projects and programs, it is imperative that each faculty member, student, and staff person believe in its worth. This often means that the faculty must work with the various publics as well as with students and staff personnel. There must be presentation of facts and figures, and intelligent analysis of situations. There is no substitute for the day-to-day, face-to-face informal contacts or communications made by every faculty member. Each has a responsibility to contribute to community committees, professional association activities, and programs designed as public services. One should carefully weigh the issues, decide how well he can contribute to the clarification of an issue, and consider personal use of time, and the timing for the discussion of a particular program or issue. The teacher should be wary of becoming more concerned about the status value of the contribution than about the contribution itself.

The teacher of nursing has a responsibility for interpreting the university's policies, programs, and activities. The teacher must also recognize that the public may need more information than has been thought regarding some of the technical aspects of higher education, but must never underestimate the public's ability to make intelligent contributions to the university once provided with the needed factual information.

Responsibilities for leadership activities

The privilege of assuming leadership roles within the teaching program carries with it the responsibility for faculty participation among diversified groups, both on the campus and at local, state, national, and international levels. Participation in groups other than nursing has significance for understanding of health and welfare or educational practices and provides teachers with opportunities to enrich their own background of knowledge and make a contribution to the university.

Teachers in part establish their reputation and that of the university by the role model they present. As a result, they may be asked to serve as consultants for professional organizational activities, as in government-sponsored projects such as Aid to International Development or World Health Organization, as delegates to learned societies in their particular field, as committee members, as speakers or writers for professional organizations, or as a member of a working group on campus, at another university, or within a community organization. Such responsibilities are not to be taken lightly. To be asked to accept a particular task is an endorsement of both the teacher and the university. One measure of a university is in the contributions its faculty make to the total society. Such responsibilities call for a maximum sharing of interests among participants and maximum contributions to complete the assigned task satisfactorily. It is true that teachers of nursing must first consider their responsibilities to the teaching and research activities in nursing and must regulate the amount of time given to other projects. However, the challenge of teaching cannot be satisfactorily met unless teachers assume responsibility for their own development of wider knowledge by sharing their scholarly pursuits with others and reflecting the image of the university as a community of scholars.

It is the responsibility of university faculty members to contribute their ideas, uphold their values, teach in accord with the basic philosophy, and advance into unknown areas to create new knowledge and propose new ideas. To be expert practitioners of nursing in the university setting, clinical teachers must be actively engaged in working with nursing colleagues and other health care workers to establish quality health care standards. They should also be involved in conducting studies seeking to improve nursing care practices along with discovering new knowledge leading to the development of creative systems of nursing. This information is communicated to students; the nursing practices arising from this result in improved nursing and health services to patients. The responsibility for maintenance of excellence in teaching, learning, and research is vested in the faculty of the university. It is these services of the universities that have assisted society in multiple achievements in the development of resources, cultural advance, quality of living, and health and welfare practices. Teachers of clinical nursing who fulfil their responsibilities toward the profession and the university contribute to both life and living.

REFERENCES

1. Darley, Ward: The professions and professional people, Nursing Forum 1:83-84, Winter, 1961-1962.
2. Standards of nursing practice, Kansas City, Missouri, 1973, American Nurses Association.
3. NSNA Convention Scrapbook, American Journal of Nursing 67:1255, June, 1967.
4. Malone, Mary F.: Research as viewed by researcher and practitioner, Nursing Forum 1: 39-59, Spring, 1962.

SUGGESTED READINGS

Abdellah, Faye G.: Frontiers in nursing research, Nursing Forum 5(1):28-38, 1966.
Cahill, I. D.: The faculty subculture in the university, Nursing Forum 12(3):218-236, 1973.
Howe, Harold, II: Responsibility and academic freedom, Adult Leadership 17:105-106, Sept., 1968.

Jacox, A.: Collective bargaining in academe: background and perspective, Nursing Outlook 21: 700-704, Nov., 1973.
Kohnke, M. F.: Do nursing educators practice what is preached, American Journal of Nursing 73:1571-1573, Sept., 1973.
Lister, Doris W.: Summer practice for nursing faculty, Nursing Outlook 15:69-70, April, 1967.
Palmer, Irene: The responsibility of the university faculty in nursing and medical education, Nursing Forum 9(2):121-129, 1970.
Pellegrino, Edmund D.: The communication crisis in nursing and medical education, Nursing Forum 5(1):45-53, 1966.
Peter, Laurence J., and Hull, Raymond: The Peter principle, New York, 1969, William Morrow & Co., Inc.
Saxton, D. F.: A personal appraisal, Nursing Outlook 21:704-707, Nov., 1973.
Schaefer, M. J.: Toward a full profession of nursing: the challenge of the educator's role, Journal of Nursing Education 11:39-45, Nov., 1972.
Schlotfeldt, Rozella M.: Nursing in the university community, Nursing Forum 5(1):22-27, 1966.
Schweer, Jean E.: Continuing education climatology, Journal of Nursing Administration 1:45-48, Jan., 1971.
Smith, D. W.: Discussion, Nursing Forum 11(4): 367-373, 1972.
Williamson, J. A.: The conflict producing role of the professionally socialized nurse-faculty member, Nursing Forum 11(4):356-366, 1972.

11 The creative teacher of clinical nursing: responsibilities to the community

Nursing functions as an integral part of the health service to the community. Schools of nursing not only seek to provide quality health services for the community but also fulfil their function as educational institutions by providing community services through programs and the contributions made by faculty members and students.

School of nursing faculty members assume responsibilities for establishing relationships with the community because (1) a part of curriculum building is based on needs of students, requiring teachers to have knowledge of the community from which students come; (2) the school of nursing provides for meeting some of the health needs of society, necessitating cooperative community planning to protect community health; (3) the nursing teacher should be thoroughly acquainted with the many learning resources available within the community in order to utilize them; and (4) teachers must be sensitive to the community and function accordingly as a role model for students.

The teacher of clinical nursing assumes a three-dimensional responsibility to the community; each component is dependent on the other in order for the teacher to function as a whole: (1) as a person, (2) as a professional nurse-teacher, and (3) as a citizen.

RESPONSIBILITIES AS A PERSON

Regardless of the position held by a nurse, the "nurse" image in the community is established by the kind of behavior each nurse displays as a person. Just as a teacher possesses individual characteristics, so each community possesses individual standards of behavior based on many facets of its heritage.

That which is judged acceptable behavior in one community may be rejected by another, while still another community may show little concern for judging its citizens. The size of the community, the cultural groups composing it, its geography and political orientation, its history, its economic foundations, all contribute to its expectations of professionals, of nurses, of teachers, of men and women. In becoming established in a community, one should study the local customs and behavior patterns. Choices available then are to accept and live within those customs and patterns, to work within the community to alter them, or to look for a place more compatible with personal beliefs. Of particular concern to many nurses today are changes in the expected role of women in the community. More and more nursing faculty members are becoming concerned with altering the social system so that women and men may more freely choose a profession, pursue it as a lifetime career, and participate in a wide range of related or unrelated activities.

Generally speaking, communities expect professional nurses to be sincere, trustworthy, honest, and objective. Personal and professional respect is *earned* as a result of one's behavior.

In fulfilling personal responsibilities the teacher of clinical nursing should consider such items as the following: (1) making a concerted effort to become acquanted with the community—housing, neighborhoods, businesses, industry, municipal services and regulations, recreation facilities, churches, theaters, art centers, educational centers, and community action centers; (2) entering into community activities willingly and with a friendly attitude; (3) learning when and how to say "no" in a way that leaves the door open for future invitations to participate in community enterprises; (4) having a record of fulfilling contractual agreements with those in the community; and (5) responding actively to expressed health needs in the community.

RESPONSIBILITIES AS A PROFESSIONAL NURSE-TEACHER

The professional nurse-teacher has two broad areas of responsibility related to creating a positive image of professional nursing in the community. The first includes those personal attributes described previously, which convey to the public that nursing is made up of persons worthy of professional status. The second is that of functioning within professional ethics and standards. This means that the professional nurse-teacher upholds established norms such as *The Code for Professional Nurses*,[1] not only in practice but also by interpreting the items to others—students, nurses, other members of the health team, patients, and other persons in the community. Every professional nurse, and teacher of nursing in particular, should use these guidelines and continually revise them to meet the changes in society. When nurses face themselves honestly in evaluating their actions, they are in a position to build the image of the professional nurse by contribution to the community well-being.

The professional nurse-teacher is in a position to assume these responsibilities because of the many contacts with others. As the teacher of nursing supervises students, the example set in professional actions and competencies serves as the model for students. In addition, all nursing personnel can strengthen professional nursing through every contact with patients and through interactions with community members.

Every time good nursing care is provided, it is a help; each instance in which we fail to fulfill our assumed responsibilities detracts. Because we have so poorly communicated our potential to the public, we are protected from much criticism, questioning, and loss of support.

The professional nurse-teacher has a legal responsibility for the protection of the public as established by the nurse practice acts of each state. These laws are minimal requirements, but they are designed to protect the public against the practices of nurses who are incompetent. As practice acts are revised, the teacher must remain informed in order to ensure that students are taught appropriately and that patient care practices are changed to comply with the law.

The professional nurse-teacher is also responsible for questioning evidence of malpractice and referring information for further investigation to the proper authorities.

The professional nurse-teacher must assume responsibility for protecting the members of the community—those who seek an educational program in nursing and the potential consumers of services from those who have pursued such a program.

The general public often considers a wide range of programs as "nursing education," including baccalaureate programs, associate degree and diploma schools, practical nursing programs, and nonacademic nursing assistant or hospital aide classes. However, it is the role of nurses to interpret roles, responsibilities, and educational preparation of various levels of nursing personnel to community members from the following two viewpoints:

1. From an educational viewpoint the professional nurse-teacher has a responsibility to keep the public informed regarding the kinds of educational programs available to those who seek some kind of nursing career, making clear distinctions among the basic purposes each kind of educational program is designed to accomplish. This in itself is a monumental task because of the diversity of educational programs. It means, further, that the nurse-teacher must reach such varied individuals or groups as: high school and college teachers and counselors;

prospective students making individual inquiries; student organizations such as Future Nurses Club, Candy-Stripers, and other volunteer groups; countless varieties of community service clubs; parents, friends, neighbors, and relatives; inactive and sometimes active nurses; alumni organizations; lay persons serving as trustees on boards of control of the schools or universities; and members of the allied health sciences.

2. From a service viewpoint the professional nurse-teacher has a responsibility to clarify what kinds of nursing services various levels of nursing personnel are equipped to provide for patients. To the average lay person the term *nurse* means any uniformed person who provides some kind of nursing care for a patient. The connotation is more in terms of the uniform and the performance of some function for the patient, regardless of the particular qualifications or label the person carries. When the quality of performance does not meet the expectations of the individual seeking care, the professional nurse-teacher, along with others, must assume responsibility for explaining or interpreting the capabilities and limitations of various levels of personnel and for altering practice patterns so that people are not attempting to practice beyond their knowledge or skill.

Articles appearing in the popular magazines serve to remind us that (1) we, as a profession, have not clarified the roles and responsibilities of various levels of nursing personnel or members of the health team; and (2) professional nurses have sometimes failed to fulfil their nursing responsibilities to the patient's satisfaction, while other levels of personnel have bridged the gap, often surpassing the professional in providing the kind of care sought by the patient.

Other evidence of the failure of professional nurses to interpret their roles to the public is seen in newspaper accounts of tragedies, legal battles, and crimes attributed to a "nurse," who, if one pursues the case, is not a professional nurse at all. However, what is called to the public mind is the professional nurse, regardless of level, and the resultant damaging publicity does little to enhance the image. This indicates a need for the professional nurse-teacher to work with the news media in order to promote an image of the professional nurse and other nursing personnel that places them in proper perspective in terms of their contributions to society. The role of interpreting functions and qualifications of various levels of personnel is a never-ending task for the professional nurse-teacher, but one that can bring satisfaction as nurses and the public begin to discuss problems and work cooperatively toward alleviating them. For every person provided with information by the nurse, the chances for informing the public are doubled, because the informed person then becomes an interpreter along with the nurse.

There are countless opportunities in which students in a school of nursing participate in community activities, either as private citizens or as a part of school activities. Each contact is evaluated by the public and can contribute to the strength of the school.

There are opportunities for schools of nursing to use lay persons to assist them in projects that provide an avenue for interpreting the education programs in schools of nursing and for giving the public a broader understanding of the nursing student and nursing. Areas suited to such involvement include providing financial support, legislative support, and recruitment into nursing.

Professional nurse-teachers also have responsibilities for contributing their own knowledge and abilities in helping non-nursing community groups develop their programs. When voluntary health and welfare agencies seek assistance from a nurse as a resource person, the professional nurse-teacher may fulfil these requests by personally accepting the assignment or by referring the agency to someone better qualified or available. We have spent years of effort gaining the right to participate in programs, policy-making, and community action groups as nurses and as citizens, and should respond when requests are made.

Professional nurse-teachers tend to rely heavily on resources within the immediate environment in providing clinical experiences for students, but at times we fail to fully use community facilities and resource persons in helping students meet health needs of patients. There are innumerable agencies whose goals in meeting society's needs are similar to those sought by nurses, but who are rarely asked to contribute to an educational program in a school of nursing. As we move into more state and regional comprehensive health planning councils, we should seek representation on these planning councils if we expect to have a voice in the kind of health care that ultimately emerges. We must also offer non-nurses from these councils opportunities to contribute to our nursing programs as consultants, lecturers, or program participants. There is a need to establish a common ground of understanding on which to build a working relationship consisting of more than that of being a member of such a group just because nursing should be represented. Comprehensive community health programs are growing; if we wish to incorporate their concepts and utilize their facilities in providing student experiences in these programs of the future, now is the time for establishing a cooperative relationship.

The emergence of multiple new health, education, and welfare programs places new responsibilities on professional nurse-teachers. For example, schools of nursing are looking at this problem in terms of assisting educationally disadvantaged students in nursing. A pioneer project of this nature was started by the Boston University School of Nursing Alumni Association in 1964[2] for the purpose of providing educationally disadvantaged persons with remedial help so that they could either qualify for entrance into schools of nursing or maintain their grade point averages once admitted to the school.

One federally funded project, VISTA volunteers, has drawn nurses of all ages deeply committed to living and working among the disadvantaged, performing broad-spectrum health services in a wide variety of settings such as: rural Appalachia, Indian reservations in the Southwest, Eskimos in Alaska, migrant workers, senior citizens' centers, and mental hospitals.[3] International programs such as the Peace Corps, Project HOPE, and others continue to attract large numbers of nurses as well. Current awareness of the complex interrelationships of life on our planet serves to make us all increasingly concerned that health become a more expected life experience for all.

RESPONSIBILITIES AS A CITIZEN

Life in a democratic society such as ours depends on the individual's knowledge and understanding of the American heritage of governmental structure and the individual's assumption to civic responsibilities within the community. To be an effective citizen one must seek to control one's actions voluntarily in terms of the public good, working for legislation designed to provide for maximum development of human resources in matters that individuals cannot accomplish for themselves. The individual functions as an informed citizen by recognizing that laws are a means of protecting individual rights, but only when laws are enacted, enforced, and useful to an informed public. For example, there is a need to conform to traffic regulations, not because a violation means infringement on one's personal rights but because violation might cause injury to another human being. Regardless of the degree of active participation pursued by citizens, recognition of the basic democratic principles on which our laws are based forces one to admit responsibility for current practices and an obligation to work toward change of those laws considered unacceptable to the individual.

The concern of many health professionals over regulation of professional practice (as through the Professional Standards Review Organizations) is based on seeing these laws as an infringement on their individual rights and professional integrity, rather than as securing and promoting the rights of patients to sound care.

When one speaks of responsibility as a citizen, it must be remembered that one was a citizen before becoming a nurse or a teacher. The teacher carries rights and responsibilities for functioning as a citizen in the community regardless of professional commitments. The teacher who functions as a responsible citizen of the community adds to the stature of the profession of nursing. The resultant role model provided by the faculty member can be as diffuse as one chooses to make it—reaching one's immediate family; neighborhood; municipal, state, national, or international government; and the community encountered in performing job functions from day to day.

The nurse as a citizen may participate in a variety of community activities, such as political, spiritual, social, educational, and health groups, community action groups, youth groups, and various voluntary agencies. While the nurse functions in any capacity in such activities as a citizen, our professional identity is an integral part. The profession of nursing should contribute to community action programs in order to gain identification and recognition, but more importantly, because nurses know something about health and how to achieve it.

Politically the nurse as a citizen exercizes the rights and responsibilities of being cognizant of current political issues and problems and their effect on individuals, groups, and the general public. Legislation is only as good or bad as it is understood and accepted or rejected by the public. The nurse who has a working knowledge and understanding of a particular matter of concern, whether in the health field or some other area, must speak and act in the interests of those who stand to be affected in the community. History reveals that some of the greatest social legislative movements were championed by nurses and women; nurses as individuals must pass on this heritage as

they function as citizens in these various capacities.

Our nursing organizations have served as role models in their efforts to speak before congressional groups, educational bodies, and other influential groups on behalf of health and welfare issues touching the nation's citizens. But nurses as individual citizens should be seeking to improve conditions in their own communities or on a larger scale. Much political action of today and tomorrow is linked with social, health, welfare, and educational movements; opportunities for nurses to participate as active citizens in any one area are multiple. As an example, Brown[4] suggests a number of ways in which nurses can work together as citizen groups or through their local professional organizations to bring about changes in existing conditions of local hospitals, nursing homes, convalescent homes, rehabilitative centers, or homes for the aged. Her suggestions are noteworthy because they emphasize the contribution of the nurse as an individual citizen, and encourage a professional group to plan their programs or project for the year in terms of promoting needed changes in existing conditions in a particular institution or health agency. When nurses assume these responsibilities by acting individually and collectively, the profession stands to be recognized as a vital force in making the community a better place in which to live.

While one cannot enumerate all the community service activities available to citizens, some examples follow: (1) sponsoring various activities of groups organized through the YWCA or YMCA; (2) volunteering services for planned parenthood programs; (3) teaching classes to community groups regarding drug abuse, sex education, family relationships, problems of adolescence, expectant parent information and other current social issues; (4) volunteering for sponsoring weekend or short-term visits with international students and underprivileged or handicapped persons; (5) volunteering services to persons in homes for the aged or blind or in rehabilitation centers; (6) functioning as camp counselors, den mothers, or comparable leaders in youth organizations; and (7) contributing services to voluntary community agencies in a variety of ways such as fund raising, public education, and public services. Participation in the foster child program, the CARE program, John Gardner's Common Cause, and others of similar nature provides one with still another dimension in serving society. Most communities have organizations whose sole purposes are related to the cultural development of the society. Some cultural activities are provided by the local governing bodies; some are sponsored by volunteer community groups made up of citizens interested in providing a particular kind of cultural activity for the community. Such organizations and activities as civic opera companies or civic symphonies, theater groups, libraries, art museums, and historical museums and societies depend on the services of interested citizens in terms of promotion, finance, and actual contributions, ranging from stage hands to the talents of those producing the music, art, plays, or exhibits. Those who participate in such activities experience the joy of sharing these cultural opportunities with others as well as the joy of self-fulfilment by contributing their own creative talents for the benefit of others.

Philosophies expressed by most schools of nursing embrace the education of the student as a "whole person." To carry out such a philosophy means that the school of nursing faculty, too, must be functioning as "whole persons" in order to serve as role models for students. One's contributions to the community are vital to this development of the whole individual. Participation in civic and cultural organizations of a local com-

munity and the world community should be viewed by school of nursing faculty members as a privilege and opportunity: (1) to bring satisfaction and self-fulfilment through sharing one's contributions with others, and (2) to fulfil the educational institutions' responsibility for bringing about desirable changes in society.

REFERENCES

1. Code for nurses with interpretive statements, New York, 1968, American Nurses Association, Committee on Ethical, Legal and Professional Standards.
2. Scheinfeldt, Jean: Opening doors wider in nursing, American Journal of Nursing **67**:1461-1464, July, 1967.
3. Wilansky, Eileen: Nursing VISTA, American Journal of Nursing **69**:991-993, May, 1969.
4. Brown, Esther L.: The nurse must know . . . the nurse must speak, Nursing Forum **5**(1):10-21, 1966.

SUGGESTED READINGS

Bernzweig, Eli P.: Liability for malpractice—its role in nursing education, Journal of Nursing Education **8**:33-40, April, 1969.

Davis, Fred, editor: The nursing profession: five sociological studies, New York, 1966, John Wiley & Sons, Inc.

DeLoughery, Grace, and Gebbie, Kristine: Political dynamics: impact on nurses and nursing, St. Louis, 1975, The C. V. Mosby Co.

De Young, Lillian: The foundations of nursing, St. Louis, 1971, The C. V. Mosby Co.

McNeil, Helen J.: How to become involved in community planning, Nursing Outlook **17**:44-47, Feb., 1969.

Miller, Carol: Nurses and the law, Danville, Ill., 1970, The Interstate Printer & Publishers, Inc.

Storlie, Frances: Nursing and the Social Conscience, Englewood Cliffs, N. J., 1970, Prentice-Hall, Inc.

Williams, Geraldine: Developing creative leadership in community services, Adult Leadership **19**:51-52, June, 1970.

Index